# COORDINATED REGULATION OF GENE EXPRESSION

# COORDINATED REGULATION OF GENE EXPRESSION

Edited by

## R. M. Clayton

and

## D. E. S. Truman

University of Edinburgh
Edinburgh, United Kingdom

PLENUM PRESS • NEW YORK AND LONDON

Library of Congress Cataloging in Publication Data

International Workshop on Coordinted Regulation of Gene Expression (1984: Edinburgh, Lothian)
    Coordinated regulation of gene expression.

    "Proceedings of an International Workshop on Coordinated Regulation of Gene Expression, held September 8–15, 1984, in Edinburgh, Scotland"—T.p. verso.
    Includes bibliographies and index.
    1. Gene expression—Congresses. 2. Genetic regulation—Congresses. I. Clayton, R. M. II. Truman, D. E. S. (Donald Ernest Samuel), 1936–    . III. Title. [DNLM: 1. Gene Expression Regulation—congresses. QH 450 I615c 1984]
    QH450.I59  1984                        574.87′322                        86-22620
    ISBN-13: 978-1-4612-9315-6      eISBN-13: 978-1-4613-2245-0
    DOI: 10.1007/ 978-1-4613-2245-0

Proceedings of an International Workshop on Coordinated Regulation of
Gene Expression, held September 8–15, 1984, in Edinburgh, Scotland

© 1986 Plenum Press, New York
Softcover reprint of the hardcover 1st edition 1986

A Division of Plenum Publishing Corporation
233 Spring Street, New York, N.Y. 10013

PREFACE

The Second Edinburgh International Workshop was held in
September, 1984 and took as its topic the coordinated regulation of
gene expression. The intention of this series of workshops is to
promote exchange of ideas and data between scientists and clinicians
whose interests span molecular and cell biology, development and
differentiation, oncology, and genetic and developmental pathologies.
It is hoped that such interdisciplinary discussions may give rise to
fruitful insights. The meetings are structured to give ample time for
discussion after each formal presentation and culminate in a session
of general discussion which is reported at the end of the volume of
proceedings.

We are very grateful to the participants, all of whom
participated in the discussion and whose contributions were essential
to the success of the meeting. Novel ideas were often put forward and
explored thoroughly from different angles.

We normally expect to achieve quite rapid publication of the
proceedings of the meeting and are grateful to authors who produced
typescripts of their contributions expeditiously, but, as may
sometimes be the case with multi-author works, some contributors had
difficulty in meeting schedules for submitting manuscripts or
corrections of the text of the discussion, and in one case we have
been unable to publish any record of the contribution. Our
committment to the publication of the discussion, allowing
participants to make corrections to the transcript of the session,
such as insertion of references and clarification of oral
contributions, has also imposed some delay. We could not omit
uncorrected parts of the discussion, since this would have made
nonsense of the dialogue, and we were finally obliged to exercise
editorial discretion over parts of the discussion, which, uncorrected,
no longer related sufficiently to other, corrected, portions.

The meeting was made possible by financial support from the following:

        Air U.K. Ltd.
        Amersham International
        Anderman and Company Ltd.
        BDH Chemicals Ltd.
        Cancer Research Campaign
        Gibco Ltd.
        ICI Bioscience and Colloid Laboratories
        ICI Pharmaceuticals Division
        International Society of Developmental Biologists
        March of Dimes Birth Defects Foundation
        Monsanto Company
        Organon International B.V.
        Sigma Chemical Company Ltd.
        Tenovus Scotland for Medical Research
        Wellcome Trust

We gratefully acknowledge their assistance without which the workshop could not have taken place.

The planning of the meeting was carried out by an organising committee consisting of A.P. Bird, R.M. Clayton, N. Maitland and D.E.S. Truman.  We should like to record our appreciation of the major contribution made to the publication of the proceedings by Mrs Louise Dobbie.

                                      R.M. Clayton
                                      D.E.S. Truman

CONTENTS

TRANSCRIPTIONAL CONTROLS

REGULATION OF GENE EXPRESSION

# CONTENTS

# INTRODUCTION

Because interdisciplinary and exploratory discussions may take unexpected directions and offer the opportunity of critical and fundamental consideration of current assumptions, we can chose topics for these meetings which we feel timely but we cannot hope for more than that we may have prepared the ground for considering the issues involved.

Different lines of investigation have over recent years contributed to our understanding of the processes of differentiation and development. These may be seen as studies which operate technically at different levels of the hierarchy of organisation of the living organism. Molecular biology, cell biology and developmental biology have each their own pattern of working. Their technologies have permitted the asking of particular types of question and the acquisition of different types of information. Although there have always been occasional convergences between investigations at the different levels, (for example, in the analysis of the pleiotropic effect on development or function of mutant genes, or in analyses of the expression of gene products within a cell), these convergences have not yet constituted a solid bridge between these disciplines.

Over the past decade our understanding of the control of single genes in eukaryotes has progressed rapidly. The existence and function of a number of cis-acting sequences important in regulating gene expression and the role of chromatin organisation, revealed by studies of sensitivity to nucleases,are instances of recent contributions to this field. Within the field of cell biology there have been notable advances in ultrastructural and functional morphology, such as mapping of the cell surface and understanding of its dynamics, and localization and identification of the functions and interrelations of cytoskeletal and extra-cellular elements. To the developmental biologist, tissues represent essentially the resultant of the behaviour of cell population. The capacity to identify a subset, or individual members, of a cell population has advanced the study of the development of tissues, using such procedures as the construction of chimaeras or the use of tagged monoclonal antibodies.

1

The study of genetic and experimental pathology also have both made
significant contributions to developmental biology.

Developments in each of these fields have an excitement and
momentum of their own. Perhaps this is why there is not much record
of investigators in one area turning to those in another for specific
advice concerning some of the very fundamental questions which are the
implicit basis of their own investigations. The intention of the
Edinburgh Workshops is to provide occasions when this can be done.
Readers of the Final Discussion chapter will see that one of the
concerns of the participants was that if we could not define the true
point at which celluar fates diverged it would be difficult to know
what kinds of signals to and from the genes one should search for.

The papers of the meeting were arranged on the basis of the level
of organisation considered. The first two sections were concerned
with transcriptional controls, the first with the structure of
chromatin and the second with regulatory sequences and their
relationship to cellular conditions influencing gene expression. The
next section considered developmental events at the cellular level and
was followed by a section relating to communication between cells and
the construction of tissues. The logical ordering of material often
seems very artificial, since the signals between cells may themselves
be, directly or indirectly, signals which affect the transcription of
particular genes. In the final section we have considered topics
which bear on the evolution of the process of differentiation, which
must depend on the evolution of structural genes and the capacity to
regulate their expression precisely and selectively.

The final discussion of the workshop is presented, with some
minor corrections and with only essential editing, so that the
questions which participants considered together on that occasion are
clearly represented. Finally three demonstrations which were put up
during the course of the meeting are included as brief reports.

## INTRODUCTION

Cellular differentiation involves the selective expression of portions of the genome in a pattern characteristic of each cell type. Apart from the rearrangement of genetic material found in immuno-globulin producing cells of vertebrates, and a few instances of selective loss or amplification of regions of DNA found in various invertebrate species, it is generally supposed that the genome is constant throughout the range of cell types of an individual. While certain regions of DNA may have a regulatory role in transcription, cell-type specificity must depend upon specific interactions between these DNA regions and factors in the nucleoplasm which vary between cell types.

One particular aspect of DNA structure has a special place in that it represents a modification which, while not irreversible, is nevertheless stable and inheritable and so parallels the stability of differentiation itself. This is the phenomenon of DNA methylation which has been for some time regarded as of special interest as a potential regulatory agency (Doerfler, 1983; Cooper and Gerber-Huber, 1985).

Various cis-acting features of DNA structure that play a role in the regulation of transcription have continued to be revealed in recent work. Initially interest centred on features 5' to the start point of transcription and within about a hundred base pairs of this point. Most of the early studies concentrated on genes which were superabundantly expressed in certain tissues and which were subject to control by agents such as hormones or heat-shock. Sequences were identified to which hormone receptors could bind specifically. It was somewhat later that genes which were weakly or constitutively expressed became available for study, and it emerged that a different pattern of upstream elements was to be found in such genes (Melton et al., 1984; Reynolds et al., 1984).

Meanwhile the term 'enhancer' had been applied to sequences originally found in viral genomes which stimulated transcription from points which might be a kilobase or more away, in either direction. In a comparatively short time the term 'enhancer' had come into more general use, and now it is frequently applied to include a variety of elements influencing transcription rates which may not necessarily be remote from the starting point of transcription (Khoury and Gruss, 1983; Serfling et al., 1985).

Associated with the active transcription of a region of chromatin there seems to be an inevitable modification of chromatin structure which leads, amongst other things, to an increased sensitivity to nucleases such as DNAase I. While the entire region of chromatin which is being transcribed may become sensitive, particular points within that region develop even greater sensitivity, that is: they become susceptible to attack by nucleases at very low concentrations, and under conditions which do not lead to hydrolysis of the remainder of the DNA. These hypersensitive sites can be mapped accurately and show changes in number during different phases of the activation of chromatin. (Burch and Weintraub, 1983: Schon et al., 1983).

While the enhancer sequences can be sharply delineated and their sequences described, much less is known about the factors in the nucleoplasm which interact with them to give rise to cell-type specificity of transcription. The factors are believed to be proteins and so they, in turn, must be encoded by genes, the expression of which would be a necessary preliminary stage in the differentiation of the cell. (Dynan and Tjian, 1985).

Whereas methylation can modify DNA in a manner which is stable but potentially reversible, there are some modifications of the genome which are clearly terminal. The ultimate in irreversible differentiation is shown by cells such as erythrocytes or lens fibres, which become enucleated. Another form of extreme terminal differentiation is shown by those cells which are programmed to die as part of the morphogenetic sequence of the whole organism.

REFERENCES

Burch, J.B.E. and Weintraub, H., 1983, Temporal order of chromatin structural changes associated with activation of the major chick vitellogenin gene, Cell 33:65
Cooper, D.N. and Gerber-Huber, S., 1985, DNA methylation and CpG suppression, Cell Differ., 17:199
Doerfler, W., 1983, DNA methylation and gene activity, Ann. Rev. Biochem., 52:93
Dynan, W.S. and Tjian, R., 1985, Control of eukaryotic messenger RNA synthesis by sequence-specific DNA-binding proteins, Nature, 316:774
Khoury, G. and Gruss, P., 1983, Enhancer elements, Cell, 33:313
Melton, D.W., Konecki, D.S., Brennaud, J. and Caskey, C.T., 1984,

Structure, expression and mutation of the hypoxanthine phospho-
ribosyltransferase gene, <u>Proc. Natl. Acad. Sci., USA,</u> 81:2147

Reynolds, G.A., Basin, S.K., Osborne, TG.F., Chin, D.J., Gil, G.,
Brown, M.S., Goldstein, J.L. and Luskey, K.L., 1984, HMG CoA
reductase:  a negatively regulated gene with unusual promoter and
5' untranslated regions, <u>Cell,</u> 38:275

Schon, E., Evan, T., Welsh, J. and Efstratiadis, A., 1983,
Conformation of promoter DNA:  Fine mapping of S1-hypersenstive
sites, <u>Cell</u> 35:837

Serfling, E., Jasin, M. and Schaffner, W., 1985, Enhancers and
eukaryotic gene transcription, <u>Trends in Genetics,</u> 1:224

# PATTERNS OF DNA METHYLATION AND EXPRESSION

# OF GENES

Adrian P. Bird

MRC Mammalian Genome Unit
King's Buildings, West Mains Road
Edinburgh, EH17 7PR, Scotland

## INTRODUCTION

The molecular approach to biological problems is incurably reductionist. If the secrets of inheritance can be uncovered by examining the structure of DNA, then should not differentiation and development also be explicable by simple molecular rules? With this outlook, molecular biologists, equipped with powerful recombinant DNA techniques, are now applying themselves to the problems of gene expression. For it is the control of gene expression that is believed to be at the heart of differentiation and development. The belief is based upon the evidence that cell types differ because of qualitative and quantitative differences in the proteins which they contain, and that differences in protein composition are primarily due to differences in gene activity at the transcriptional level.

DNA methylation is an attractive candidate for a genetic control mechanism, as it has several features that make it potentially suitable for such a role. First, it is known that the presence or absence of methylation in bacteria can determine whether a protein (i.e. a restriction endonuclease) interacts productively or unproductively with its recognition sequence on DNA. This raises the possibility that eukaryotic methylation is also involved in switching DNA-protein interactions. Secondly, the process of methylation has the properties of a replication system that is capable of perpetuating a pattern of methylation through many cell generations (Wigler, 1981). The idea of a heritable, but reversible, signal on the DNA, whose presence or absence does not affect genetic coding, has obvious attractions.

The methylated base in animals, 5-methyl cytosine (5mC,)

up to 5% of all cytosine (Wyatt, 1951). Early work
two points that have been reinforced by later results:
the act of methylation follows synthesis of the DNA
NA replication (Scarano et al, 1965; Burdon and Adams,
.r and Potter, 1969; Kappler, 1970); and second, that the
'equence is 5'XCGY, where X and Y can be any of the four
(Doskocil and Sorm, 1962; Grippo et al, 1968). Not all
:hylated, and it is possible to partially map the
.s of methylated and non-methylated CpGs both at specific
nd in the genome as a whole. This is achieved by using
:riction endonucleases whose recognition sequences
sequence CpG, but which are blocked from cutting by
of the C (Bird and Southern, 1978).


OF ACTIVE AND INACTIVE GENES

lation is involved in controlling gene expression, there
.fferences between the methylation pattern of a gene in
the gene is expressed compared with cells where it is
 genes that are exressed tissue-specifically have now
.ly analysed. Although the results are not uniform, the
 t finding is that the gene in question is less methylated
g tissues than in non-expressing tissues, and is most
ylated in sperm (Felsenfeld and McGhee, 1982; Bird,
 is an intriguing result which invites the speculation
: methylation at a gene is a step in activation.

' of methylation at an expressed gene, however, has an
 explanation since it may be a consequence, rather than a
:anscription. Recent experiments have addressed this
 asking whether methylated genes can be expressed in
 y systems. Unfortunately most genes must be methyl-
:ally, as they can only be purified by cloning, which
)genous patterns of methylation. The problem has been
.n some cases (notably the human globin gene; Busslinger
 and it has been found that usually transcription is
1ibited or abolished by methylation (reviewed in Bird,


studies of DNA methylation have utilised the genes for
:A. In the amphibian Xenopus laevis, there are about
nal RNA genes per cell arranged as a head-to-tail array.
.ng unit comprises a non-transcribed spacer that contains
1ich influence transcription, and a transcribed region.
:ells, the genes are heavily methylated at CpG (Dawid et
)ut there is a region of undermethylation in the non-
 spacer which maps to a cluster of repeated 60bp
3ird and Southern, 1978). Copies of the 60bp repeat have
:o be required for expression of ribosomal RNA genes in

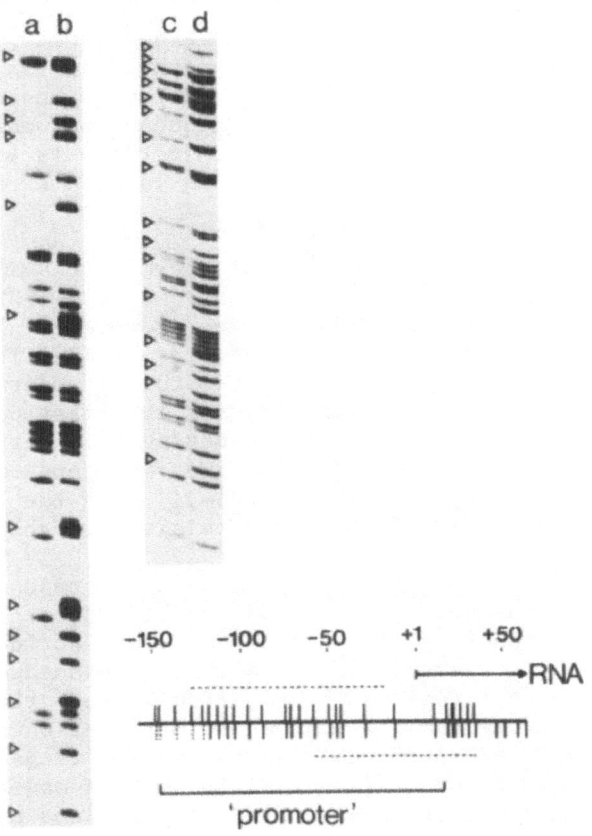

Fig. 1.   Methylation at all C–Gs in the promoter of **X.laevis** rDNA.
The figure shows examples of Maxam–Gilbert sequencing gels
of sperm (lanes a and c) and cloned (pXlr108c, lanes b and
d) rDNA fragments after partial cleavage at C residues.
Missing bands in the sperm track (arrow heads) indicate 5–
methyl C residues.   Complete sequencing of the sperm rDNA
promoter region showed that each missing band is opposite a
G on the other strand, and is part of the sequence 5' C–G.
The regions covered in the examples are from overlapping
segments on opposite strands as shown by the lower (lanes a
and b) and upper (lanes d and e) broken lines on the
diagram.   The diagram shows the promoter region (bracket)
and the position of 5–methyl C residues on each strand
(vertical lines).   All the C–Gs that were encountered on
both strands were methylated.   Methyl C residues marked by
broken lines are in a region where the sequence could not
be read properly on this strand. Their positions were
inferred from missing C bands in sperm tracks, and from the
sequence on the other strand. Figure from Macleod and Bird
(1983) with permission.

Xenopus embryos (Busby and Reeder, 1983). Furthermore, this
sequence is highly conserved (and under-methylated) in the rDNA of
Xenopus borealis (La Volpe et al, 1982), although most other
regions of the spacer have diverged in sequence between X.laevis
and X.borealis (Forsheit et al, 1974). Thus there is strong
evidence that the undermethylated CpGs are located at sequence of
regulatory significance.

     Unlike somatic tissues, the rDNA of sperm is heavily methylated
in this and other parts of the spacer (Bird et al, 1981), and direct
sequencing shows that all 19 CpGs in the "promoter region" are
methylated on both strands (Macleod and Bird, 1983). The transition
from the fully methylated spacer of sperm to the undermethylated
spacer of somatic cells takes place during the first day of embryonic
development (Bird et al, 1981).  It is during this period that
nucleoli appear in embryonic cells and the rRNA genes are transcriptionally activated (Brown and Littna, 1964).  Thus the loss of spacer
methylation and the onset of rRNA synthesis are roughly coincident.

     If loss of methylation is a prerequisite for transcription of
the rRNA genes, then sperm rDNA should not be transcribed upon
injection into the nucleus of a Xenopus oocyte.  Fortunately
this can be directly tested, as a significant advantage of the
Xenopus system is that rDNA can be purified without recourse to
cloning, and therefore has its endogenous methylation pattern
intact.  When purified sperm rDNA was tested for transcription in
oocytes we were surprised to find that sperm rDNA and non-methylated
rDNA were transcribed with equal efficiency (Macleod and Bird,
1983).  DNA replication does not occur in the oocyte, and no loss of
methylation was detected. The conclusion is that a high degree of
methylation does not interfere with rDNA transcription in oocytes.
The simplest conclusion from the data, therefore, is that loss of
methylation in the spacer is likely to be a consequence of transcription.

     There are now several examples in the literature of genes whose
expression does not appear to be accompanied by changing patterns of
methylation, as well as genes showing a clear correlation (reviewed
by Bird, 1984).  This variability can be put in perspective by considering patterns of DNA methylation in the animal kingdom as a
whole.  Levels of methylation vary from little or none in
Drosophila, through intermediate levels in other invertebrates,
to the unusually high levels found in vertebrates.  Most
significant, however, is the absence, so far, of any example of a
methylated gene in the invertebrates, whereas in vertebrates non-
methylated genes are the exception rather than the rule.
Vertebrates, then, appear to be unusual among animals in possessing
methylated genes.

     Based on this evolutionary variability in DNA methylation and

upon results with artifically methylated genes, it has been
speculated that DNA methylation normally interferes with gene
expression, and has spread throughout the genome during vertebrate
evolution (Bird, 1984). We can envisage three ways in which genes
could cope with the spread of such a repressive influence:

(1) <u>Ignore</u>  the gene's regulatory sequences could evolve in
    such a way that methylation no longer interfered with
    transcription.
(2) <u>Prevent</u>  regulatory regions could be rendered immune to
    methylation.
(3) <u>Use</u>  genes that are methylated (and thereby inactive)
    in a non-expressing tissue might selectively lose
    methylation in tissues where expression is required, as
    part of a developmentally controlled switch.


Surprisingly, potential examples of all three responses are
known already: the ribosomal RNA genes of **Xenopus** and, perhaps,
the vitellogenin genes of **Xenopus** and chicken qualify for
category 1; several housekeeping genes qualify for category 2, as
they maintain "methylation free zones" near their 5' ends (see
below); globin genes may qualify for category 3, although this is
not yet completely clear (Busslinger et al, 1984).


METHYLATION AND MUTATION

The dinucleotide CpG occurs at about 20% of its expected
frequency in vertebrate DNA. Since CpG is also the predominant
methylated sequence, it has been suggested that methylation and the
CpG deficiency are related phenomena. In bacteria it is known that
5mC is a hotspot for mutation through deamination to T . Deamination
of unmodified C, by contrast, gives U which, unlike T, is recognised
as abnormal and excised from the DNA. Three lines of evidence
implicate a similar 5mC to T transition as the source of the CpG
deficiency in vertebrates (Bird, 1980). First, the extent of the CpG
deficiency in different animals is proportional to the extent of
methylation of the genome. Insects, for example, have undetectable
CpG methylation and have no significant CpG deficiency. Secondly,
the deficiency of CpG is matched by a corresponding excess of TpG
and CpA, as would be expected if mCG mutates to TpG. Animals with no
CpG deficiency have no TpG + CpA excess. Thirdly, there are
indications that restriction sites that include CpG are unusually
polymorphic between individuals of the same species. These results
imply that cytosine methylation imposes a burden of increased
mutability. Presumably the advantages conferred by the presence of
5mC outweigh this attendant disadvantage.

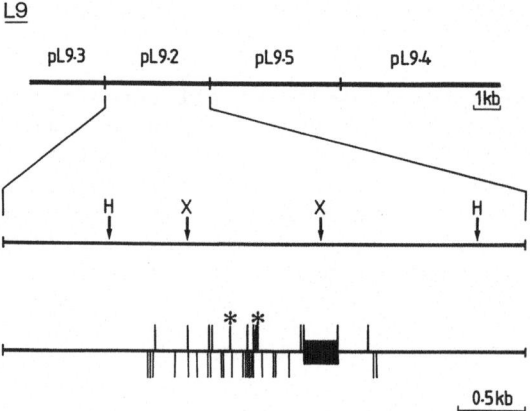

Fig. 2.   An HTF island from mouse DNA. A map of EcoRI fragments of a
          genomic clone is shown (top) together with a blow up of the
          island-containing fragment.  Arrows represent sites for
          HindIII (H) and XhoI(X).  The bottom map shows sites for
          the CpG enzymes HpaII (above the line) and HhaI (below the
          line).  The black box is the fragment that was originally
          cloned from mouse DNA (see Bird et al, 1985).

## NON-METHYLATED, CpG-RICH DNA IN VERTEBRATES

In the past we have analysed the distribution of methyl-C in various animal genomes and have observed wide variations. Most invertebrates have a fraction of the genome (less than one-third) that is heavily methylated while the remainder is not methylated at all (Bird and Taggart, 1980). In the heavily methylated genome of vertebrates, on the other hand, no non-methylated fraction could at first be detected. The fact that non-methylated DNA does occur in vertebrates was first shown by our experiments on the rDNA of mice (Bird et al, 1981) and we were later able to detect a discrete fraction of vertebrate DNA that contained other non-methylated sequences (Cooper et al, 1983). This "HpaII tiny fragment" (HTF) fraction was present in somatic and sperm cells, and amounted to about 1% of the genome. When HTF sequences were cloned, it emerged that about 25% of the fraction was indeed rDNA, with the remainder comprising a complex mixture of unrelated sequences. The striking finding (Bird et al, 1985) was that each of the non-ribosomal sequences that were mapped in detail was derived from a separate island of genomic DNA (for example, Figure 2) which had three distinctive properties: HTF island DNA was non-methylated at testable CpGs, high in G+C content, and not deficient in the dinucleotide CpG. The nucleotide sequences in different islands did not appear to be related. The absence of a CpG deficiency could be accounted for by our previous argument that CpG should only be deficient in methylated DNA (see above).

Having identified HTF islands as a distinctive fraction of mouse DNA, we sought examples in the literature of sequences with these properties. All candidates proved to be associated with genes and often with their 5' ends. In fact, all genes belonging to the "prevent" category (see above) appear to have HTF islands surrounding the transcription start site. The possibility of a consistent relationship between HTF islands and genes was made more likely by the preliminary finding that our three HTF islands hybridised to discrete transcripts in mouse RNA.

## ACKNOWLEDGEMENTS

I wish to acknowledge my collaborators in the work cited here: Marianne Frommer, Donald Macleod, Jack Miller and Mary Taggart. I also thank Anne Deane for typing the manuscript. The research was funded by the Medical Research Council (London).

## REFERENCES

Bird, A.P. and Southern, E.M., 1978, Use of restriction enzymes to study eukaryotic DNA methylation: I The methylation pattern in ribosomal DNA from Xenopus. J.Mol.Biol. 118:27.

Bird, A.P., 1980, DNA methylation and the frequency of CpG in animal
    DNA. Nucl. Acids Res. 8:1499.

Bird, A.P. and Taggart, M.H., 1980, Variable patterns of total DNA
    and rDNA methylation in animals. Nucl. Acids Res. 8:1485.

Bird, A.P., Taggart, M.H. and Gehring, C., 1981a, Methylated and
    unmethylated ribosomal RNA genes in the mouse. J.Mol.Biol.
    152:1.

Bird, A.P., Taggart, M.H. and Macleod, D., 1981b, Loss of rDNA
    methylation accompanies the onset of ribosomal gene activity in
    early development of X.laevis. Cell 26:381.

Bird. A.P., 1984, DNA methylation - how important in gene control?
    Nature 307:503.

Brown, D.D. and Littna, E., 1964, RNA synthesised during the
    development of Xenopus laevis, The South African clawed toad. J.
    Mol. Biol. 8:669.

Burdon, R.H. and Adams, R,L.P., 1969, The in vivo methylation of DNA
    in mouse fibroblasts. Biochim. Biophys. Acta 174:322.

Busslinger, M., Hurst, J. and Flavell, R.A., 1983, DNA Methylation
    and the regulation of globin gene expression. Cell 34:107.

Cooper, D.N., Taggart, M.H. and Bird, A.P., 1983, Unmethylated
    domains in vertebrate DNA. Nucl. Acids Res. 11:647.

Dawid, I.B., Brown, D.D. and Reeder, R.H., 1970, Composition and
    structure of chromosomal and amplified ribosomal DNAs of Xenopus
    laevis. Mol. Biol. 51:341.

Doscocil, J. and Sorm, F., 1962, Distribution of 5- methylcytosine
    in pyrimidine sequences of deoxyribonucleic acids. Biochim.
    Biophys. Acta 55:953.

Felsenfeld, G. and McGhee, J., 1982, Methylation and gene control.
    Nature 296:602.

Forsheit, A.B., Davidson, N. and Brown, D.D., 1974, An electron
    microscope heteroduplex study of the ribosomal DNAs of Xenopus
    laevis and Xenopus mulleri. J. Mol. Biol. 90:301.

Grippo, P., Iaccarino, M., Parisi, E. and Scarano, E., 1968,
    Methylation of DNA in developing sea urchin embryos. J. Mol.
    Biol. 36:196.

Kappler, J.W., 1970, The kinetics of DNA methylation in cultures of
    a mouse adrenal cell line. J. Cell Physiol. 75:21.

La Volpe, A., Taggart, M.H., Macleod, D. and Bird, A.P., 1982,
    Coupled demethylation of sites in a conserved sequence of
    Xenopus ribosomal DNA. Cold Spring Harbor Symp. Quant. Biol.
    46:585.

Macleod, D. and Bird, A., 1982, DNase I sensitivity and methylation
    of active versus inactive rRNA genes in Xenopus species hybrids.
    Cell 29, 211-218.

Scarano, E., Iaccarino, M., Grippo, P. and Winckelmans, D., 1965,
    On methylation of DNA during development of the sea urchin
    embryo. J. Mol. Biol. 14:603.

Sneider, T.W. and Potter, V.R., 1969, Methylation of mammalian DNA:
    Studies on Novikoff Hepatoma cells in tissue culutre. J. Mol.
    Biol. 42:271.

Wigler, M.H., 1981, The inheritance of methylation patterns in
    vertebrates.  Cell 24:285.
Wyatt, G.R., 1951, The purine and pyrimidine composition of
    deoxypentose nucleic acids.  Biochem. J. 48:584.

# CHROMATIN STRUCTURE AND PROTEIN-DNA INTERACTIONS IN THE 5'-FLANKING REGION OF THE CHICKEN LYSOZYME GENE

Albrecht E. Sippel,* Joachim Nowock,* Manfred Theisen,*
Uwe Borgmeyer,* Ute Strech-Jurk,* Conny Bonifer,*
Tibor Igo-Kemenes,[†] and Hans P. Fritton[†]

*Zentrum für Molekulare Biologie der Universität (ZMBH)
Im Neuenheimer Feld 364, D-6900 Heidelberg, FRG
[†]Institut für Physiologische Chemie, Physikalische
Biochemie und Zellbiologie der Universität
Goethestraße 33, D-8000 München 2, FRG

## INTRODUCTION

The exact mechanisms which ensure that a eukaryotic gene is expressed at a specific time in a specific cell are presently unknown. It is, however, generally assumed that the structural organization of chromatin determines the state of differentiation and activity of eukaryotic genes. Our work is aimed at understanding the molecular details of the processes which prepare genes to be differentially and coordinately expressed.

To answer this question, we have - in a first approach - examined the pattern of DNAase hypersensitivity in the 5' upstream chromatin region of the chicken lysozyme gene. Different sets of DNAase I hypersensitive sites have been revealed, depending on whether the gene is constitutively expressed (in cultured macrophages) or active in a steroid controlled manner (in oviduct cells). As a second step, we looked for specific DNA binding proteins which interact with the DNA of hypersensitive chromatin sites and which could therefore function as regulatory trans-acting factors. We have found two proteins of this kind: The TGGCA binding protein, which seems to have a more general function in gene expression, and the progesterone receptor protein, which is involved directly in promoter action.

RESULTS

## The Lysozyme Gene Is Constitutively Expressed in Mature Chicken Macrophages

Lysozyme is one of the major egg white proteins synthesized in the presence of steroid hormones in the tubular gland cells of the developed avian oviduct (Palmiter, 1972; Sippel, 1983). Regulation of lysozyme in this tissue follows the general pattern for steroid

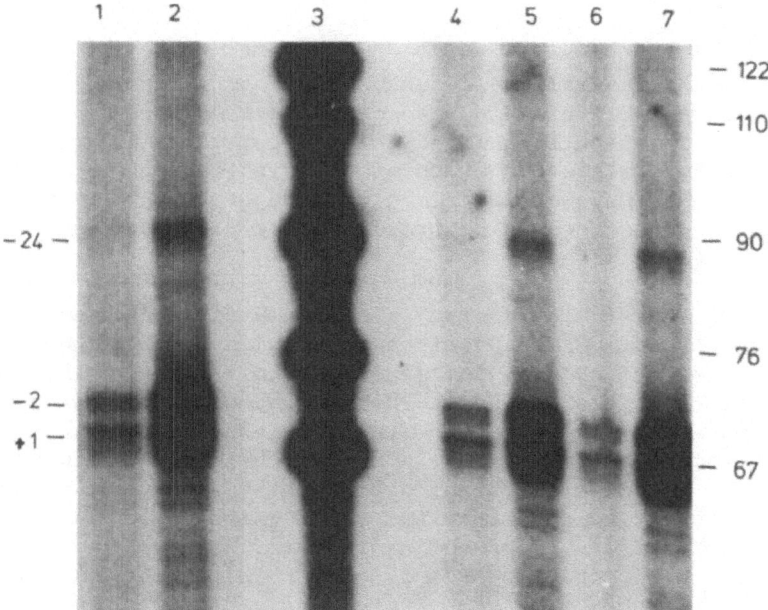

Fig. 1.   S1 mapping of lysozyme gene transcripts in mature chicken macrophages. Peripheral blood derived macrophages were cultured for 5 days at 41°C in MEM Iscove, 8% fetal calf serum, 2% chicken serum (slots 1 and 2) and the same medium was freed of steroids by treatment with charcoal in the absence (slots 4 and 5) and presence of $10^{-8}$ M diethylstilbestrol (DES). After cells were harvested total RNA was isolated and S1 mapping was performed as previously described for oviduct RNA (Grez et al., 1981). 2 µg RNA was used for hybridization in slots 1, 4, and 6; 10 µg RNA in slots 2, 5, and 7. Specific transcripts are indicated as +1, -2, and -24 according to their point of transcriptional initiation (Grez et al., 1981); single-stranded DNA size markers (slot 3) are given in nucleotide lengths.

hormone action (Schütz et al., 1978). Steroids raise specific mRNA
levels by increasing transcriptional activity as well as by differential mRNA stabilization in the cytoplasm (Hynes et al., 1979;
Sippel et al., 1980). Lysozyme is also synthesized in chicken macrophages (Hauser et al., 1981) and is most likely involved in the bac-
tericidal strategy of these cells. Fully mature cultured macrophages
derived from peripheral blood contain steady-state levels of lysozyme
specific mRNA sequences two orders of magnitudes lower than in laying hen oviduct cells (Fig. 1). In addition, S1 mapping shows that
the lysozyme specific transcripts are initiated at nucleotides +1,
-2, and -24 of the lysozyme gene. The result demonstrates that the
same initiation sites are used as in chicken oviduct cells and that
the relative proportions of transcripts initiated at the three closely
located start sites are unchanged. However, there is a characteristic
difference in the mode of expression of lysozyme transcripts in the
two tissues. Figure 1 shows that the same level of transcripts is
present in cultured macrophages whether they grow in the absence of
steroid hormone, at the low steroid hormone concentrations of normal
fetal calf serum, or in $10^{-8}$ M diethylstilbestrol containing medium.
The tissue specific molecular mechanisms of lysozyme expression can
therefore be studied under different regulatory states, a considerable advantage over the situation for other widely studied genes such
as ovalbumin, vitellogenin, and hemoglobin, which are expressed,
according to current knowledge, only in one regulatory mode.


## Alternative Sets of DNAase Hypersensitive Sites Characterize the Various Functional States of the Chicken Lysozyme Gene

     The various modes of regulation of the lysozyme gene raised two
basic questions:
1. How does chromatin structure change when we deinduce and reinduce
   the transcriptional activity of this gene in the oviduct by estrogen withdrawal and reapplication?
2. What is the chromatin structure of the same gene in inactive tissue
   or in macrophages in which the gene is constitutively expressed?

     We have studied the chromatin structure of the chicken lysozyme
gene domain in different tissues. Using the indirect endlabeling
method (Wu, 1980; Nedospasov et al., 1980), we mapped DNAase hypersensitive sites in chromatin of isolated nuclei.

     Eight DNAase I hypersensitive sites cluster around the chicken
lysozyme gene within a chromatin region of 16.1 kb in laying hen
oviduct cells, five upstream from the promoter and three downstream
from the poly(A) addition signal (Fritton et al., 1983). Figure 2
shows a summary of the pattern of DNAase I hypersensitive sites in
the chromatin of the 5' flanking region of the lysozyme gene from 12
different hormone responsive, nonresponsive, and dormant cell types.

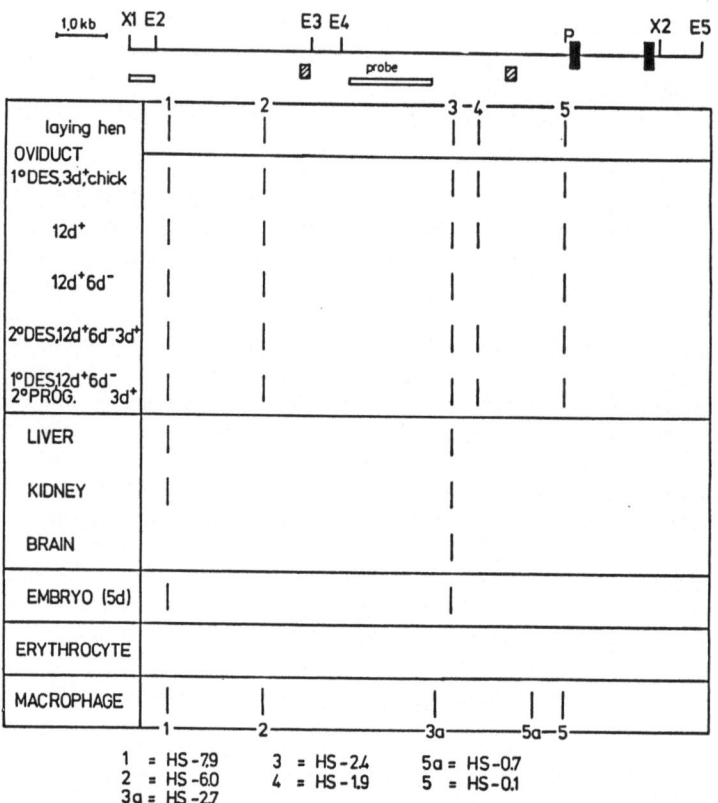

Fig. 2.  DNAase I hypersensitive sites in the 5' flanking chromatin
region of the chicken lysozyme gene. The map shows 8.7 kb
of DNA upstream of the promoter (P) and the first 2.7 kb of
the gene including four EcoRI sites (E2 to E5; Nowock and
Sippel, 1982), two Xba I sites (X1 and X2), the first two
exons of the gene (black boxes) and the location of two
approximately 200 bp long middle repetitive sequence
elements (hatched boxes; Witte, 1984). The DNAase I hypersensitive sites, indicated as vertical lines, were mapped
with radioactively labelled DNA probes derived from subcloned regions marked as open bars. Methods are described
in and results are partly taken from earlier publications
(Fritton et al., 1983, 1984). Immature chick oviducts were
primarily induced (1°) with diethylstilbestrol (DES) for
the indicated number of days (d), withdrawn, and secondarily
reinduced (2°) with DES or progesterone (PROG). Hypersensitive sites (HS) were numbered from left to right and
named according to their position in kilobases upstream
from the cap site of the gene.

These data suggest that the pattern of DNAase I hypersensitive
sites upstream from the cap site must contribute to the way this gene

is transcriptionally expressed. Different modes of regulation correlate with alternative chromatin structures (Fritton et al., 1984). The following features are noteworthy: (1) The hypersensitive site immediately upstream of the cap site, HS -0.1, is only present in cells which either express or have the potential to express the lysozyme gene. (2) A close correlation could be demonstrated between the presence of the steroid hormone and the formation of the DNAase I hypersensitive site at -1.9 kb (HS -1.9) in the oviduct. (3) In liver, as in other nonexpressing tissues, HS -0.1 and HS -1.9 are absent. This remarkable difference in chromatin structure must be responsible for the fact that the lysozyme gene cannot be activated even though the liver is a pronounced estrogen target organ with a competent steroid receptor (Burch and Weintraub, 1983). (4) The most striking outcome is that marked differences exist in the structural organization of chromatin between nuclei from two lysozyme producing cell types. In macrophages, HS -1.9 and HS -2.4 are absent. However, two new sites, HS -0.7 and HS -2.7, can be mapped. (5) The absence or presence of HS -2.4 indicates that this site might play a role in suppressing lysozyme gene activity. Such a function would be required in the oviduct in which transcription is reversibly changed depending on the hormonal state. (6) HS -6.0 is the only hypersensitive site which is strictly correlated with the state of the promoter (HS -0.1). In all 12 cases, the chromatin at -6.0 kb is in an open or closed configuration whenever the same is true for the chromatin at -0.1 kb.

These findings show for the first time that different modes of transcriptional regulation of an eukaryotic gene correlate with a different chromatin organization and support the notion that the hypersensitive structures themselves determine the functional state of a gene (Fritton et al., 1984). It remains to be shown how chromatin structural changes observed kilobases away from the transcriptional initiation point can regulate promoter activity.

## The TGGCA Protein Binds to DNA Sequences at the DNAase Hypersensitive Region 6 kb Upstream from the Promoter

DNAase hypersensitive sites are believed to be short nucleosomefree regions which mark sites where access is required for regulatory proteins to specific DNA sequences (McGhee et al., 1981). Analogous to the situation in prokaryotes, we therefore assume that the recognition of specific signal sequences by DNA binding proteins must be at the basis of the regulatory protein complexes in chromatin.

Using low salt nuclear protein extracts in nitrocellulose filter binding assays with labeled subcloned DNA fragments we have detected specific protein-DNA interactions at several sites in the lysozyme gene domain (Nowock and Sippel, 1982; Sippel and Nowock, 1982). Exact mapping of several DNA binding sequences by in vitro DNAase I protection experiments ("footprinting") led to a consensus recognition

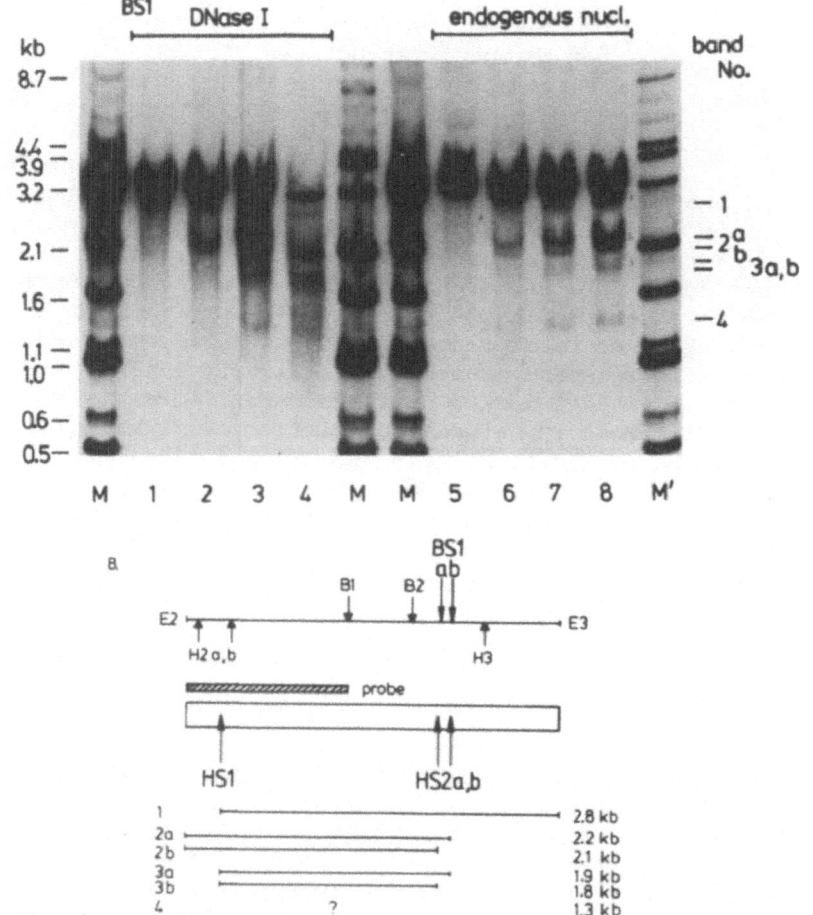

Fig. 3.   Mapping of DNAase hypersensitive sites i  the chromatin re-
          gion 8.2 to 5.1 kb upstream from the gene. A: Isolated lay-
          ing hen oviduct nuclei were digested either with increasing
          concentrations of DNAase I (slots 1 to 4) or autodigested by
          endogenous nucleases with increasing incubation times at 20°C
          (slots 5 to 8) as described previously (Fritton et al.,
          1983). After DNAase digestion DNA was isolated, cut by EcoRI,
          and Southern blots were probed by radioactive, subcloned DNA
          between restriction sites E2 and B1 as indicated in B. Stan-
          dard DNAs (slots M and M') are marked by their lengths in kb
          and individual bands of subfragmented nuclear DNAs are num-
          bered at the righthand margin. B: The schematic diagram
          shows the DNA region between EcoRI site E2 and E3 8.2 to 5.1
          kb upstream from the lysozyme gene. Bam H1 (B), Hind III (H)
          restriction sites and the TGGCA-protein binding sites BS1a
          and BS1b are indicated according to previous results (Borg-
          meyer et al., 1984). Arrows from below mark the positions of
          the DNAase hypersensitive sites HS1 (= HS -7.9) and HS2a and
          b (= HS -6.0) as deduced from the subbands 1, 2a, 2b, 3a,
          and 3b.

sequence for the newly discovered nuclear DNA binding protein (Borgmeyer et al., 1984). The protein was named TGGCA-binding protein
after its recognition consensus sequence.

We concluded that, if this protein acts on the level of genomic
DNA in vivo, we might observe an imprint of this interaction in the
structure of the chromatin. We therefore compared the pattern of in
vitro DNA-binding sites with that of the DNAase hypersensitive sites.
Fig. 3 presents the digestions of the chromatin region of hen oviduct.
In particular, the digest with endogenous endonucleases shows striking identity for the map positions of the in vitro TGGCA-protein
binding sites BS1a and BS1b (92 bp mean distance) and the DNAase
hypersensitive site 2 (= HS -6.0), which actually is a doublet of two
closely located sites with an approximate distance of 100 bp (HS2a
and HS2b). We consider this to be a strong indication that the TGGCA-
binding protein is involved in the DNAase hypersensitive chromatin
structure at -6.0 kb, the region for which we found a strict correlation with the state of the promoter in 12 different types of
nuclei. Since only two out of five TGGCA-binding sites map with a
DNAase hypersensitive structure, the effect of this binding must be
exerted in concert with additional specific DNA-protein interactions.

## The TGGCA Protein Binds Directly to the Promoter on the LTR of the Mouse Mammary Tumor Virus Proviral DNA

We have shown that the TGGCA protein is not only present in
avian oviduct cells, where it was initially detected, but that it is
most likely a ubiquitous protein of vertebrate cells (Borgmeyer et
al., 1984; Nowock et al., 1985). This general cellular distribution
made it unlikely to be a protein factor involved exclusively in the
regulation of egg white protein gene activity. In order to approach
the biological function of this newly discovered protein-DNA interaction from a different angle, we searched for homologous DNA binding
sites in a DNA data bank by sequence comparison with the consensus
recognition sequence.

A potentially elucidating example is the proviral DNA of the
mouse mammary tumor virus (MMTV). Nitrocellulose filter binding
assays with protein extracts from either mouse liver of chicken oviduct nuclei yielded preferential binding of fragments containing sequences of the long terminal repeats (Nowock et al., 1985). Figure
4 shows the fine mapping of the TGGCA-protein binding site to the
promoter region of the MMTV right-LTR by two methods. In Figure 4A
an endlabeled DNA fragment was partially digested with two frequently
cutting restriction enzymes and differential protein binding to subfragments was assayed in nitrocellulose filter binding assays. As a
result, a 459 bp AluI subfragment can still be retained on the filter
whereas a 425 bp Hin F1 subfragment cannot. This indicates the presence of a protein binding site on the DNA between the respective
AluI site and the Hin f1 site 425 bp upstream from the EcoRI site.

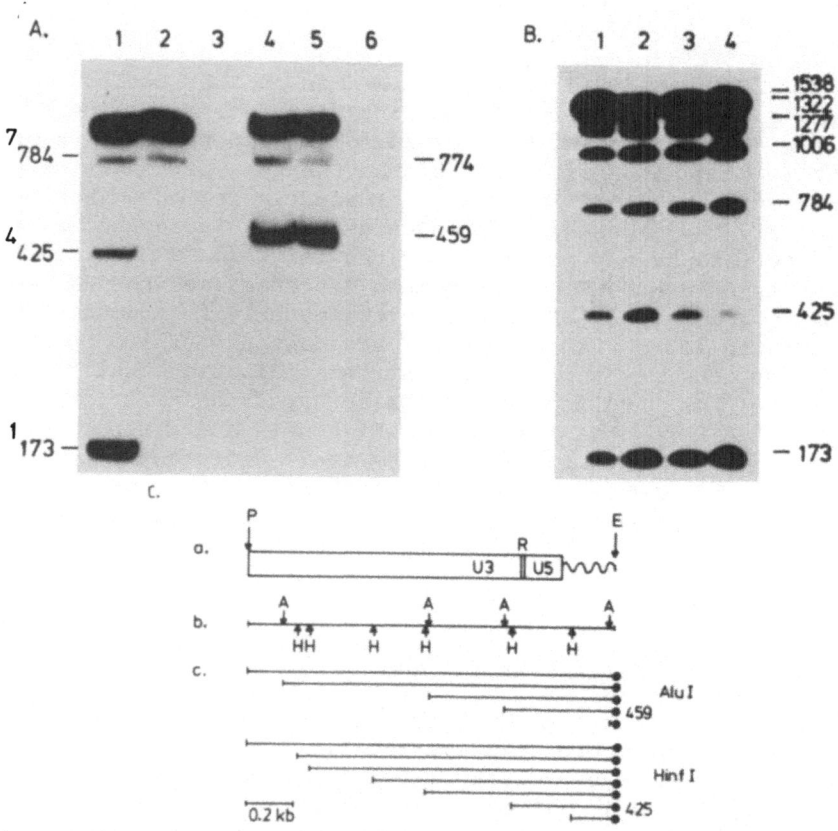

Fig. 4.   Mapping of TGGCA binding site on the 3' LTR of MMTV DNA. The
          DNA fragment (shown in Ca) containing nearly the entire 3'
          LTR plus 218 bp of the adjacent mouse genomic DNA (P = PstI,
          E = EcoRI) of GR16 (Hynes et al., 1983) was asymmetrically
          endlabeled at the EcoRI site by "fill in" with E. coli DNA
          polymerase (large fragment). The two procedures used for
          binding site mapping were previously described (Borgmeyer
          et al., 1984). A: The DNA was partially digested with Hin f1
          (H in Cb and Cc) or AluI (A in Cb and Cc), incubated with
          nuclear protein extracts from oviduct cells and passed
          through NC filters. Retained DNA was analyzed on an agarose
          gel (slot 2 for Hin f1 and slot 5 for AluI). Respective con-
          trols of DNA incubated with binding protein extract but used
          directly for analysis (slots 1 and 4) or incubated with BSA
          and filtered (slots 3 and 6) are shown. B: The DNA was in-
          cubated with BSA (slot 1) or inreasing amounts of oviduct
          nuclear extract (slots 2 to 4), then Hin f1 was added and the
          DNA partially digested. Resulting DNA fragments were analyzed
          on an agarose gel. Numbers give DNA length in bp.

In order to further map the DNA binding site, a so-called "restriction enzyme protection experiment" (Borgmeyer et al., 1984) was performed. As can be seen in Figure 4B preincubation with increasing amounts of nuclear extract leads to a direct protection of the Hin f1 site at 425 bp. The schematic diagrams in Figure 4C point out that the DNA binding site must fall very close to the left of the R sequence at the border between the U3 and U5 parts of the LTR. In DNAase I protection experiments, to be published elsewhere (Nowock et al., 1985), we could show that the TGGCA protein protects the noncoding strand DNA from DNAase digestion in the promoter region from positions -85 to -58 upstream from the transcriptional initiation site. The protected sequence GTTCTTTTGGAATCTATCCAAGTCTT includes a sequence related to the TGGCA-protein consensus sequence with its center at -70 bp (second C from the left) and includes the above-mentioned central Hin f1 site GAATC.

Figure 5 shows a summary of the protein recognition sequences of the three binding sites 5' to the chicken lysozyme gene (Borgmeyer et al., 1984) and the MMTV binding site (Nowock et al., 1985). The result stregthens our previous finding that the consensus recognition sequence includes a short palindromic DNA sequence, a

A: 0 3 1 1 1 0 0 0 0 1 4 2 0 1 1 0 0 0 3 3 1 1 1 0 1

G: 1 0 1 0 1 0 0 4 4 0 0 0 1 0 0 3 0 0 0 0 3 1 1 1 0

C: 1 0 2 1 1 2 0 0 0 3 0 1 1 2 0 0 3 4 1 1 0 1 2 2 1

T: 2 1 0 2 1 2 4 0 0 0 0 1 2 1 3 1 1 0 0 0 0 1 1 1 2

```
┌──────────────────────────────────┐
│ A · · · Py TGGCA · · · TGCCAAG · · · · · │
└──────────────────────────────────┘
        ←——— * ———→
```

Fig. 5 Summary of the TGGCA protein recognition sequences on lysozyme gene and MMTV DNA. The protein protected sequences of the three binding sites upstream from the chicken lysozyme gene (Borgmeyer et al., 1984) and the single homologous binding site on the MMTB LTR (Nowock et al., 1985) are aligned for maximal homology. The numbers give frequencies for each base, Py = pyrimidine. The boxed consensus sequence includes a region of two fold rotational symmetry marked by arrows.

feature reminiscent of procaryotic protein recognition sites on operator DNA (Pabo and Sauer, 1984). Future work must show whether the homology of the protein-DNA interaction between the region 6.0 kb upstream from the cap site of the chicken lysozyme gene and 70 bp upstream from the cap site of the MMTV LTR indicates a functional homology as well.

## A Highly Purified Fraction of Progesterone Receptor A Subunit Binds to the Promoter Region of the Chicken Lysozyme Gene

Steroid hormones act via a common molecular mechanism (Yamamoto and Alberts, 1976). Target cells are characterized by the presence of a highly specific steroid binding protein, the so-called receptor. It is generally believed that, upon binding of the hormone, the receptor translocates to a chromatin position close to the promoter of those genes the transcriptional activity of which is regulated. Direct in vitro binding of receptor to promoter DNA could thus far only be shown in case of the rat liver glucocorticoid receptor to the promoter of the MMTV LTR, the human metallothionein II gene and the chicken lysozyme gene (Scheidereit et al., 1983; Payvar et al., 1983; Karin et al., 1984; Renkawitz et al., 1984) and for the chicken progesterone receptor to the promoter region of the ovalbumin gene (Compton et al., 1983). Gene transfer experiments using a lysozyme-SV40 T-antigen fusion gene have shown that the regulatory DNA sites for glucocorticoid and progesterone action are located in a region between -200 and -50 bp 5' to the cap site of the lysozyme gene (Renkawitz et al., 1984).

We have purified the progesterone receptor A subunit from laying hen oviduct more than 50,000 times by chromatography on ion exchange and DNA-affinity columns (Bonifer et al., in preparation). In fractions in which the 76 KDa subunit A is 10 to 30% pure and the level of an unspecific DNA-binding protein component low, we could detect specific in vitro protein binding activity to the promoter region of the lysozyme gene. Figure 6 shows the result of a nitrocellulose filter binding experiment with the highly purified receptor fraction and a PstI fragment spanning the region from -460 to +310 bp. As can be seen from the pattern of filter-retained DNA, there is highly significant preferential binding to the PstI-Hin f1 subfragment -460 to -53 bp. The result is in full agreement with the mapping of the progesterone responsive site by gene transfer experiments (Renkawitz et al., 1984). Again, as in the case of the TGGCA protein and the DNAase hypersensitive site at -6.0 kb in the lysozyme gene domain, the steroid receptors bind to a region of increased DNAase sensitivity in active or potentially active oviduct chromatin (HS -0.1).

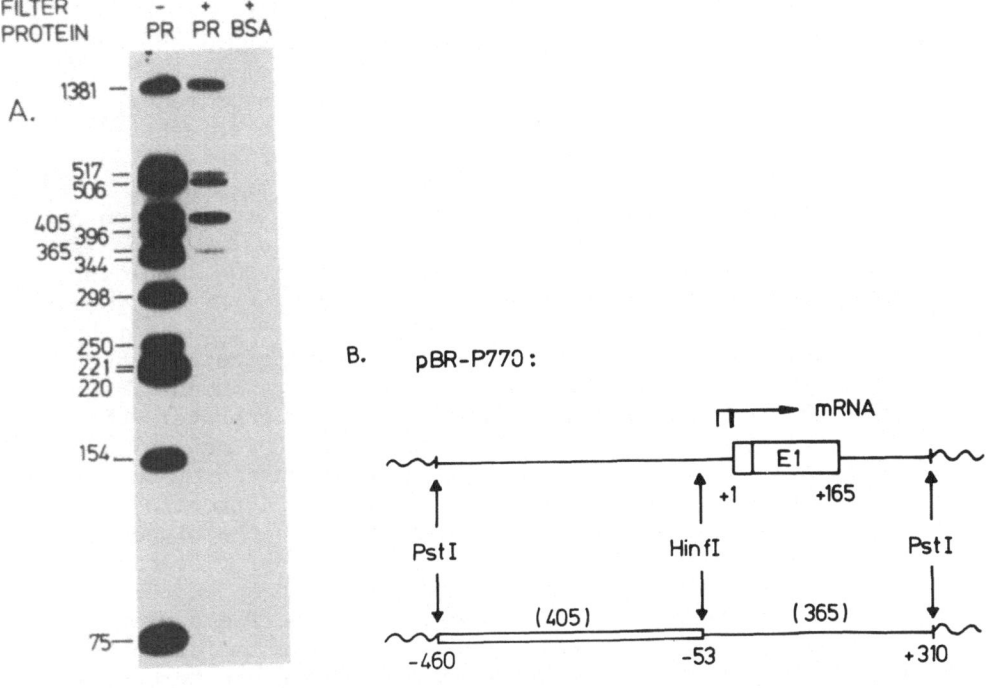

Fig. 6. Binding of a fraction of highly enriched progesterone receptor A subunit to the promoter region of the lysozyme gene.
A: The lysozyme gene PstI fragment from –460 to +310 bp was
subcloned in pBR322 (pBR-P770) restricted with Hin f1 and
labeled by "fill in" with E. coli DNA polymerase (large
fragment). In 50 µl reaction volume 17.6 ng digested plasmid
DNA (100 pM binding site) were incubated at 37°C with 1.3 nM
10% pure progesterone A subunit from laying hen oviduct
(Bonifer et al., in preparation). DNA was analyzed either
directly (filter –) or after filtration as nitrocellulose
retained fraction (filter +) on 5% acrylamide gels. Numbers
give the length of DNA fragments in bp. B: Schematic diagram
showing a map of the relevant chicken DNA region including
restriction sites, location of the first exon (E1) and
transcriptional initiation sites. PR = progesterone receptor.

Conclusions

The results of our extensive mapping of DNAase hypersensitive
sites 5' to the chicken lysozyme gene in the chromatin of various
tissues and at different regulatory states of the gene provide strong

support for a regulatory function of these sites. Since only a
single lysozyme gene is present per haploid genome and since no
indications for gross rearrangements on the DNA level could be found
(Sippel et al., 1980), it appears that diverse modes of regulation
of the same gene are associated solely with discrete epigenetic protein structures. The results presented here add to the existing evidence that DNAase hypersensitive chromatin regions mark sites of
nonhistone protein-DNA complexes. Specific sequence recognition by
DNA binding proteins is most likely one of the molecular mechanisms
involved in the formation of nonnucleosomal protein-DNA complexes.
These nonhistone DNA complexes could be necessary for RNA polymerase
II function as the transcription factor TFIIIA-DNA complex for RNA
polymerase III (Brown, 1984). Our two DNA binding proteins, the
TGGCA protein as well as the progesterone receptor A subunit, are
most likely involved in the construction of specific protein-DNA
complexes in eukaryotic chromatin. Another feature of nonnucleosomal
protein-DNA complexes is that they might be constructed by more than
one protein component. The binding site of the TGGCA protein on the
MMTV LTR is 3' adjacent and partially overlaps with the glucocorticoid receptor binding site (Scheidereit et al., 1983). The binding
site is also located close to the TATA motive of the promoter (-32
to -26). This in-between position suggests that the TGGCA protein can
make protein-protein contacts with other components to form a multifactorial stable complex at the promoter DNA. The progesterone receptor protein which binds close upstream from the conserved sequence
motives of the promoter of the lysozyme gene could again be part of
a multifactorial protein complex together with other steroid receptors and the proposed TATA-binding protein (Davison et al., 1983).
Similar to RNA polymerase III, RNA polymerase II would not have to
recognize naked DNA sequences or DNA packaged around nucleosomes,
but could interact with preformed regulatory protein-DNA complexes.

There are observations from our work which point to yet another
feature of the nonhistone protein DNA complexes. If the TGGCA protein
can form protein-protein contacts with the other protein components
at the MMTV LTR promoter, can it also do so in case of the lysozyme
promoter? It is striking that from our chromatin studies in 12 different types of nuclei (see Fig. 2) the TGGCA protein connected
DNAase hypersensitive site (HS -6.0) is the only one whose state
of chromatin coincided strictly with the state of the chromatin at
the promoter (HS -0.1). Protein-protein contact between the TGGCA
protein placed at -6.0 kb and proteins in complex with promoter DNA
could only be achieved if the long DNA stretch in between formed a
folded structure.

Theoretically, stable protein-DNA complexes could be composed
via protein-protein contacts whether their individual DNA binding
sites are located adjacent or apart from each other. Such "DNA loop
out" regulatory structures would have great evolutionary advantages.
It would not be necessary to align individual signal sequences along

the DNA in a strict order and at fixed distances. If protein-protein contacts can form a stable complex, varying lengths and orientations of DNA loops might be of minor importance. In this respect, the "loop out" model extends the evolutionary advantage of the exon-intron structure of eukaryotic genes (Gilbert, 1978) also to their regulatory sites in flanking DNA regions.

This work was supported by the Deutsche Forschungsgemeinschaft (SFB 74 and Forschergruppe Genomorganisation) and the Bundesministerium für Forschung und Technologie (BCT 0364/1).

REFERENCES

Borgmeyer, U., Nowock, J., and Sippel, A.E., 1984, The TGGCA-binding protein: a eukaryotic nuclear protein recognizing a symmetrical sequence on double-stranded linear DNA, Nucl. Acids Res. 12:4295.

Brown, D., 1984, The role of stable complexes that repress and activate eukaryotic genes, Cell 37:359.

Burch, J.B.E. and Weintraub, H., 1983, Temporal order of chromatin structural changes associated with activation of the major chicken vitellogenin gene. Cell 33:65.

Compton, J.G., Schrader, W.T., and O'Malley, B.W., 1983, DNA sequence preference of the progesterone receptor, Proc. Natl. Acad. Sci. USA 80:16.

Davison, B.L., Egly, J.-M., Mulvihill, E.R., and Chambon, P., 1983, Formation of stable preinitiation complexes between eukaryotic class B transcription factor and promoter sequences, Nature 301:680.

Fritton, H.P., Sippel, A.E., and Igo-Kemenes, T., 1983, Nuclease hypersensitive sites in the chromatin domain of the chicken lysozyme gene, Nucl. Acids Res. 11:3467.

Fritton, H.P., Igo-Kemenes, T., Nowock, J., Strech-Jurk, U., Theisen, M., and Sippel, A.E., 1984, Alternative sets of DNase I-hypersensitive sites characterize the various functional states of the chicken lysozyme gene, Nature 311:163.

Gilbert, W., 1978, Why genes in pieces? Nature 271:501.

Grez, M., Land, H., Giesecke, K., Schütz, G., Jung, A., and Sippel, A.E., 1981, Multiple mRNAs are generated from the chicken lysozyme gene. Cell 25:743.

Hauser, H., Graf, T., Beug, H., Greiser-Wilke, I., Lindenmaier, W., Grez, M., Land, H., Giesecke, K., and Schütz, G., Structure of the lysozyme gene and expression in the oviduct and macrophages, in: "Haematology and Blood Transfusion," Vol. 26, R. Neth, R.C. Gallo, T. Graf, K. Mannweiler, and K. Winkler, eds., Springer, Berlin (1981).

Hynes, N.E., Groner, B., Sippel, A.E., Jeep, S., Wurtz, T., Nguyen-Huu, M.C., Giesecke, K., and Schütz, G., 1979, Control of cellular content of chicken egg white protein specific RNA during estrogen administration and withdrawal, Biochemistry 18:616.

Hynes, N., van Ooyen, A.J.J., Herrlich, P., Ponta, H., and Groner, B., 1983, Subfragments of the large terminal repeat cause gluco-corticoid-responsive expression of mouse mammary tumor virus and of an adjacent gene. Proc. Natl. Acad. Sci. USA 80:3637.

Karin, M., Haslinger, A., Holtgreve, H., Richards, R.I., Krauter, P., Westphal, H.M., and Beato, M., 1984, Characterization of DNA sequences through which cadmium and glucocorticoid hormones induce human metallothionein $II_A$ gene, Nature 308:513.

McGhee, J.K., Wood, W.I., Dolan, M., Engel, J.D., and Felsenfeld, G., 1981, A 200 base pair region at the 5' end of the chicken adult ß-globin gene is accessible to nuclease digestion, Cell 27:45.

Nedospasov, S.A. and Georgiev, G.P., 1980, Non-random cleavage of SV40 DNA in the compact mini-chromosome and free in solution by micrococcal nuclease, Biochem. Biophys. Res. Commun. 92: 532.

Nowock, J. and Sippel, A.E., 1982, Specific protein-DNA interaction at four sites flanking the chicken lysozyme gene, Cell 30:607.

Nowock, J., Borgmeyer, U., Püschel, A.W., Rupp, R.A.W., and Sippel, A.E., 1985, The TGGCA protein binds to the MMTV LTR, the adenovirus origin of replication and the BK virus enhancer, submitted.

Pabo, C.O. and Sauer, R.T., 1984, Protein-DNA recognition, Ann. Rev. Biochem. 53:293.

Palmiter, R., 1972, Regulation of protein synthesis in chick oviduct. I. Independent regulation of ovalbumin, conalbumin, ovomucoid and lysozyme induction, J. Biol. Chem. 274:6450.

Payvar, F., DeFranco, D., Firestone, G.L., Edgar, B., Wrange, Ö., Okret, S., Gustafsson, J.-A., and Yamamoto, K.R., 1983, Se-quence-specific binding of the glucocorticoid receptor to MTV DNA at sites within and upstream of the transcribed re-gion, Cell 35:381.

Renkawitz, R., Schütz, G., von der Ahe, D., and Beato, M., 1984, Sequences in the promoter region of the chicken lysozyme gene required for steroid regulation and receptor binding, Cell 37:503.

Scheidereit, C., Geisse, S., Westphal, H.M., and Beato, M., 1983, The glucocorticoid receptor binds to defined nucleotide se-quences near the promoter of mouse mammary tumour virus, Nature 304:749.

Schütz, G., Nguyen-Huu, M.C., Giesecke, K., Hynes, N.E., Groner, B., Wurtz, T., and Sippel, A.E., 1978, Hormonal control of egg white protein messenger RNA synthesis in the chicken oviduct, Cold Spring Harbor Symp. Quant. Biol. 42:617.

Sippel, A.E., Nguyen-Huu, M.C., Lindenmaier, W., Blin, N., Lurz, R., Hauser, H., Giesecke, K., Land, H., Grez, M., and Schütz, G., Mechanism of induction of egg white protein by steroid hor-mones, in: "Steroid induced uterine proteins," M. Beato, ed.,

Elsevier/North-Holland Biomedical Press, Amsterdam, New York (1980).

Sippel, A.E. and Nowock, J., The gene for chicken lysozyme: Structure and expression, in: "Biochemistry of Differentiation and Morphogenesis, 33rd Colloquium - Mosbach," L. Jaenicke, ed., Springer-Verlag, Berlin, Heidelberg (1982).

Sippel, A.E., The egg white protein genes, in: "Eukaryotic Genes: Their Structure, Activity and Regulation," N. McLean, S.O. Gregory, and R.A. Flavell, eds., Butterworths, London (1983).

Witte, V., 1984, Mittelrepetitive Sequenzelemente in der Region des Gens für Hühnerlysozym, Diploma thesis, University of Cologne.

Wu, C., 1980, The 5' ends of Drosophila heat shock genes in the chromatin are hypersensitive to DNAase I, Nature 286:854.

Yamamoto, K.R. and Alberts, B.M., 1976, Steroid receptors: elements for modulation of eukaryotic transcription, Ann. Rev. Biochem. 45:721.

# NUCLEASE ACTIVATION IN PROGRAMMED CELL DEATH

A.H. Wyllie, R.G. Morris, M.J. Arends and A.E. Watt

Department of Pathology
University of Edinburgh Medical School
Teviot Place
Edinburgh EH8 9AG

The subject of cell death has always had a following amongst developmental biologists (Glucksmann, 1951). It is not difficult to see why, for the programmed deletion of cells in specific sites is a prominent and apparently necessary feature of development of most structures, and abnormalities in the pattern and quantity of cell death lead to malformations. Early studies included impressive descriptions of the unusual morphology of cell death in this context (Bellairs, 1961). It became clear that at least some of the deaths were intrinsically programmed – that is they occurred on schedule even when the cells in question were removed from their natural environment and grafted elsewhere (Saunders, 1966). In a number of cell systems, notably the avian wing bud (Fallon & Saunders, 1968; Hinchliffe & Griffiths, 1984), the palatal shelves during fusion (Pratt & Greene, 1976; Hassell & Pratt, 1977), and the motor neurones supplying skeletal muscle (O'Connor & Wyttenbach 1974; Oppenheim, 1984), information continues to accumulate on the stimuli which initiate the programme of death, or can modify it once it is under way.

The organised deletion of cells within living tissues is not the exclusive prerogative of developmental biology, however. Cells are constantly deleted from mature labile tissues, balancing the cell gain by mitosis. Endocrine target tissues in particular show phases of cell death, apparently as a result of alteration in the prevailing levels of trophic hormones (Wyllie et al., 1973; Kerr & Searle, 1973; Hopwood & Levison, 1974; Sandow et al., 1979; Anderson, Ferguson & Raab, 1982). An outstanding but still poorly explained property of the majority of tumour cell populations is their high rate of cell loss (Steel, 1977; Kerr & Lamb, 1984). In these varied circumstances the stimuli for death are most unlikely to be closely similar, but

33

there are reasons for believing that the intracellular effector
pathways share many features.  This chapter attempts to define
discrete molecular events within these pathways.  Our principal
emphasis will be on changes within the nucleus, but to place them in
context we begin with a summary of the major structural changes in
both nucleus and cytoplasm during programmed cell death.


MORPHOLOGICAL CHANGES IN PROGRAMMED CELL DEATH

     Only a summary of the morphological changes in cell death is
given here, as detailed descriptions have been published elsewhere
(Kerr, Wyllie & Currie, 1972; Wyllie, Kerr & Currie, 1980).  The dying
cells undergo an initial phase of reduction in volume.  This is
associated with convolution of the cell membrane, compaction of
cytoplasmic organelles and dilatation of endoplasmic reticulum.
Vesicles of endoplasmic reticulum appear to fuse with the plasma
membrane, and scanning electron micrographs show bizarre cratered
surfaces (Morris et al., 1984).  In general, the structure of
cytoplasmic organelles is conserved, although on occasion unusual
semi-crystalline arrays of free ribosomes have been observed
(Ballairs, 1961; O'Connor & Wyttenbach, 1974).  The most dramatic
changes, however, occur in the nucleus.  Chromatin undergoes a
characteristic peripheral condensation, producing hemilunar or
toroidal deposits of granular, osmiophilic material underneath the
nuclear membrane.  Initially the centre of the nucleus remains
electron lucent, with the exception of the remnants of the nucleolus.
This organelle shows segregation of its fibrillar and granular
components.  The fibrillar centre tends to lie close to the peripheral
condensed chromatin, whilst the granular component disaggregates into
coarse osmiophilic particles.  The nuclear membrane remains intact,
although pore structures are not observed adjacent to the condensed
peripheral chromatin.  At this stage the nucleus may fragment into
several portions.  There is progressive compaction, with loss of the
central electron lucent zones, until the nuclear material is
represented only by globular masses of densely osmiophilic material.
The nuclear fibrillar centre is identifiable until late in the
process.

     These changes in the nucleus are sometimes accompanied by
fragmentation of the whole cell into a series of membrane-bounded
bodies each containing an assortment of organelles or nuclear
fragments.  The dying cells and their fragments at this stage exclude
vital dyes and retain enzymic activities, but they are recognised by
adjacent cells which bind to and phagocytose them.  The identity of
these phagocytic cells varies according to circumstances, but they may
be either resident members of the monocyte/macrophage series, or on
occasion, adjacent parenchymal cells.  Once within the phagosome of
the digesting cell, the fragments of the dying cells undergo a series
of degradative changes, and their ultimate appearance is that of any
large lysosomal residual body.

This distinctive series of events contrasts with the swelling and rupture which are commonly observed when cells are killed through abrupt cessation of oxygen or substrate supply, or by membrane-active agents including complement, detergents or lytic virus infection at high multiplicity (Wyllie, 1986). The morphological changes are, however, widespread in biology (Kerr, Wyllie & Currie, 1972; Wyllie, Kerr & Currie, 1980), and occur in essentially similar form in cell death in development, endocrine-induced atrophy, normal tissue turnover, tumour populations during growth and regression, and in the targets of cell killing by T cells and NK cells (Russell, 1983). To distinguish this mode of cell death from others, it has been called apoptosis.

In the remainder of this article we attempt to clarify the nuclear events which underlie the unique morphological changes of apoptosis.


INTRANUCLEAR EVENTS IN APOPTOSIS

Despite their obvious importance, developmental systems are poorly suited to detailed study of the cell biology of apoptosis, as the affected cells are surrounded and usually greatly out-numbered by their viable neighbours. Accordingly, we adopted as our experimental model, systems in which a high proportion of the cells could be induced to undergo apoptosis on application of a defined stimulus. Certain lymphoid cell lines provide suitable material, as they are readily cultured in suspension in vitro, and undergo apoptosis on application of glucocorticoid hormones. Rodent cortical thymocytes, in short term culture, also undergo apoptosis after a few hours' exposure to glucocorticoid, and afford the further advantage that the early apoptotic cells can be purified by density centrifugation (Wyllie & Morris, 1982). Using these systems, we have reached the following conclusions about the nuclear events in apoptosis.

The characteristic chromatin condensation is always associated with cleavage of DNA at dispersed, internucleosomal sites, apparently through the action of an endogenous endonuclease (Wyllie 1980; Wyllie et al., 1984). It is clear that this cleavage is responsible for the morphological changes, because isolated nuclei, treated with purified nucleases in the presence of high concentrations of protease inhibitors, show nearly identical changes. The chromatin fragments in the nuclei of apoptotic cells consist of well-organised nucleosome chains which, by the criteria of nucleosome sedimentation rates, buoyant density in caesium chloride after formaldehyde fixation, digestion kinetics with exogenous nucleases, and SDS gel electrophoresis of the constituent proteins, show the normal complement and arrangement of the most abundant chromatin proteins, including histones and HMG 1 and 2 (Wyllie, Morris & Arands, unpublished work). Morphological studies on proteinaceous nuclear residues after treatment with high salt and exogenous nuclease (i.e. 'nuclear matrices') show normal peripheral structures in apoptotic nuclei also (Wyllie, Duvall & Blow, 1984). However, these lymphoid cells proved very fragile and our studies did not permit good visualisation of the centre of the nuclear matrix, which could have been altered.

Further analysis of the chromatin fragments indicates that they are of two types: a majority (approx. 70% in thymocytes) retaining attachment to the matrix, and a minority in which there is a higher proportion of mono- and lower order oligonucleosomes, which separates freely from the nucleus. Studies to determine whether these two fractions of chromatin include distinctive DNA sequences are in process, but it appears likely that the free oligonucleosomes derive from chromatin that was in an unfolded conformation prior to the onset of apoptosis.

These observations suggest that a major determinant of the changes of apoptosis within the nucleus is the activation of endonuclease enzymes, apparently in the absence of substantial proteolytic activity. We therefore set about attempting to isolate the enzymes responsible.

## NUCLEAR ENDONUCLEASE ACTIVITY IN APOPTOSIS

Rodent and human thymocytes contain an endonuclease, active at neutral pH, which is dependent on the coincident presence of calcium and magnesium, and which cleaves chromatin at dispersed inter-nucleosomal sites (Cohen & Duke, 1984; Wyllie, Morris & Watt, 1986). The enzyme appears to prefer such dispersed sites of action; when exposed to purified SV40 DNA as substrate it does not generate substantial quantities of acid soluble material even after prolonged digestion. The enzyme activity can be recovered from both cytoplasm and nucleus, and elutes optimally from the nucleus at salt concentrations above 200 mM, suggesting that it may normally be bound to nuclear DNA. In thymocytes it appears to be a protein of rapid turnover, as the recovered activity is much lower in cells previously treated for a few hours with cyclo-heximide or emetine.

Nuclei of several cultured cell lines contain little similar nuclease activity, including those of the rodent S49 lymphoma and the human lymphoid line CCRF CEM C7, both T-cell derived glucocorticoid sensitive lines. However, in these two cell lines, the enzyme activity rises after treatment with glucocorticoid, in parallel with evidence of endogenous chromatin cleavage and the appearance of the morphological changes of apoptosis (Fig. 1). In contrast, steroid treatment does not induce the enzyme in sublines of CCRF CEM C7 which

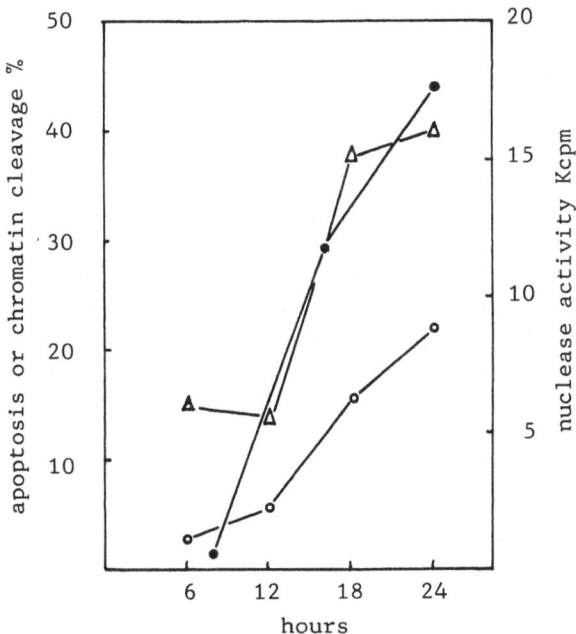

Fig. 1    Changes in nuclear morphology (O), chromatin cleavage (▲) and
          extractable endonuclease activity (●) in S49 murine lymphoma
          cells during the induction of apoptosis by treatment with $10^{-6}$
          M methyl- prednisolone in vitro.  Changes in nuclear
          morphology were quantified by scoring the percentage of cells
          showing apoptosis.  Chromatin cleavage was measured as the
          proportion of total chromatin failing to sediment after
          centrifugation at 27,000g for 20 mins. of cell lysates in 10mM
          Tris, 5mM EDTA, 0.5% Triton.  Extractable nuclease was
          measured by co-incubating S49 nuclei with a suspension of
          heptoma nuclei, labelled with tritiated thymidine during
          growth in culture, and recording the counts released into the
          supernatant.

were selected for resistance to the lethal effects of glucocorticoid.

     By virtue of its mode of cleavage, nuclear location, and
association with terminally differentiated cells and cells about to
undergo apoptosis, we feel that this calcium/magnesium dependent
endonuclease is likely to be responsible for the chromatin changes
in apoptosis.  More definitive proof is difficult to acquire without
further purification and intervention studies.  It is of interest,
however, that endonucleases with some of these properties have been
isolated previously from cells of the thymus gland (Nakamura et al.,
1981) in which apoptosis is normally plentiful; in liver (Stratling,
Grade & Horz, 1984) in which it is readily induced (Kerr, 1971); and

in lens cells in the course of their differentiation (Herve, Jacquemin
& Lescure, 1983), in which chromatin condensation associated with
internucleoscmal cleavage also occurs (Appleby & Modak, 1977) and
appears to be dependent upon protein synthesis (Counis et al., 1980).
It has been postulated that such enzymes would remain inactive within
the nucleus until application of a calcium pulse as the magnesium (but
not the calcium) concentration in the nucleus is probably in the
millimolar range (Duke, Cherniak & Cohen, 1983).  The suggestion has
also been made by these workers that such nuclear endonucleases may be
inhibited by zinc, a metal ion present in relatively high
concentration within the nucleus.  There is much attraction in this
proposition, since zinc depletion appears to cause cell deletion in
several different cell systems (Fraker, Haas & Luecke, 1977; Elmes,
1977; Elmes & Gwyn Jones, 1980; Donahoe et al., 1982).

In conclusion it may be asked why terminal differentiation and
programmed cell death should be associated with the capacity for
endogenous chromatin cleavage of this sort.  Three possible answers
may be proffered.  Firstly, it is known that transcription is very
greatly reduced when DNA is altered from a supercoiled to a relaxed
conformation, even in the presence of identical chromatin packaging
proteins (Harland, Weintraub & McKnight, 1983).  Dispersed cleavage
events would destroy supercoiling and so might be expected to cause a
swift decline of transcription to low levels.  In fact, the uridine
incorporation in apoptotic cells is a barely detectable fraction of
that of normal thymocytes (Wyllie & Morris, 1982).  Secondly, the
efficient handling of potentially re-cyclable cellular material may be
facilitated by nuclease action as this would reduce the high viscosity
of high molecular weight DNA and chromatin.  Finally, since the
chromatin of apoptotic cells normally finds itself within the endosome
compartment cf an adjacent viable cell, there is at least a
theoretical possibility that some of the DNA sequences might become
available for reinsertion into the genome of the phagocytic cell - a
type of in vivo "transfection".  Multiple cleavage events within the
apoptotic chromatin may serve the function of reducing the possibility
that active and potentially damaging genes may be transferred from
cell to cell by this route.

ACKNOWLEDGEMENT

The authors' work was supported by the Cancer Research Campaign
and the Wellcome Trust.

REFERENCES

Anderson, T.J., Ferguson, D.J.P. and Raab, G.M., 1982, Cell turnover
     in the "resting" human breast:  influence of parity,
          contraceptive pill, age and laterality.  Br. J.Cancer, 46: 376.

Appleby, D.W. and Modal, S.P., 1977,  DNA degradation in terminally
        differentiating lens fibre cells from chick embryos. Proc.
        Natl. Acad. Sci. USA, 74: 5579.
Bellairs, R., 1961, Cell death in chick embryos as studied by electron
        microscopy. J. Anat. 95: 54.
Cohen, J.J. and Duke, R.C., 1984, Glucocorticoid activation of a
        calcium-dependent endonuclease in thymic nuclei leads to cell
        death. J. Immunol., 132: 38.
Counis, M.F., Chaudun, E., Carreau, J.P. and Courtois, Y., 1980,
        Cycloheximide effects on DNA degradation and δ-crystallin
        synthesis in terminally differentiating lens cells. Biochem.
        Biophys. Acta. 607: 43.
Donahue, P.K., Budzik, G.P., Trelstad, R., Mudgett-Hunter, M., Fuller,
        A., Hutson, J.M., Ikawa, H., Hayashi, A. and MacLaughlin, D.,
        1982, Mullerian-inhibitory substances:  an update. Rec.Progr.
        Horm. Res. 38: 279.
Duke, R.C., Cherniak, R. and Cohen, J.J., 1983, Endogenous endo
        nuclease-induced DNA fragmentation: an early event in cell-
        mediated cytolysis. Proc. Natl. Acad. Sci. USA 80: 6361.
Elmes, M.E., 1977, Apoptosis in the small intestine of zinc-deficient
        and fasted rats. J. Pathol. 123: 219.
Elmes, M.E. and Gwyn Jones, J., 1980, Ultrastructural studies on
        paneth cell apoptosis in zinc deficient rats. Cell TissueRes.,
        208: 57.
Fallon, J.F. and Saunders, J.W., 1968, In vitro analysis of the
        control of cell death in a zone of prospective necosis from the
        chick wing bud. Dev. Biol. 18: 553.
Fraker, P.J., Haas, S.M. and Luecke, R.W., 1977, Effect of zinc
        deficiency on the immune response of the young adult A/J mouse.
        J. Nutr. 107: 1889.
Glucksmann, A., 1951, Cell deaths in normal vertebrate ontogeny. Biol.
        Rev. 26: 59.
Harland, R.M., Weintraub, H. and McKnight, S.L., 1983, Transcription
        of DNA injected into Xenopus oocytes is influenced by template
        topology. Nature 302: 38.
Hassell, J.R. and Pratt, R.M., 1977, Elevated levels of cAMP alter the
        effect of epidermal growth factor in vitro on programmed cell
        death in the secondary palate epithelium. Exp. Cell Res. 106:
        55
Herve, B., Jacquemin, E. and Lescure, B., 1983, Endogenous endo
        nuclease activity in chick embryo lens cells. Cell Differ.,12:
        265.
Hinchliffe, J.R. and Griffiths, P.J., 1984, Experimental analysis of
        the control of cell death in chick limb bud development. in
        "Cell Ageing and Cell Death" I. Davies and D.C. Sigee, eds.,
        Cambridge University Press, pp223
Hopwood, D. and Levison, D.A., 1974, Atrophy and apoptosis in the
        cyclical human endometrium. J. Pathol. 119: 159
Kerr, J.F.R., 1971, Shrinkage necrosis, a distinct mode of cellular
        death. J. Pathol. 105: 13-20.

Kerr, J.F.R. and Searle, J., 1973, Deletion of cells by apoptosis
    during castration-induced involution of the rat prostate.
    Virchows Arch. B. 13: 87.

Kerr, J.F.R., Wyllie, A.H. and Currie, A.R., 1972, Apoptosis: a basic
    biological phenomenon with wide-ranging implications in tissue
    kinetics. Br. J. Cancer, 26: 239.

Kerr, K.M. and Lamb, D., 1984, Actual growth rate and tumour cell
    proliferation in human pulmonary neoplasms. Br. J. Cancer, 50:
    343.

Morris, R.G., Duvall, E., Hargreaves, A.D. and Wyllie, A.H., 1984,
    Hormone-induced cell death 2.  Changes in the cell surface
    of apoptotic thymocytes. Am. J. Pathol. 115: 426.

Nakamura, M., Saraki, Y., Watanabe, N. and Takagi, Y., 1981,
    Purification and characterization of the $Ca^{2+}$ plus $Mg^{2+}$-
    dependent endonucleases from calf thymus chromatin. J.Biochem.
    (Tokyo), 89: 143.

O'Connor, T.M. and Wyttenbach, C.R., 1974, Cell death in the embryonic
    chick spinal cord.  J. Cell Biol. 60: 448.

Oppenheim, R.W., 1984, Cell death in motoneurones in the chick embryo
    spinal cord VIII.  Motoneurones prevented from dying in the
    embryo persist after hatching. Dev. Biol., 101: 35.

Pratt, R.B. and Greene, R.M., 1976, Inhibition of palatal epithelial
    cell death by altered protein synthesis. Dev.Biol. 54: 135.

Russell, J.H., 1983, Internal disintegration model of cytotoxic
    lymphocyte-induced target damage. Immunol. Rev. 72: 97.

Sandow, B.A., West, N.B., Norman, R.L. and Brenner, R.M., 1979,
    Hormonal control of apoptosis in hamster uterine lumen
    epithelium. Am. J. Anat. 156: 15.

Saunders, J.W., 1966, Death in embryonic systems. Science 154: 604

Steel, G.G., 1977, Growth kinetics of tumours.  Cell population
    kinetics in relation to the growth and treatment of cancer.
    Clarendon, Oxford.

Stratling, W.H., Grade, C. and Horz, W., 1984, Ca/Mg-dependent
    endonuclease from porcine liver. J. Biol. Chem., 259: 5893

Wyllie, A.H., 1980, Glucocorticoid-induced thymocyte apoptosis is
    associated with endogenous endonuclease activation. Nature,
    284: 555

Wyllie, A.H., 1986, Cell Death, Int. Rev. Cytol. (in press).

Wyllie, A.H., Duvall, E. and Blow, J.J., 1984, Intracellular
    mechanisms in cell death in normal and pathological tissues.
    in: "Cell Ageing and Cell Death" I. Davies and D.S. Sigee,
    eds., Cambridge University Press, pp269.

Wyllie, A.H., Kerr, J.F.R. and Currie, A.R., 1980, Cell death:  the
    significance of apoptosis. Int. Rev. Cytol. 68: 251.

Wyllie, A.H., Kerr, J.F.R., Macaskill, I.A.M. and Currie, A.R., 1973,
    Adrenocortical cell deletion: the role of ACTH. J. Pathol.
    111: 85.

Wyllie, A.H. and Morris, R.G., 1982, Hormone-induced cell death.
    Purification and properties of thymocytes undergoing apoptosis
    after glucocorticoid treatment. Am. J. Pathol. 109: 78.

Wyllie, A.H., Morris, R.G., Smith, A.L. and Dunlop, D., 1984,
        Chromatin cleavage in apoptosis:  association with condensed
        chromatin morphology and dependence on macromolecular
        synthesis.  J. Pathol. 142: 67.
Wyllie, A.H., Morris, R.G. and Watt, A.E.  Terminally differentiated
        and dying lymphoid cells contain nuclear endonuclease
        potentially responsible for chromatin changes of apoptosis.
        J. Path, 148:94A.

# REGULATION OF GENE EXPRESSION

## INTRODUCTION

Continuing the theme of transcriptional controls begun in a general way in the first section, we can now turn to the more responsive and selective transcriptional controls exemplified by the papers in this section dealing with specific genes. In this context we consider both specific sequences which may respond to particular factors present in differentiated cells and cellular environments for signals which elicit such responses.

The role of upstream elements in specific transcriptional control has been indicated by experiments involving constructs with reporter sequences inserted into specific cell types (Walker et al., 1983), by deletion experiments associated with switchable gene expression, as in work on the heat-shock proteins (Pelham, 1982), or by studies of binding of regulatory proteins to specific DNA sequences (Payvar et al., 1981). Other technical approaches include inserting the gene or a range of constructs into a cytoplasmic environment wholly novel to the gene in question such as an oocyte, a teratocarcinoma cell, or cells of a different species. Further possibilities of regulation of transcription involve alternative promotors and alternative starting points of transcription.

While there is no doubt that the interactions between DNA and its molecular environment, by regulating transcription, have a key role in cellular differentiation, it is clear that a full understanding of the regulation of the cellular phenotype involves a number of other levels of regulation. The processing of the primary transcript to mature messenger RNA by splicing, capping and polyadenylation and the transport of the mRNA to the cytoplasm are some of the stages at which regulation can occur which affects mRNA availability for translation in tissue-specific manner (Young et al., 1981; Capetaneki et al., 1983; Rosenfeld et al., 1984). In addition to these stages which affect the production of messages, their cellular concentration can also be affected by sequestration (Showman et al., 1982; Moon et al., 1983), or by changes of stability, and there are a number of systems in which both production of mRNA and its breakdown are regulated so as to affect protein synthesis, as in the control of ovalbumin by oestrogen (Palmiter and Carey, 1974).

43

Selective control of translation of messenger RNA that is present in the cell has been demonstrated in a number of instances (Rosenthal, et al., 1980). After the synthesis of proteins there are several types of modification that can occur to convert the initial polypeptide chain into its biologically active form, including cleavage, addition of prosthetic groups or interaction with other polypeptide chains.

While many studies of molecular aspects of development and differentiation have been based on analyses of populations of cells within tissues, it must be remembered that within a cell population there can be distinct heterogeneities, with varying levels of cellular components found in adjacent cells, which may appear to be similar morphologically (Jeanny et al., 1985).

From some of the earliest experiments in embryology it is evident that the DNA in different portions of the embryo comes to occupy different cellular environments. This heterogeneity originated in the spatial organisation of the undivided egg; but disparities in the cellular environment are self-increasing with successive cell divisions. Part of the heterogeneity is intrinsic to the cell, and some may reside in the differential capacity to be exposed to, to accept, and to respond to external signals of various kinds. The task of the developmental biologist is to identify the factors which control transcription specifically, the sequences of DNA which recognise them, and their mode of action.

The study of oncogenes has provided us with a powerful tool for the analysis of gene expression in two different ways: the investigation of cellular pathology may be expected to illuminate specifically the processes which are disturbed, (as does the investigation of pathology at any level), but it has become evident recently that the oncogenes have specific roles to play in normal differentiation. One of the classes of oncogenes is thought to have a specific role in regulating the transcription of other genes, and it has been suggested that there may also be a class which regulates DNA replication. The function of some oncogenes in normal cells may be to encode growth factors or growth factor receptors, (reviewed by Hamlyn and Dyson, 1984, Bishop, 1985).

REFERENCES

Bishop, J.M., 1985, Trends in oncogenes, Trends in Genetics, 1:245.
Capetaneki, Y.G., Ngai, J., Flytzanis, C.N. and Lazarides, E., 1983.
    Tissue-specific expression of two mRNA species transcribed from a
    single vimentin gene, Cell, 35:411
Hamlyn, P.A. and Dyson, P.J., 1984, Oncogenes, in, Molecular Biology

and Human Disease, 1984, A. MacLeod and K. Sikorz, p150,
Blackwell Scientific Publishers, Oxford, London, Edinburgh.

Jeanny, J-C., Bower, D.J., Errington, L.H., Morris, S. and Clayton,
R.M., 1985, Cellular heterogeneity in the expression of the δ-
crystallin gene in non lens tissues, Dev. Biol., 112:94.

Moon, R.T., Nicosia, R.F., Olsen, C., Hille, M.B. and Jeffery, W.R.,
1983, The cytoskeletal framework of sea urchin eggs and embryos:
developmental changes in the association of messenger RNA,
Dev. Biol., 95:447.

Palmiter, R.D. and Carey, N.H., 1974, Rapid inactivation of ovalbumin
messenger ribonucleic acid after acute withdrawal of estrogen.
Proc. Natl. Acad. Sci. U.S.A., 71:2357.

Payvar, F., DeFranco, D., Firestone, G.L., Edgar, B., Wrange O.,
Okret, S., Gustafsson, S-A. and Yamamoto, K.R., 1981, Sequence-
specific binding of glucocorticoid receptor of MTV DNA at sites
within and upstream of the transcribed region, Cell, 35:381.

Pelham, H.R.B., 1982, A regulatory upstream promoter element in the
Drosophila hsp70 heat-shock gene, Cell, 30:517.

Rosenfeld, M.G., Amara, S.G., and Evans, R.M., 1984, Alternative RNA
processing:  determining neuronal phenotype, Science, 225:1315.

Rosenthal, E.T., Hunt, T. and Ruderman, J.V., 1980, Selective
translation of mRNA controls the pattern of protein synthesis
during early development of the surf clan spisula solidissima,
Cell, 20:487.

Showman, R.M., Wells, D.E., Anstrom, J., Hursh, D.A. and Raff, R.A.,
1982, Message-specific sequestration of maternal histone mRNA in
the sea urchin egg, Proc. Natl. Acad. Sci. U.S.A., 79:5944.

Walker, M.D., Edlund, T., Boulet, A.M. and Rutter, W.J., 1983, Cell-
specific expression controlled by the 5'-flanking region of
insulin and chymotrypsin genes, Nature, 306:557.

Young, R.A., Hagenbuchle, O. and Schibler, U., 1981, A single mouse
alpha-anylase gene specifies two different tissue specific mRNAs.
Cell, 23:451.

# REGULATION OF ALPHA-AMYLASE GENE EXPRESSION

H.C. Hurst, O. Hagenbüchle, U. Schibler, P.H. Shaw, D.L. Cribbs and P.K. Wellauer

I.S.R.E.C., 1066 Epalinges, Switzerland

## INTRODUCTION

The aim of our studies is to elucidate in molecular detail the principles underlying the tissue specific expression of eucaryotic genes. It is hoped that by understanding how a particular gene becomes activated in one (or a few), but not other tissues we may gain more insight into the complex processes that govern cellular differentiation. The alpha-amylase multigene family of mouse has proven a suitable model system to study tissue specific modulation of gene expression since members of this gene family are expressed with different efficiencies in the pancreas, parotid gland and liver.

## Structure of alpha-amylase genes

In rodents alpha-amylase proteins and mRNA's accumulate to very different concentrations in the exocrine pancreas, the parotid gland and the liver (Takeuchi et al., 1975; Ray et al., 1979). Typical levels of alpha-amylase mRNA within the cytoplasmic $p(A)^+$ RNA of each of these tissues in mouse are : pancreas, $10^5$ molecules/cell (23%); parotid gland, $10^4$ molecules/cell (2%); liver $10^2$ molecules/cell (0.02%), (Schibler et al., 1980). The alpha-amylase structural genes are located at two closely linked, but distinct genetic loci, Amy-1 (parotid-like) and Amy-2 (pancreas-like) on mouse chromosome 3 (Sick and Nielsen, 1964; Eicher and Lane, 1980). We have cloned and characterized these genes from the inbred mouse strain A/J which expresses only a single isozyme species for each form of alpha-amylase. The structure of the mouse alpha-amylase genes Amy-1[a] and Amy-2[a] is depicted in Figure 1.

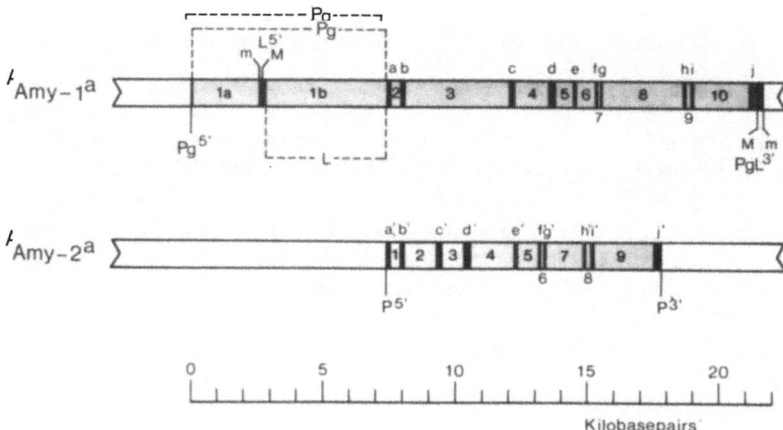

**Figure 1.** Sequence organization of mouse alpha-amylase genes, Amy-1ᵃ and Amy-2ᵃ.

These maps are based on restriction enzyme mapping, electron microscopy and sequence analysis. Introns are shown as shaded boxes and are numbered. Exons are represented with black boxes with comparable exons between the two genes lettered according-ly. Flanking sequences are shown as open boxes. The cap (5') and polyadenylation (3') sites are marked for the pancreatic (P) and for the major (M) and minor (m) liver (L) and parotid gland (Pg) alpha-amylase mRNA's. Dashed lines indicate the tissue-specific RNA splicing events that occur to generate Amy-1ᵃ transcripts with the tissue specific parotid gland (Pg) and liver (L) leader sequences.

The Amy-1$^a$ gene is present at only one copy per haploid genome and specifies both parotid gland and liver alpha-amylase mRNAs which have identical coding regions, but different 5' noncoding leader sequences (Hagenbüchle et al., 1981; Young et al., 1981). These tissue specific leader sequences are encoded by separate exons that map 2.9 kb apart in the genome (Young et al., 1981; Schibler et al., 1982). Both of these exons have their own cap sites and a distinct promoter. Expression from the parotid promoter, producing an alpha-amylase mRNAs with a parotid specific 47 nucleotide leader sequence, is detected solely in the acinar cells of the parotid gland. However, transcripton from the liver promoter is observed in all three amylase producing tissues resulting in an mRNA species possessing the liver-specific 158 nucleotide leader sequence (Schibler et al., 1983).

The Amy-2$^a$ locus, which specifies pancreatic alpha-amylase mRNA and which is active exclusively within this tissue, is composed of multiple (four) similar genes that exhibit minor differences in their restriction enzyme maps. The coding sequences of all four genes appear to be identical, producing a mRNA species 89% homologous to the Amy-1$^a$ transcripts (Hagenbüchle et al., 1980). With the exception of the tissue specific first exons and the first intron in Amy-1$^a$, which have no counterpart in Amy-2$^a$, the coding region of both loci are divided between 10 exons with the introns being located at similar if not identical positions within comparable regions of the two genes (Schibler et al., 1982). Some introns also exhibit considerable (50%) sequence homology. This suggests that the two loci evolved by duplication of a common, split ancestor gene. Recent genomic cloning has led to the isolation of a 106 kb region which contains the single Amy-1$^a$ gene, 23 kb of intervening DNA and one member of the Amy-2$^a$ multigene family, denoted Amy-2$^{a1}$ (Pittet and Schibler, submitted). Presumably the other Amy-2$^a$ genes are linked further downstream to this copy, but cloning in cosmids has so far failed to yield two linked copies. Therefore, these genes are spaced at greater that 40 kb (S. Bodary, unpublished observation).

In addition to Amy-1$^a$ and Amy-2$^a$ several other amylase-like sequences exist in the mouse genome. One of these sequences, designated Amy-X, has been cloned and analyzed in some detail, showing it to be closely related to Amy-2$^a$. However, expression from Amy-X is undetectable within all mouse tissues examined. Therefore, Amy-X is most likely a pseudogene, although it cannot be ruled out that it is expressed during early development or within mouse tissues not yet examined (Schibler et al., 1982).

<u>Tissue-specific expression of alpha-amylase genes</u>

A variety of techniques have been used to examine the
expression of the alpha-amylase genes, including S1 mapping of
steady state nuclear RNA and analysis of nascent alpha-amylase
transcripts within nuclei isolated from mouse tissues.

The most important finding is that transcription from the
alpha-amylase genes is absolutely tissue specific, only occurring
in the tissues that accumulate the native mRNA's. Transcription
from all three amylase promoters initiates at the cap sites while
termination has been found to occur several kb downstream of the
polyadenylation sites of both <u>Amy</u>-1$^a$ and <u>Amy</u>-2$^a$. RNA molecules
that map within this downstream region are not polyadenylated and
contain heterogeneous 3' termini (Hagenbüchle et al., 1984;
Pittet and Schibler, submitted). Therefore, transcription termin-
ates at multiple sites producing primary transcripts that must,
in addition to splicing, be processed at their 3' ends and poly
adenylated to produce mature mRNA. At present we are investigating the nature of these transcription termination regions within
the downstream sequences of alpha-amylase genes.

As there are four copies of the <u>Amy</u>-2$^a$ gene, the question
arises as to how many of these sequences constitute functional
genes. Only the gene most proximal to the <u>Amy</u>-1$^a$ locus, namely
<u>Amy</u>-2$^{a1}$, is sufficiently distinct to allow a primary transcript
to be unambiguously assigned to it. This gene has two deletions
(relative to the other three <u>Amy</u>-2$^a$ genes) of 100 bp and 300 bp
that both map within the last intron. The 100 bp deletion was
exploited in an S1 mapping experiment that showed the pancreas to
contain primary amylase transcripts with and without this
sequence in roughly equivalent amounts (Pittet and Schibler,
submitted). Thus, at least two of the four <u>Amy</u>-2$^a$ genes are
active, including the one proximal to the <u>Amy</u>-1$^a$ locus.

The relative efficiencies, or strengths of the three amylase promoters present in <u>Amy</u>-1$^a$ and <u>Amy</u>-2$^a$ have been examined by quanti-
tation of nascent RNA transcripts radiolabelled <u>in vitro</u> using
nuclei from the three amylase producing tissues (Schibler et al.,
1983 and unpublished work). It is not possible to directly compare the strengths of the <u>Amy</u>-1$^a$ promoters with an individual
<u>Amy</u>-2$^a$ promoter because of the gene duplication of the latter.
However, considering the <u>Amy</u>-2$^a$ promoters as an entity, the
relative efficiencies of the liver, parotid and pancreas
promoters are 1 : 30 : 550, respectively. These numbers closely
reflect the relative abundance of alpha-amylase mRNA in each of
the three tissues on a per cell basis, implying that the accumulation of this mRNA is regulated mainly at the transciptional

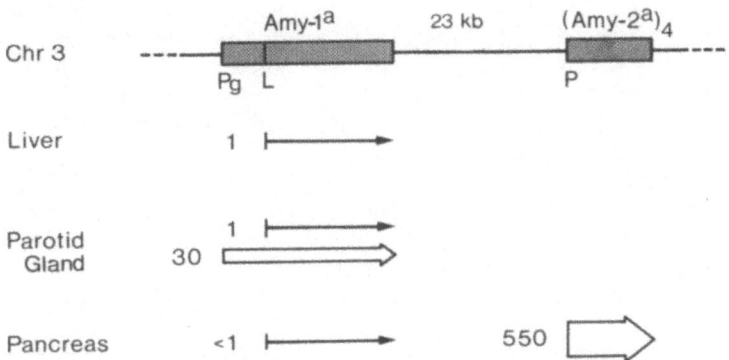

<u>Figure 2</u>. Relative transcription efficiencies from alpha-amylase gene promoters.

The genetic link between the <u>Amy-1</u>ª and <u>Amy-2</u>ª loci is depicted schematically. Below each gene the relative promoter efficiencies within the three amylase producing tissues are indicated by numbered arrows. As the <u>Amy-2</u>ª locus contains four identical genes only the sum of their relative transcripional efficiencies is given.

level in each case. Also it is apparent that even if all the Amy-2ᵃ sequences are transcriptionally active in the pancreas, each must be at least as efficient as the parotid promoter. Hence, the rigidly tissues specific parotid and pancreas promoters are strong relative to the more ubiquitous liver promoter (Fig. 2). The liver promoter is also active in cell free in vitro transcription assays (O. Hagenbüchle, unpublished) and upon transfection of the cloned DNA into cultured mouse L-cells (U. Schibler, unpublished). Neither of the strong promoters are active under these conditions. This implies that they require a tissue-specific factor for activity. In contrast the weak liver promoter, which is active in all three amylase producing tissues, may only require transcription competent chromatin for activity. This general view of alpha-amylase promoter activation may be an over simplification though. While most mouse tissues (e.g. spleen) show no transcription of the Amy-1ᵃ gene some tissues examined (e.g. brain, kidney exhibit low levels of transcripts that initiate well upstream (>7.5 kb) of the parotid cap site, but extend into the Amy-1ᵃ transcription unit. These transcripts are not processed to form alpha-amylase mRNA. However, this result shows that the Amy-1ᵃ locus can be transcriptionally active in some tisues without either of the tissue-specific promoters being recognized and used (Schibler et al., 1983).

It is intriguing how the distinct tissue-specific pattern of expression of two such closely linked genes as Amy-1ᵃ and Amy-2ᵃ becomes established during development. Recently we had studied parotid development, since the acinar cells of this tissue only proliferate and differentiate after birth. Cellular levels of alpha-amylase mRNA increase more than a 100 fold during the first three weeks after birth. Analysis of run off transcripts from isolated nuclei has shown this increase to be transcriptionally controlled and that the liver promoter is active before the parotid promoter. This observation was examined in terms of cellular commitment within the parotid gland using in situ hybridization of frozen tissue sections at different stages of development. At early stages (2 weeks after birth) all acinar cells are using the liver promoter while only a fraction use the parotid-specific promoter. This fraction of cells increases with time (Shaw, Sordat and Schibler, submitted).

These results may be explained in terms of a two-step activation of Amy-1ᵃ during differentiation of the parotid gland. Initially the Amy-1ᵃ locus becomes transcriptionally competent allowing activity of the liver promoter alone. Later a parotid-specific factor accumulates and allows the strong, parotid promoter to function. A similar scenario may be proposed for pancreatic differentiation. Again the Amy-1 locus becomes permissive for transcription allowing the liver promoter to function and a pancreas-specific factor is then synthesized, activating the Amy-2$^a$ promoters.

If indeed tissue-specific transcription factors are essential for activation of the strong Amy-1$^a$ and Amy-2$^a$ promoters, then these may interact with a tissue-specific enhancer element within the gene. Such sequences have been identified within mouse immunoglobulin genes (Gillies et al., 1983; Banerji et al., 1983; Queen and Baltimore, 1983) and rat chymotrypsin and insulin genes (Walker et al., 1983). Indeed, within any one tissue, the genes for the abundant products might be expected to carry an equivalent enhancer sequence to bind a common tissue-specific factor. Such functionally equivalent sequences may be identified by transfection of the cloned genes into primary cells or differentiated cell lines. This type of experiment is at present in progress in our laboratory in an attempt to identify the cis- and trans-acting elements required for the tissue-specific regulation of mouse genes.

## ACKNOWLEDGEMENTS

We thank Dr. B. Hirt for his continuing support and S. Cherpillod for typing the manuscript. This work was supported by grants from the Swiss national Science Foundation.

## REFERENCES

Banerji, J., Olson, L. and Schaffner, W. (1983) Cell 33, 729-740.

Eicher, E.M. and Lane, P.W. (1980) J. Hered. 71, 315-318.

Gillies, S.D., Morrison, S.L., Oi, V.T. and Tonegawa, S. (1983) Cell 33, 717-728.

Hagenbüchle, O., Bovey, R. and Young, R.A. (1980) Cell 211, 179-187.

Hagenbüchle, O., Tosi, M., Schibler, U., Bovey, R., Wellauer, P.K. and Young, R.A. (1981) Nature 289, 643-646.

Hagenbüchle, O., Wellauer, P.K., Cribbs, D.L. and Schibler, U. (1984) Cell, in press.

Queen, C. and Baltimore, D. (1983) Cell 33, 741-748.

Ray, S.B., Rothenberg, B.E. and Rosenfeld, M.G. (1979) J. Biol. Chem. 254, 1196-1204.

Schibler, U., Tosi, M., Pittet, A.-C., Fabiani, L. and Wellauer, P.K. (1980) J. Mol. Biol. 142, 93-116.

Schibler, U., Pittet, A.-C., Young, R.,A., Hagenbüchle, O., Tosi, M., Gellman, S. and Wellauer, P.K. (1982) J. Mol. Biol. 155, 247-266.

Schibler, U., Hagenbüchle, O., Wellauer, P.K. and Pittet, A.C. (1983) Cell 33, 501-508.

Sick, K. and Nielsen, J.T. (1964) Hereditas 51, 291-296.

Takeuchi, T., Matsushima, T. and Sugimura, T. (1975) Biochim. Biophys. Acta 403, 122-130.

Walker, M.D., Edlund, T., Boulet, A.M. and Rutter, W.J. (1983) Nature 306, 557-561.

Young, R.A., Hagenbüchle, O. and Schibler, U. (1981) Cell 23, 451-458.

# MULTIPLE CONTROL ELEMENTS ASSOCIATED WITH THE HUMAN ε-GLOBIN GENE

Maggi Allan, Paul Montague, G. Joan Grindlay, Zhu Jing-de
and John Paul

The Beatson Institute for Cancer Research
Garscube Estate
Switchback Road
Glasgow, G61 1BD

## SUMMARY

The human ε-globin gene has multiple transcription initiation
sites located far upstream of the major cap site.  These alternative
promoters are located within regions of erythroid specific DNAseI
hypersensitivity.  There is also a prominent DNAseI hypersensitive
site 6.5 kb upstream of the major cap site which corresponds to an
unusual nucleotide sequence.  The upstream promoters can be regulated
independently of the major cap site in response to a number of cis and
trans controls.  Several lines of evidence suggest that the upstream
promoters are transcribed early in differentiation prior to activation
of the major cap site.  The switch to cap site transcription occurs in
response to embryonic erythroid trans factors.  The upstream promoter
located 4.5 kb upstream of the major cap site is located within a
region which reduces transcription of the ε-globin cap site by
approximately 10-fold.  A fragment containing the ε-globin -200 cap
site can in certain circumstances act as a positive regulator of
transcription.  Possible mechanisms by which these distant regulatory
sequences exert their effect are discussed.

## INTRODUCTION

The paradoxical relationship between the amount of DNA needed to
code for polypeptides and the size of the genome has stood as a
challenge for many years.  In each mammalian globin gene the 1.5 kb or
so of DNA needed to code for the major RNA precursor is embedded
within a 10-15 kb sequence.  Is the extra DNA "junk"; does it simply

function as spacer or does it have regulatory functions? In view of
the complexity of regulation of different globins during normal
ontogeny it is reasonable to postulate that some of it is functionally
important yet most detailed investigations of control sequences have
concentrated on the coding region itself and the 100 bp or so upstream
of the major cap site (Dierks et al., 1983; Grosveld et al., 1982;
Chao et al., 1983; Wright et al., 1984) despite the fact that evidence
from HPFH and thalassemia studies has indicated that some control
regions may be located at long distances from it. Moreover, studies
on some other genes have clearly implicated more distant sequences
(Shermoen and Beckendorf, 1982; McGinnis et al., 1983; Guarente and
Mason, 1983).                                     .

These and other considerations have prompted us to investigate
the possible regulatory roles of distant DNA sequences in relation to
genes of the β-globin cluster and in this communication we summarise
some findings which show potential regulatory function for sequences
upstream of the human ε-globin gene.

We initially approached this problem by searching for minor
transcription initiation sites at locations upstream of the canonical
mRNA cap site of the human ε-globin gene. Somewhat controversial
evidence over the years had suggested that long transcripts might be
made (Bastos and Aviv, 1977; Reynaud et al., 1980; Shaul et al., 1981)
and we reasoned that if this was true, such alternative initiation
sites might serve as landmarks for distant regions involved in control
of the gene. These experiments were subsequently extended by studying
the expression of recombinant DNA molecules transfected into erythroid
and non-erythroid cells to gain information about the functions of
these loci.

## Multiple Transcription Initiation Sites Occur Upstream of the ε-Globin Gene;  Most of them Correspond to Nuclease Hypersensitive Sites in Chromatin

Using S1 mapping, primer extension and direct cap analysis we have
identified a number of specific sites of transcription initiation
considerably upstream of the human ε-globin gene both in normal
embryonic erythroblasts and in RNA from the K562 erythroleukaemic cell
line (Allan et al., 1982; Allan et al., 1983). The most distant site
is located -4500 bp upstream of the gene and represents the
transcriptional boundary not only of the ε-globin gene but of the
human β-globin cluster. Other initiation sites are positioned -1480,
-900 and -200 bp upstream of the cap site (Figure 1). Transcripts
derived from upstream sites extend to the 3' end of the ε-globin gene
and are polyadenylated (Allan et al., 1983). The two longest ε-globin
transcripts contain both Alu repeat sequences and coding sequences.
Interestingly, we have also detected another class of Alu transcript
associated with transcription of the gene (Allan and Paul 1984). This
transcript originates from a PolIII promoter in the more distal Alu

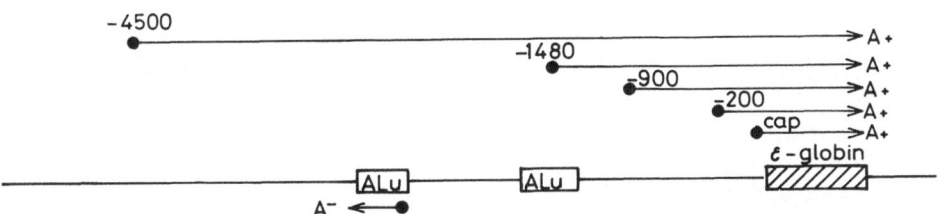

Fig. 1   Transcription initiation sites were located by a combination
         of S1 mapping, primer extension and direct cap analysis (see
         Allan et al., 1983), and are represented by closed circles.
         Distance from the major cap site is indicated, and the
         direction of transcription is represented by arrows.

element shown in Figure 1 whose activity has previously been
demonstrated in vitro (di Segni et al., 1981). It is 350 bp in
length, non-polyadenylated, nucleus confined and is transcribed from
the opposite DNA strand and in the opposite orientation to the $\varepsilon$-
-globin gene. This transcript has been detected only in cells where
the $\varepsilon$-globin gene is also transcribed. We are currently investigating
whether the pattern of transcription of Alu repetitive sequences in
association with the $\varepsilon$-globin gene has any significance for regulation
of the gene.

    One possible explanation for low level initiation events at
locations other than the cap site would be the occurrence at these
sites of sequences approximating to CAAT and TATA regulatory signals.
However, inspection of sequences adjacent to the upstream promoters
suggested that this was extremely unlikely. We then asked if the
upstream promoters coincided with some physical aspect of chromatin.
As summarized in Figure 2, there is indeed a striking correlation
between upstream $\varepsilon$-globin promoters and regions of erythroid specific
nuclease hypersensitivity (Zhu et al., 1984). There are two
exceptions to this correlation. Firstly, a DHS located at -6.5 kb
upstream of the $\varepsilon$-globin does not correspond to any known promoter
associated with the $\varepsilon$-globin gene. Secondly, the PolIII distal Alu
promoter apparently does not occur within a region of nuclease
hypersensitivity. The significance of these findings is not clear at
present.

## $\varepsilon$-Globin Upstream Promoters can be Regulated Independently of the Major Cap Site

    The finding that transcriptional activity of one of the upstream
promoters (the -200 cap site) and the major cap site can be uncoupled
(Allan et al., 1983) suggests that these upstream promoters are

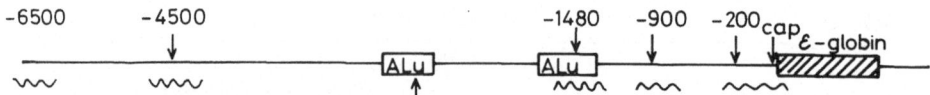

Fig. 2   Data summarised from Allan et al., (1983) and Zhu et al.,
         (1984).  Transcription initiation sites are indicated by
         arrows and DNase1 hypersensitive regions are represented by
         wavy lines.

mechanistically different from the cap site promoter.  Thus, although
the upstream promoters are not used in normal embryonic non-erythroid
tissues, the -200 cap site is used to the exclusion of the cap site in
certain established non-erythroid cell lines in which "leaky" ε-globin
gene activity has been observed (Allan et al., 1983).  Moreover, the
ratio of upstream to major cap site ε-globin transcripts is greater
prior to induction of differentiation of the K562 erythroid cell line;
induction of differentiation stimulates only major cap site
transcription (Young et al., 1984).  These findings, together with the
fact that the upstream promoters are located within DHS, encourage the
speculation that the upstream promoters may be active in erythroid
precursor cells and may be involved in early events in regulating the
ε-globin gene.

To examine the details of how the upstream promoters differ from
the major cap site and to identify the factors influencing transcription from each site, we have used a transient cellular transformation assay.  We have specifically examined the relationship between
the -200 cap and the major cap.  When a 3.7 kb fragment containing the
ε-globin gene is transiently introduced into a variety of non-
erythroid cell lines, transcription initiation almost exclusively
derives from the -200 cap site (Allan et al., 1984, and Figure 3), and
therefore mimics the pattern of "leaky" ε-globin transcription in non-
erythroid cell lines.  Under these conditions, stimulation of
replication of the gene in the transfected plasmid (by inclusion of an
SV40 origin of replication in the construct and transfection into Cos
7 cells) increases transcription from the -200 cap site while the
major cap site is unaffected (Figure 3).  In contrast, only the major
cap site promoter responds to SV40 enhancer sequences in cis.

The fact that transcription initiation from the major cap site
can be stimulated by the presence of an active enhancer suggested that
either the 3.7 kb EcoRI fragment used in transfections did not contain
an appropriate enhancer or that an erythroid specific enhancer was
involved.  To test this, we have transfected the 3.7 kb ε-globin

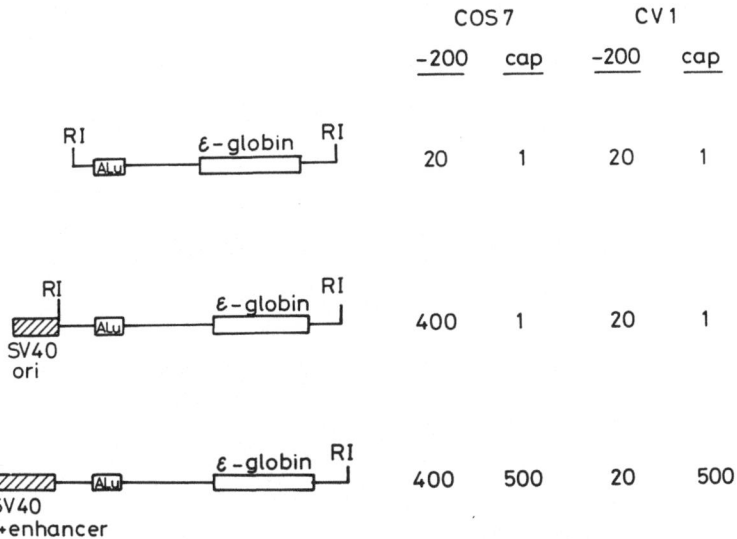

Fig. 3   Effect of 'cis' factors on transcription from different ℰ-
         -globin promoters.  Data summarized from Allan et al., (1984).
         Constructs indicated by line drawings were transfected into
         Cos7 or Cv1 cells.  RNA was prepared 48 hours later and
         quantitative S1 mapped.  Relative amounts of transcription are
         shown.

fragment into the K562 erythroid cell line on the assumption that
these cells should possess appropriate trans factors.  As shown in
Figure 4B, following transfection of the ℰ-globin gene into K562
cells, transcription initiation occurs maximally from the major cap
site.  This is in striking contrast to our findings with every non-
erythroid cell line examined to date, and implies the existence in
K562 cells of a specific transacting factor responsible for switching
the gene from a pre-terminal to a terminal state of activation.

    Interestingly, co-transfecting an ℰ-globin plasmid with a plasmid
containing the adenovirus E1A gene into Cos 7 cells similarly has the
effect of redirecting transcription from the -200 cap site to the
major cap site (Figure 4A).  In this case, comparison of similar
amounts of steady state RNA suggests that E1A in 'trans' reduces
transcription from the -200 cap site by around 20-fold, and
correspondingly increases transcription from the major cap site
though the total number of transcripts does not change.  This finding
suggests a relationship these two cap sites which can be altered
depending on the availability of certain control signals acting in
trans, and would predict that the -200 cap and major cap may compete
for transcription complexes.  To test this we have constructed a
plasmid in which a 350 bp Xba/Bam fragment containing the -200 cap

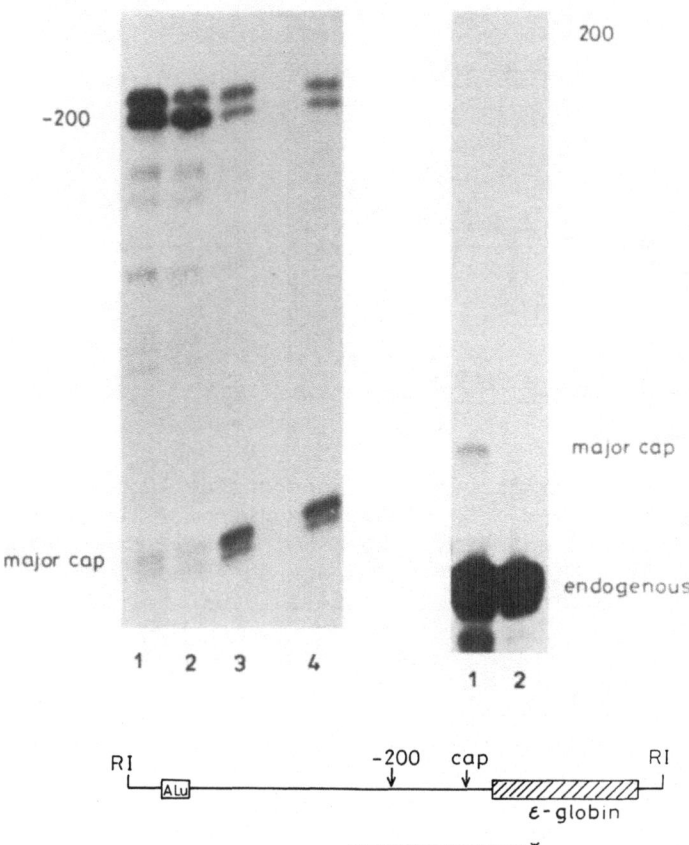

Fig. 4   (A) 40 µg of a plasmid containing the Є-globin gene and 1.5 kb
         of 5' flanking sequence (see line drawing) was transfected in
         Cos7 cells either alone (lanes 1 and 2) or in the presence of
         a plasmid containing the Ad5 E1A gene (lane 3).  The same
         plasmid was also transfected into 293 cells (lane d4) and into
         K562 cells (B. lane 1).
         (B) Lane 2 - K562 cells without plasmid. RNA was made 48 hours
         after transfection and quantitative S1 analysis carried out.

site was inserted in front of a CAT gene driven by the HSV immediate
early promoter and assayed for CAT activity 48 hours following
transfection into Cos 7 cells. The baseline level of CAT protein in

Cos 7 cells was given an arbitrary value of 10 (Figure 5).    Addition
of E1A in trans increases CAT levels to 200.   Inclusion of the 350 bp
Xba/Bam fragment containing the ε-globin cap site has no effect on CAT
activity either in the presence or absence of E1A when in the direct
orientation.   However, in the reverse orientation, the presence of
this fragment reduces CAT activity to below baseline.   Thus when a
small fragment containing the -200 cap site is inserted in front of a
CAT gene such that the direction of transcription from the ε-globin
promoter would be away from the CAT gene, the activity of the CAT gene
is reduced 200 fold.   This implies that the -200 cap site is a
powerful competitor for some component/s of the transcriptional
machinery.   In the direct orientation this can result in the delivery
of such components to the cap site where they may be used to initiate
transcription or else the upstream derived transcripts themselves give
rise to CAT protein.   In the reverse orientation, the direction of
transcription components would be away from the CAT gene and therefore
unavailable to the HSV promoter.   Alternatively, the findings might be
explained by a strong stop signal or a repressor binding site located
upstream of the -200 site.   We are currently analysing transcripts
from these constructs to test these hypotheses.

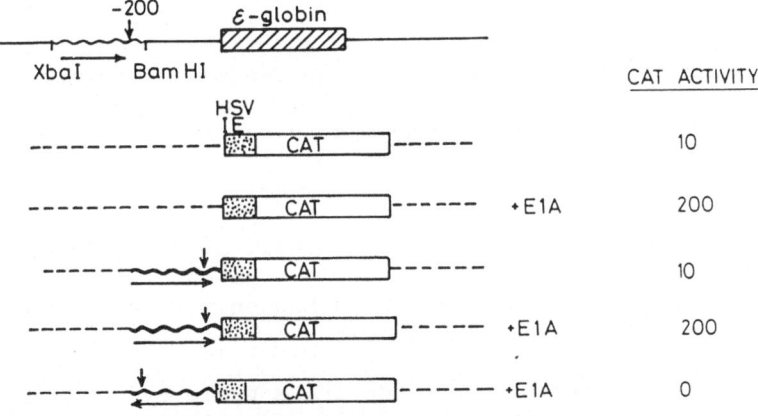

Fig. 5    A 350 bp XbaI/BamHI fragment containing the ε-globin -200 cap
          site was inserted, as shown on the line drawing, into a
          plasmid containing the chloramphenicol acetyl transferase gene
          driven by the Herpes Simplex Virus immediate early promoter.
          The -200 cap site is indicated by a vertical arrow, and
          direction of transcription from this promoter by a horizontal
          arrow.   The constructs shown were transfected into Cos7 cells
          either in the presence or absence of the adenovirus 5 E1A gene
          and CAT activity measured 48 hours later.

Significance of Upstream Regulatory Sequences

Our experiments clearly imply the existence of sequences with
control functions considerably more than 100 bp upstream of the major
cap site of the human ε-gene.  Our major conclusions may be summarised
as follows:
1.  All globin genes so far studied have multiple discrete minor cap
sites extending for several kilobases upstream from the major cap
site.  All in the human ε-globin gene are associated with DNaseI
hypersensitive sites.  The most likely explanation is that these
regions represent regular perturbations of chromatin structure which
make DNA more accessible.  Such DNaseI hypersensitive regions of
chromatin have been formally shown to be implicated in control of
their associated gene (Elgin, 1981).
2.  Some of these upstream initiation sites can be uncoupled from the
major cap site and in particular the -200 cap site of the human
ε-globin gene appears to function independently of the major cap site.
These two sites respond differently to the presence of an enhancer in
cis, the presence of trans-operating factors and to replication.
There are strong similarities between the behaviour of the -200 site
in response to the adenovirus E1A product and the -300 initiation site
of the adenovirus E1A gene itself.  It is of interest that in
adenovirus this sequence has an enhancer function and that the
ε-globin -200 site contains an enhancer core sequence.  This invites
the speculation that this region may contain an enhancer which
responds to a diffusible molecule, a speculation which is strengthened
by our observation that the switch from -200 to major cap site
initiation seems to be effected by a trans factor in erythroid cell
cytoplasm.
3.  The -200 site in the ε-globin gene appears to act in a markedly
polarised manner as shown by the experiment in Fig. 5 and in this it
is distinct from other enhancer-like sequences.
4.  In the longer transcripts, upstream Alu sequences are
co-transcribed with the ε-globin gene probably by RNA polymerase II.
A 350 bp RNA molecule is also transcribed, apparently by RNA
polymerase III, from the opposite strand but only in erythroid cells.
We have no information about its function.

These findings apparently provide prima facie evidence for
controls at some distance from the protein-encoding sequences of
the ε-globin genes.  The main weakness of the evidence we present is,
however, that much of it is derived from rather artificial
experiments.  This objection does not, of course, apply to the
evidence for naturally-occurring upstream starts (which we have
shown in normal embryonic tissue) nor to the evidence for nuclease-
hypersensitive sites which was derived from studies on the intact
cells but one has to assess cell transfection experiments particularly
critically.  Probably the most important consideration is the extent
to which transferred genes, usually present as head-tail concatamers
either located extrachromosomally or integrated more-or-less randomly

into the genome, can be equated with the behaviour of genes in the normal chromosomal location.  Though the evidence bearing on the point is sparse it seems likely that at least some aspects of normal regulatory behaviour are exhibited in transfected cell systems. Hence, while opportunities must be sought for checking the findings in intact normal cells and the validity of the observations in relation to normal behaviour should be regarded only as suggestive till this is done nevertheless the findings can be seen as useful clues to what may happen normally.

Bearing these reservations in mind we would  therefore like to offer some speculations about our findings.  First, the notion that each gene occupies its own domain is attractive and our findings suggest that for the $\epsilon$-globin gene this may be at least 10 kb long, including the 1.5 kb of coding region, the 6.5 kb up to the strong DNaseI hypersensitive site at the extremity of the region and probably 2-3 kb downstream of the gene.  To activate the entire region in erythroid cells would require an unwinding mechanism and, although there are many other candidates the B-Z transition of a long stretch of DNA, such as we have shown in association with the $\beta$-major globin gene of the mouse (Gilmour et al., 1984) is an interesting possibility.  As we have pointed out there is a similar region near the -6.5 kb site in the human $\epsilon$-globin gene.

Once unwound it is easy to envisage cis-acting regulatory sequences which themselves may be subject to diffusible factors.  The -200 site in the $\epsilon$-globin gene region is interesting in this connection in that by the use of surrogate genetics we do have some evidence that it may act as a polarised enhancer, influenced by trans factors.  An indication that this may not simply be a phenomenon due entirely to the artificial systems used is given by the differential usage of -200 and major cap sites in uninduced and induced K562 cells and in some other cultured non-erythroid cells in which the -200 site gives rise to transcripts whereas the major cap site does not.

We also have preliminary evidence that a 1 kb region surrounding the -4500 $\epsilon$-globin initiation site is involved in transcriptional regulation of the major cap site.  The possible involvement of two of the $\epsilon$-globin initiation sites in regulation of the gene supports our original premise that such sites would serve as landmarks for regulatory sequences.  It also raises the interesting possibility that the process of transcription per se may be a vital component of the mechanism by which at least one class of distant control elements may exert their effect.  There are a number of ways in which we might envisage this happening.  For example, 1) transcription from a distant control site may serve to increase the accessibility of chromatin to regulatory molecules.
2) Distant control regions may serve as entry sites for the transcriptional machinery and depending on the nature and availability of 'trans' regulators an initiated complex may be formed at the

upstream site or alternatively the complex may directionally scan the
DNA until the major cap site is encountered.  3) Read-through
transcripts from upstream sites could potentially inhibit
transcription from the major cap site as has been shown for the
bacterial IS1 insertion element (Machida et al., 1983).  This
speculation is supported by the finding that the fragment containing
the $\mathcal{E}$-globin -4500 cap site down-regulates transcription of the major
cap site in non-erythroid cells.  In order to transcribe the gene at
full activity in terminally differentiated erythroid cells there is
presumably a requirement either to reduce transcription from the
upstream site or to block the passage of upstream-derived transcripts.
A candidate for the latter mechanism might conceivably be provided by
the erythroid specific transcription of the distal Alu repetitive
element in the opposite direction (see Figure 1).

Current experiments are directed towards understanding how the
$\mathcal{E}$-globin upstream control elements function, whether and how they
interact with each other, and how they act to regulate gene activity
during differentiation.


ACKNOWLEDGEMENTS

The Beatson Institute is supported by Cancer Research Campaign of
Great Britain.


REFERENCES

Allan, M., Grindlay, G.J., Stefani, L., Paul, J., 1982, Epsilon globin
    gene transcripts originating upstream of the mRNA cap site in
    K562 cells and normal human embryos.  Nucl. Acids Res. 10: 5133.
Allan, M., Lanyon, W.G., Paul, J., 1983, Multiple origins of
    transcription in the 4.5 Kb upstream of the $\mathcal{E}$-globin gene. Cell,
    35: 187.
Allan, M., Paul, J., 1984, Transcription in vivo of an Alu family
    member upstream from the human $\mathcal{E}$-globin gene.  Nucl. Acids Res.,
    12: 1193.
Allan, M., Zhu, J-D., Montague, P., Paul, J., 1984, Differential
    response of multiple $\mathcal{E}$-globin cap sites to cis and transacting
    controls.  Cell, 38: 399.
Bastos, R.N., Aviv, H., 1977, Globin RNA precursor molecules: bio-
    synthesis and processing in erythroid cells.  Cell, 11: 641.
Chao, M.V., Mellon, P., Charnay, P., Maniatis, T., Axd, R., 1983,  The
    regulated expression of $\beta$-globin genes introduced into mouse
    erythroleukaemia cells.  Cell, 32: 483.
Di Segni, A., Carrara, G., Tocchini-Valentini, G.R., Shoulders, C.C.
    Baralle, F.E., 1981, Selective in vitro transcription of one of
    the two Alu family repeats present in the 5' flanking region of
    the human $\mathcal{E}$-globin gene.  Nucl. Acids Res., 9: 6709.

Dierks, P., van Ooyen, A., Cochran, M.D., Dobkin, C., Reiser, J., Weissman, C., 1983, Three regions upstream from the cap site are required for efficient and accurate transcription of the rabbit β-globin gene in mouse 3T6 cells. Cell, 32: 695.

Elgin, S.R.C., 1981, DNaseI hypersensitive sites of chromatin. Cell, 27: 413.

Gilmour, R.S., Spandidos, D.A., Vass, J.K., Gow, J.W., Paul, J., 1984, A negative regulatory sequence near the mouse β-major globin gene associated with a region of potential Z-DNA. EMBO J., 3: 1263.

Grosveld, G.C., de Baer, E., Shewmaker, C.K., Flavel, R.A., 1982, DNA sequences necessary for transcription of the rabbit β-globin gene in vivo. Nature, 295: 120.

Guarente, L., Mason, T., 1983, Heme regulates transcription of the CYC1 gene of S. cerevisiae via an upstream activation site. Cell, 32: 1279.

McGinnis, W., Shermoen, A.W., Heemskerk, J., Beckendorf, S.K., 1983 DNA sequence changes in an upstream DNAaseI hypersensitive region are correlated with reduced gene expression. Proc.Natl. Acad. Sci., 80: 1063.

Machida, C., Machida, Y., Wang, H-C., Ishizaki, K., Ohtsubo, E., 1983, Repression of cointegration ability of insertion element IS1 by transcriptional readthrough from flanking regions. Cell, 34: 135.

Reynand, C., Imaizumi-Scherrer, M., Scherrer, K., 1980, The size of the transcriptional units of the avian globin genes defined at the pre-messenger RNA level. J. Mol. Biol., 140: 481.

Shaul, Y., Kaminchik, J., Aviv, H., 1981, Large globin RNA molecules and their processing. Eur. J. Biochem., 116: 461.

Shermoen, A.W., Beckendorf, S.K., 1982, A complex of interacting DNAseI-hypersensitive sites near the Drosophila glue protein gene Sgs4. Cell, 29: 601.

Wright, S., Rosenthal, A., Flavell, R.A., Grosveld, F.G., 1984, DNA sequences required for regulated expression of β-globin genes in MEL cells. Cell, 38: 265.

Young, K., Donovan-Peluso, M., Bloom, K., Allan, M., Paul, J., Bank, A., 1984, Stable transfer and expression of exogenous human globin genes in human erythroleukemia (K562) cells. Proc. Natl. Acad. Sci. USA, 81: 5315.

Zhu, J-D., Allan, M., Paul, J., 1984, The chromatin structure of the human ε-globin gene: nuclease hypersensitive sites correlate with multiple initiation sites of transcription. Nucl. Acids Res., 12: 9191.

# COORDINATE GENOTYPIC AND PHENOTYPIC EXPRESSION AS DIFFERENTIATION MARKERS IN HUMAN LYMPHOID MALIGNANCIES

C.C. Bird

Department of Pathology
University of Leeds
Leeds LS2 9JT

Although lymphoid malignancies comprise a relatively rare form of human cancer (~3-4%), the pivotal role of the immune system in most biological processes has led to disproportionate interest in malignancies derived from the lymphoreticular system. The ready access to material for investigation in blood and superficial lymphoid tissue has also provided further stimulus to investigation of these malignancies. Nonetheless studies of lymphoid malignancies have revealed important new concepts governing tumour differentiation and behaviour that have much wider application.

## CLASSIFICATION LEUKAEMIAS AND LYMPHOMAS

Human lymphoid malignancies can be broadly divided into the acute and chronic forms of leukaemia and the solid lymphomas: Hodgkin's disease and non-Hodgkin's lymphoma (Table 1). The solid lymphomas occur with roughly twice the frequency of leukaemias with non-Hodgkin's lymphoma (NHL) and chronic lymphocytic leukaemia (CLL) comprising the commonest of these malignancies. It should be appreciated however, that considerable overlap exists between lymphocytic leukaemias and NHL and these may merely represent differing expressions in blood and lymphoid tissues of the same basic neoplastic process. Moreover, during the natural history of these malignancies transitions from one form of malignancy to another may be observed not infrequently. The origin of malignant cells in Hodgkin's disease (presumed to be the Reed-Sternberg cell) remains controversial with differing protagonists advocating a lymphocytic (B- or T-cell), histiocytic or reticulum cell derivation (Stein et al., 1983; Dorreen et al., 1984). For this reason Hodgkin's disease will not be considered further.

Table 1.  Relative Frequency of Leukaemia and Lymphoma

| Malignancy | | No. Cases | (%) |
|---|---|---|---|
| Leukaemia | acute lymphocytic | 47 | ( 4) |
| | acute myeloid | 109 | ( 9) |
| | chronic lymphocytic | 236 | ( 19) |
| | chronic myeloid | 83 | ( 7) |
| Lymphoma | Hodgkin's disease | 243 | ( 20) |
| | Non-Hodgkin's lymphoma | 525 | ( 41) |
| | | 1243 | (100) |

* Frequency in Yorkshire Health Region (population - 3.5 million) during 1982-84.

DIFFERENTIATION OF NORMAL LYMPHOID CELLS

    An understanding of the nature of differentiation in lymphoid malignancies requires consideration of the current state of knowledge of the differentiation sequence in normal human lymphoid cells. Lymphoid cells may be broadly divided into two main categories:  T- and B-cells (Fig. 1), derived from a common terminal deoxynucleotidyl transferase (Tdt)-positive stem cell in the foetal yolk sac and liver (Vogler, 1982; Janossy & Prentice, 1982).  Thereafter development takes place separately, T-cells in the thymus and B-cells in the bone marrow, although controversy still exists as to whether the earliest recognisable T cells - prothymocytes - undergo some development in bone marrow.  During the course of differentiation B- and T-cells manifest differing antigenic profiles that are readily demonstrable by immunocytochemical techniques employing monoclonal and polyclonal antibodies.  The expression of surface membrane antigens however, is complex and as yet inadequately understood.  In our own studies of surface membrane glycoproteins of normal and malignant lymphoid cells we have observed marked heterogeneity of expression in both B- and T- cells (Fig. 2).  Only four of over 30 glycoproteins identified in a series of B-cell lines were found to be shared and each cell line appeared to express a unique glycoprotein profile.  Similar findings were made in a series of T-cell lines with only two glycoproteins (61 and 100 Kd molecular weight) being shared with the B-cell lines. Comparable results were obtained with leukaemic cells derived from a series of patients with CLL (data not shown).  Much has yet to be

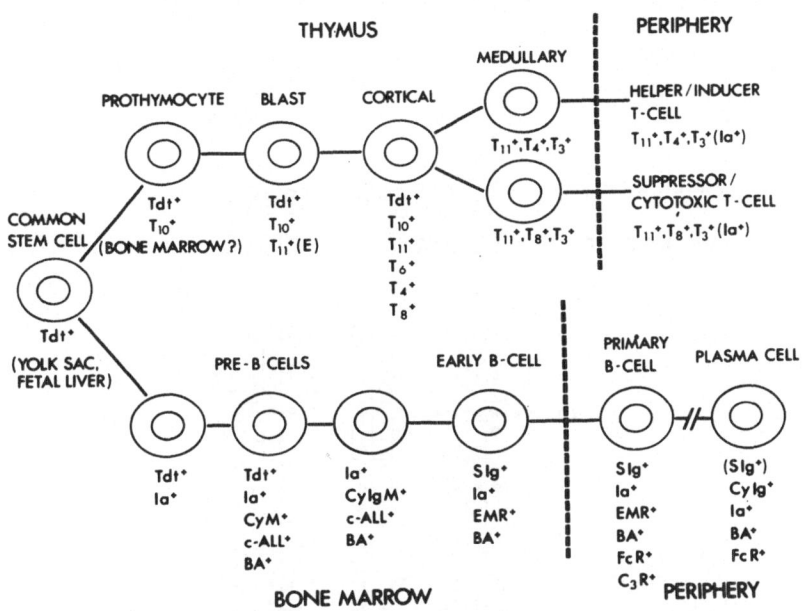

Fig. 1    Phenotypic expression during differentiation of normal T- and
          B-cells in thymus and bone marrow.  Mature phenotypes are
          expressed on release to periphery.

learnt therefore, of the range of surface membrane antigens in human
lymphoid cells and their function.

As T- and B-cells differentiate within the thymus and bone marrow
fairly consistent patterns of antigen expression have been delineated
with the ultimate release of functionally mature lymphoid cells into
the peripheral tissues (Fig. 1).   Mature T-cell forms are composed of
T-helper/inducer and T-suppressor/cytotoxic subsets circulating
between blood and lymphoid tissues (Janossy & Prentice, 1982).   B-
cells on release however, require a further series of differentiation
steps before they assume fully mature antibody-secreting status
(Galton & Maclennan, 1982).   These further differentiation steps may
be divided into two parts:   one antigen-independent and the other
antigen-dependent.

In the antigen-independent sequence (Fig. 3) primary B-cells
differentiate to form recirculating B-cells and static B-cells.
Together these comprise the memory and virgin B-cells.  Recirculating

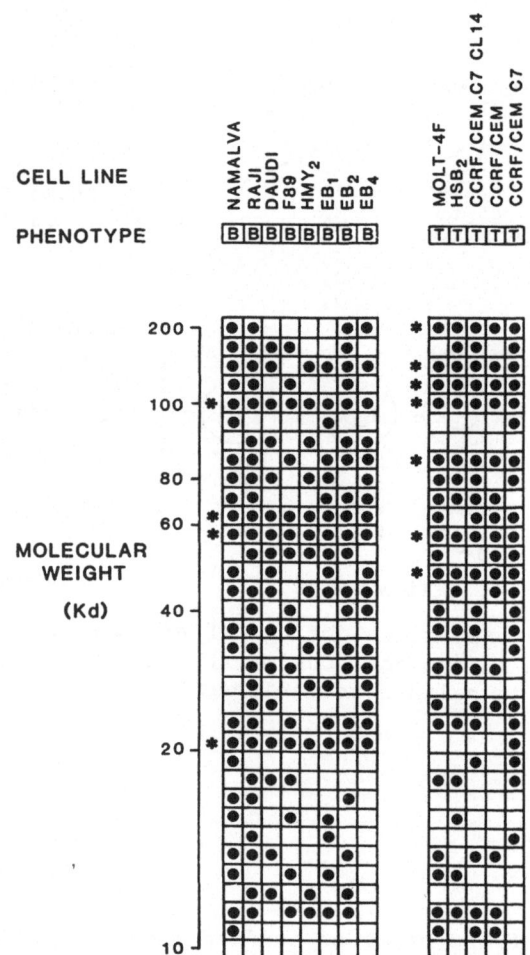

Fig. 2    Surface membrane glycoprotein profiles of B- and T-cell human
          lymphoid cell lines.  Cells were radiolabelled with $^{125}$I by
          iodogen method and membrane extracts separated by SDS
          polyacrylamide gel electrophoresis and autoradiographed MW of
          each band detected (●) represents mean of at least three
          separate determinations.  Common bands are indicated by an
          asterisk.  For details of cell lines see Burrow et al., 1981
          and Blewitt et al., 1983.

B-cells make up >95% of lymph node follicle cells and >85% of peripheral blood B-lymphocytes. Static B-cells comprise a small proportion of lymph node follicular cells and peripheral B-lymphocytes but over one-third of spleen lymphocytes. These recirculating and static B-cells probably represent different classes of B-cells with potential for responding to different forms of antigen of protein and carbohydrate nature.

Antigen-dependent maturation (Fig. 4) on the other hand depends on the influence of various antigens and requires the cooperation of T-helper cells and antigen presenting cells. Under their influence the recirculating and static B-cells differentiate both in germinal centres of lymph node follicles to form centroblasts and centrocytes and give rise to interfollicular immunoblasts which in turn mature to form the antibody secreting plasma and lymphoplasmacytoid cells. The type of antibody produced depends on the antigen stimulus and the biological activity specified.

Using the antigen profiles of normal lymphoid cells as a guide, it is possible in most instances to define the lineage origins and differentiation status of the different B- and T-cell malignancies.


T-CELL MALIGNANCIES

T-cell malignancies may be divided into two major categories - thymic and peripheral types (Catovsky et al., 1982). Thymic types comprise T-cell forms of acute lymphoblastic leukaemia (ALL) and the lymphoblastic lymphomas. All show the early thymic markers: Tdt, $T_{10}$ and $T_{11}$. However, whereas T-cell ALL lacks any of the later T-cell markers some of the lymphoblastic lymphomas show more mature thymic markers: $T_4$, $T_6$ and $T_3$. The latter comprise the more common forms of lymphoblastic lymphoma. The peripheral forms of T-cell malignancy all lack Tdt but show $T_{11}$ and $T_3$ positivity. In addition the adult T-cell leukaemia/lymphoma (associated with HTLV I and II viruses) and the cutaneous lymphomas (mycosis fungoides and Sezary syndrome) generally also show the T-helper ($T_4$) phenotype whereas T-CLL normally expresses the T-suppressor ($T_8$) phenotype. T-cell forms of prolymphocytic leukaemia (PLL) may express either the helper or suppressor phenotype. Considering these phenotypes in the context of normal T-cell differentiation (Fig. 5) we see that the various forms of T-cell malignancy appear to represent cells frozen at differing stages of normal T-cell differentiation with T-cell forms of ALL and lymphoblastic lymphoma

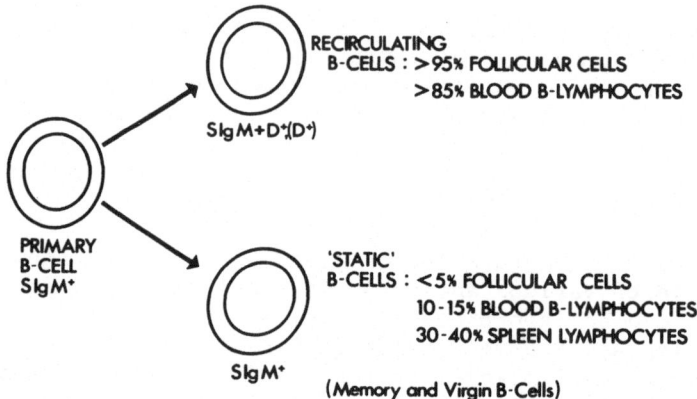

Fig. 3    Antigen independent maturation of B-cells in peripheral
          tissues.

representing the most primitive tumours whilst cutaneous lymphomas,
T-cell leukaemia/lymphoma and chronic leukaemias (T-CLL and T-PLL)
represent the most mature forms.

B-CELL MALIGNANCIES

     The antigenic profiles observed in B-cell malignancies delineate
essentially four patterns of malignancy (Table 2) (Galton and
Maclennan, 1982).  The common form of ALL (cALL) and Burkitt's
lymphoma appear to correspond to pre-B cells whilst B-CLL, B-PLL,
hairy cell leukaemia (HCL) and small cell lymphocytic lymphoma
resemble peripheral circulating B-cells.  Malignancies corresponding
to peripheral activated B-cells are represented by multiple myeloma,
immunoblastic sarcoma and Waldenström's macroglobulinaemia.  Finally,
the solid lymphomas of follicular centre cell (FCC) origin may be
deemed to represent peripheral activated germinal centre cells.
Comparison with the normal B-cell maturation sequence (Fig. 6)
indicates that B-cell malignancies correspond closely to normal B-
cells frozen at different stages of B-cell differentiation from early
pre-B cells through to the most mature B-cell forms: plasma cells.

     It is of some interest that the most common B-cell malignancies
(FCC forms of NHL, multiple myeloma and CLL) appear to represent cells
frozen at the more mature end of the B-cell spectrum.  It is possible
to speculate that this could result either from selective transform-

Table 2.   Patterns of B-cell Malignancy

| Normal equivalent | Malignancy |
|---|---|
| Early pre-B cells | cALL<br>Burkitt's lymphoma |
| Peripheral circulating B-cells | B-CLL<br>B-PLL<br>HCL<br>Small cell lymphocytic<br>lymphoma |
| Peripheral activated B-cells | Myeloma<br>Plasma cell leukaemia<br>Immunoblastic sarcoma<br>Lymphoplasmacytoid lymphoma<br>Waldenström's macroglobulin-<br>aemia |
| Peripheral activated germinal centre cells | Centroblastic/centrocytic<br>lymphoma<br>Centrocytic lymphoma<br>Centroblastic lymphoma |

cALL = common form acute lymphoblastic leukaemia
CLL  = chronic lymphocytic leukaemia
PLL  = prolymphocytic leukaemia
HCL  = hairy cell leukaemia

Follicular centre cell (FCC) lymphoma

ation of cells at the mature end of the B-cell spectrum or from continued differentiation (but with subsequent arrest of more primitive transformed cells.  At present it is not possible to determine with certainty which of these is the correct explanation but recent studies of immunoglobulin gene status in B-cell tumours suggests the latter is the more likely explanation.

IMMUNOGLOBULIN GENES

Immunoglobulins are composed of four polypeptide chains with two light chains and two heavy chains in each molecule.  Only one light chain and one heavy chain type is expressed in each molecule. Neoplastic proliferations of B-lymphocytes are characterised by restricted light chain production with all cells in the neoplastic clone producing either kappa (K) or lambda (L) light chains, but not

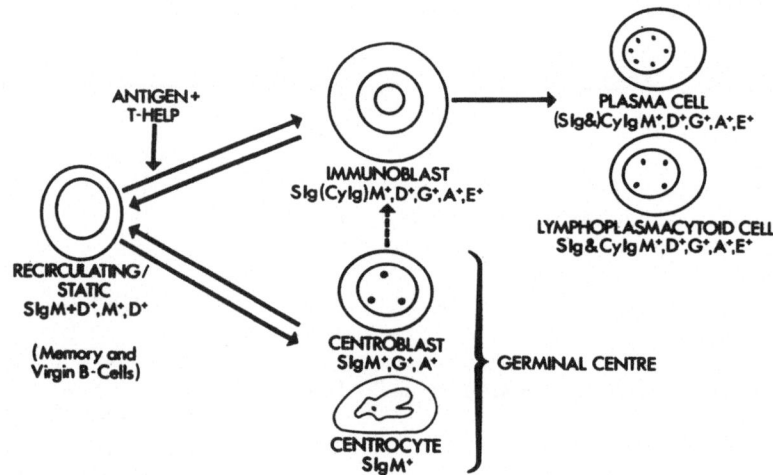

Fig. 4    Antigen dependent maturation of peripheral B-cells.

both.   Reactive (non-neoplastic) B-cell proliferations on the other
hand are polyclonal in nature and composed of mixtures of lymphocytes
expressing K or L light chains usually in a 60/40 ratio (Calton and
Maclennan, 1982).   Each light and heavy chain is coded at the genomic
level by a series of discontinuous segments of DNA.   In the case of
heavy chains there are four gene sub-segments; variable, diversity,
joining and constant regions whereas light chains contain only three
gene sub-segments:   variable, joining and constant regions (Honjo,
1983).   The precise number of genes in the different sub-segments is
not yet known with certainty but there are likely to be hundreds of
variable genes with much fewer numbers of the others.   In man, heavy
chain genes are located in chromosome 14, K light chains on chromosome
2 and L light chains on chromosome 22.   Antibody diversity is normally
generated during rearrangement and recombination of these gene sub-
segments in appropriately primed B-cells with somatic mutation
occurring at the time of recombination adding to this diversity
(Tonegawa, 1983).   This process is known as gene shuffling and by this
means B-lymphocytes are capable of generating several million
different antibodies from a relatively limited repertoire of genes.
The rearrangement of immunoglobulin genes in B-cells can be demonstrated by a change in position of the restriction enzyme cleavage sites
normally existing in the germ line state and visualised in Southern
blots.   This sensitive technique permits detection of as little as 1%
of the cell population manifesting such clonal rearrangements (Cleary
et al., 1984a).

Table 3. Immunoglobulin Gene Rearrangements in Leukaemia[1]

| Type[2] | No. Cases | Immunophenotype[3] | Genotype[4] Heavy chain | K | L |
|---|---|---|---|---|---|
| Non-B non-T-ALL | 14 | cALL⁻, Ia⁺, T⁻, B⁻ | R | G | G |
| Non-B non-T-ALL | 14 | cALL⁺, Ia⁺, T⁻, B⁻ | R(13/14) | R(13/14) | R(4/14) |
| B-CLL | 11 | cALL⁻, Ia⁺, T⁻, B⁺ | R | R(8/11) | R(5/11) |
| B-PLL | 4 | cALL⁻, Ia⁺, T⁻, B⁺ | R | R | R(2/4) |
| HCL | 10 | cALL⁻, Ia⁺, T⁻, B± | R | R(7/10) | R(6/10) |
| LBC. CML | 11 | cALL⁺, Ia⁺, T⁻, B± | R(9/11) | R(3/11) | R(1/11) |
| T-ALL | 12 | cALL⁻, Ia⁻, T⁺, B⁻ | G | G | G |
| T-CLL | 4 | cALL⁻, Ia⁻, T⁺, B⁻ | G | G | G |

[1] Data derived from Kosmeyer et al, 1983a and b, Bakhshi et al, 1983; Foroni et al, 1984

[2] ALL = acute lymphoblastic leukaemia; CLL = chronic lymphocytic leukaemia; PLL = prolymphocytic leukaemia; HCL = hairy cell leukaemia; LBC.CML = lymphoblastic crisis of chronic myeloid leukaemia

[3] + = usually positive; − = usually negative; ± = either positive or negative

[4] R = rearranged or deleted gene; G = germ line gene

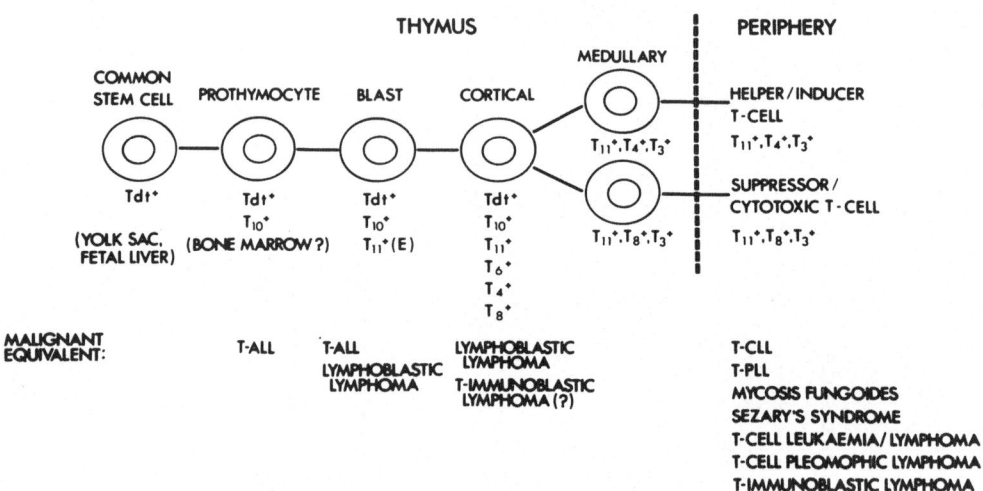

Fig. 5    Phenotypic expression of T-cell malignancies in relation to
          normal T-cell differentiation.


## IMMUNOGLOBULIN GENES IN LEUKAEMIA AND LYMPHOMA

Employing these techniques phenotypic T-cell ALL and CLL have
normally been shown to lack evidence of immunoglobulin gene rearrangements (Table 3).  On the other hand non-B-non-T ALL's show
unequivocal evidence of B-cell origin with those lacking the cALL
antigen usually showing only heavy chain rearrangements whereas those
with the cALL antigen demonstrate both heavy and light chain
rearrangements.  B-CLL and B-PLL similarly show heavy and light chain
rearrangements.  HCL whose origin has been disputed for some time also
shows clear evidence of heavy and light chain rearrangements in most
cases in keeping with a B-cell origin. Likewise, cases of chronic
myeloid leukaemia terminating in lymphoblastic crisis manifest a
B-cell origin by virtue of the immunoglobulin gene rearrangements
present.  As yet few lymphomas have been examined by these techniques
(Table 4) but those marking phenotypically as B-cells have had their
B-cell lineage confirmed by the presence of immunoglobulin gene
rearrangements.  Lymphomas lacking B-cell markers but suspected on
morphological grounds of B-cell derivation have also been found to
demonstrate B-cell immunoglobulin gene configurations in most
instances.  Immunoglobulin gene configuration therefore, provides
another useful marker of B-cell origin and helps define the stage of
tumour differentiation by virtue of the rearrangements present (Fig.
6).  However, some caution must be exercised in assigning tumours to a
B-cell lineage purely on the basis of immunoglobulin gene rearrange-

Table 4. Immunoglobulin Gene Rearrangements in Lymphoma[1]

| Type | No. cases | Immunophenotype[2] | | | Genotype[3] | | |
| --- | --- | --- | --- | --- | --- | --- | --- |
| | | Heavy chain | K | L | Heavy chain | K | L |
| Large cell | 3 | + | + | - | R | R | G |
| Large cell | 17 | - | - | - | R(16/17) | R(10/17) | R(4/17) |
| Small cell | 4 | + | + | - | R | R | R(1/4) |
| Small cell | 2 | - | - | - | R | R | R(1/2) |

[1]Data from Cleary et al., 1984a and b and Arnold et al., 1983.

[2] + = positive;  - = negative

[3] R = rearranged or deleted gene;  G = germ line gene

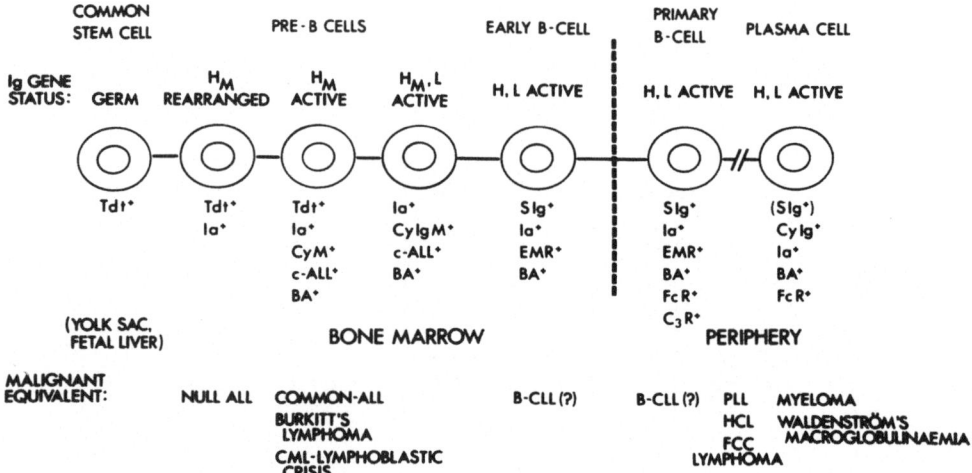

Fig. 6   Phenotypic expression and immunoglobulin gene status of
         malignant and normal B-cells.

ments since recent reports indicate that occasional T-cell
malignancies and myeloid leukaemias can manifest heavy chain
rearrangements (Ha et al., 1984a and b).


COORDINATE GENE AND ANTIGEN EXPRESSION

     Studies of gene rearrangements appear also to show a coordinate
sequence of gene and surface antigen expression in some B-cell
malignancies (Korsmeyer et al., 1983a).  In B-cell forms of ALL
immunoglobulin heavy chains have been shown to rearrange before light
chains and K light chains before L light chains.  These rearrangements
occur coincidentally with the expression of different surface antigens
commencing with the MHC-class II (Ia) antigens, then the B-series of
differentiation antigens and finally the cALL antigen.  These studies
have also suggested that many immunoglobulin gene rearrangements are
ineffective and when this occurs alternative recombinations are
attempted in a predefined sequence commencing first with the different
heavy chain classes, then K light chains and finally L light chains.
Moreover, it has been suggested that cells become trapped at different
stages within the B-cell precursor series either because these
rearrangements are ineffective or the possibilities become exhausted
(Korsmeyer et al., 1983a).

Table 5.   Correlation of Heavy and Light Chain Expression with Lymphoma
Grade

| Light chain | Heavy chain isotype | | | |
| | MD | | MG | |
| | LG[1] | HG | LG | HG |
|---|---|---|---|---|
| K | 4 | 3 | 10 | 0 |
| L | 3 | 7 | 5 | 4 |
| | 7 | 10 | 15 | 4 |

[1]LG = low grade;  HG = high grade
P = <0.025> 0.01

CLINICAL SIGNIFICANCE OF IMMUNOGLOBULIN EXPRESSION

        Whilst such findings are of considerable theoretical and
biological interest it is necessary to consider also whether they have
any prognostic or therapeutic significance.  As yet, little has been
done to resolve such questions although we have recently begun to
consider the clinical value of immunoglobulin expression in B-cell
lymphomas (Lauder et al., 1984).  In a prospective series of over a
hundred lymphoma cases, approximately 60 B-cell NHL's were available
for investigation.  The great majority produced more than one heavy
chain class and when the largest groups, producing MD and MG heavy
chains, were considered it was found that a significantly greater
proportion of morphologically defined (Lennert, 1978) high grade
tumours produced M and D heavy chains whereas low grade tumours more
commonly produced M and G heavy chains (Table 5).  Also when light
chain expression was considered in relation to grade in the same
tumours, it was found that significantly more low grade tumours
produced K than L light chains wherease the reverse was true for high
grade tumours.  Both these findings are in keeping with the
hierarchial sequence of immunoglobulin gene expression described
previously and might relate to the biological potential of tumours.
That this was indeed the case was confirmed when the clinical
responsiveness of tumours to treatment was examined.  Irrespective of
morphological grade it was found that patients with tumours expressing
K light chains did much better than those whose tumours expressed L
light chains (Table 6).  Treatment responsiveness was assessed bv the
completeness of initial therapeutic response and survival of patients
for a minimum of one year from the time of diagnosis.  Thus the
phenotypic properties of lymphomas and their related genotypic status
appear to reflect their biological potential and may provide important
therapeutic indicators.

Table 6.   Light Chain Expression in Relation to Treatment Response

| Light chain | Treatment Response[1] | |
| | Good | Poor |
| --- | --- | --- |
| K | 15 | 7 |
| L | 11 | 17 |
| | 26 | 24 |

[1] Good = Complete remission;   Poor = Incomplete or no remission
p = <0.05> 0.025

FUTURE PERSPECTIVES

This brief overview serves to illustrate that human lymphoid
malignancies closely parallel their normal non-neoplastic cellular
counterparts in phenotypic and genotypic expression.  Most
malignancies, whether of B- or T-cell origin appear to represent
lymphoic cells frozen at varying stages of the normal differentiation
sequence and genotypic and phenotypic expression remains essentially
coordinated even in the malignant state.  As yet, a fairly limited
repertoire of antigenic determinants have been explored as differentiation markers although the extensive range of surface membrane
glycoproteins indicates the great potential for further investigation.
So too, the recent acquisition of gene probes for lymphoid cells adds
a new dimension to studies of differentiation in normal and malignant
lymphoid cells.  This is especially the case in regard to probes for
T-cell antigen receptors and oncogenes and exciting new concepts will
no doubt emerge when these have been more extensively explored.  To
this may be added refinements in chromosomal analysis of malignant
cells where already links between well established karyotypic
abnormalities and oncogene locations in chromosomes of leukaemias and
lymphomas have been established (LeBeau and Rowley, 1984).  However,
as yet few attempts have been made to translate these findings to
practical value in the clinical sphere.  A carefully devised strategy
is now urgently required to bring genotypic and phenotypic aspects
together in a more rational form so that the diagnostic and clinical
relevance of these findings may be ascertained.

ACKNOWLEDGEMENT

This work was supported by a grant from the Yorkshire Cancer
Research Campaign.

REFERENCES

Arnold, A., Cossman, J., Bahkshi, A., Jaffe, E.S., Waldmann, T.A. and
    Korsmeyer, S.J., 1983, Immunoglobulin-gene rearrangements as
    unique clonal markers in human lymphoid neoplasms, New Eng.J.
    Med., 309: 1593-1599.
Bakhshi, A., Minowada, J., Arnold, A., Cossman, J., Jensen, J.P.,
    Whang-Peng, J., Waldmann, T.A. and Korsmeyer, S.J., 1983,
    Lymphoid blast crises of chronic myelogenous leukaemia represent
    stages in the development of B-cell precursors. New Eng. J.
    Med., 309: 826-831.
Blewitt, R.W., Abbott, A.C. and Bird, C.C., 1983, Mode of cell death
    induced in human lymphoid cells by high and low doses of gluco-
    corticoid, Br. J. Cancer, 47: 477-486.
Burrow, H.M., Bird, C.C., Warren, J.V., Steel, C.M., Barrett, I.D.,
    and Panesar, N.S., 1981, Human lymphoid cell lines and gluco-
    corticoids: I. Characterization and cytolethal responses of
    lymphoblastoid, leukaemia and lymphoma lines, Diag. Histopath.
    4: 175-188.
Catovsky, D., Linch, D.C. and Beverley, P.C.L., 1982, T cell disorders
    in haematological diseases, Clinics in Haematology,11: 661-695.
Cleary, M.L., Chao, J., Warnke, R., and Sklar, J., 1984a, Immuno
    globulin gene rearrangement as a diagnostic criterion in B-cell
    lymphoma, Proc. Natl. Acad. Sci. USA, 81: 593-597.
Cleary, M.L., Warnke, R., and Sklar, J., 1984b, Monoclonality of
    lymphoproliferative lesions in cardiac-transplant recipients,
    New Engl. J. Med., 310: 477-482.
Dorreen, M.S., Habeshaw, J.A., Stansfeld, A.G., Wrigley, P.F.M., and
    Lister, T.A., 1984, Characteristics of Sternberg-Reed, and
    related cells in Hodgkin's disease: An immunohistological study
    Br. J. Cancer, 49: 465-476.
Foroni. L., Catovsky. D., Rabbitts, T.H., and Luzzatto, L., 1984,
    Immunoglobulin gene rearrangement in lymphotic leukemia,
    Br. J. Haem., 58:101.
Galton, D.A.G., and MacLennan, I.C.M., 1982, Clinical patterns in B
    lymphoid Malignancy, Clinics in Haematology, 11: 561-587.
Ha, K., Minden, M., Hozumi, N., and Gelfand, E.W., 1984a, Immunoglobin
    chain gene rearrangement in a patient with T cell acute
    lymphocytic leukaemia, J. Clin. Invest., 73: 1232-1236.
Ha, K., Minden, M., Hozumi, N. and Gelfand, E.W., 1984b, Immuno-
    globulin gene rearrangement in acute myelogenous leukemia,
    Cancer Res., 44: 4658-4660.
Honjo, T., 1983, Immunoglobulin genes, Ann. Rev. Immunol.. 1: 499-529.
Janossy, G. and Prentice. H.G., 1982, T cell subpopulations, mono
    clonal antibodies and their therapeutic applications. Clinics in
    Haematology. 11: 631-660.
Korsmeyer, S.J., Arnold. A., Bakhshi, A., Ravetch, J.V., Siebenlist,

U., Hieter, P.A., Sharrow, S.O., Lebien, T.W. and Waldmann, T.A 1983a, Immunoglobulin gene rearrangement and cell surface antigen expression in acute lymphocytic leukaemias of T cell and B cell precursor origins. J. Clin. Invest., 71: 301-313.

Korsmeyer, S.J., Greene, W.C., Cossman, J., Hsu, S., Jensen, J.P., Neckers, L.M., Marshall, S.L., Bakhshi, A., Deper, J.M., Leonard. W.J., Jaffe, E.S. and Waldmann, T.A., 1983b, Rearrangement and expression of immunoglobulin genes and expression of Tac antigen in hairy cell leukaemia, Proc. Natl.Acad. Sci. USA, 80:4522-4526.

Lauder, I., Bird, C.C., Child, J.A. and Grigor, I., 1984, Surface membrane phenotypic expression and treatment response of malignant lymphomas. J. Path., 142:517.

LeBeau, M.M., and Rowley, J.D., 1984, Heritable fragile sites in cancer, Nature, 308: 607-608.

Lennert, K., 1978, Malignant lymphomas other than Hodgkin's disease. in: Handbuck der Spezillen Anatomie und Histologie, Uehlinger, E., ed., Springer, New York and Berlin. 1:3.

Stein, H., Gerdes, J., Schwab, U., Lemke, H., Diehl. V., Mason, D.Y. Bartels, H. and Ziegler, A., 1983, Evidence for the detection of the normal counterpart of Hodgkin's and Sternberg-Reed cells Haematol. Oncol., 1: 21-29.

Tonegawa, S., 1983, Somatic generation of antibody diversity, Nature, 302: 575-581.

Vogler, L.B., 1982, Bone Marrow B cell development, Clinics in Haematology, 11: 509-529.

# ACTIVATION OF RAS ONCOGENES IN MULTISTAGE CARCINOGENESIS OF MOUSE SKIN

Martin Ramsden, Miguel Quintanilla and Allan Balmain

Beatson Institute for Cancer Research
Garscube Estate
Bearsden
Glasgow G61 1BD, Scotland

## INTRODUCTION

The vast majority of human tumours arise in cells of epithelial origin, probably as a result of exposure to a range of environmental factors, and appear after a multistage sequence of events. Clarification of the molecular events involved in the various stages of tumour development is obviously crucial to the understanding of cancer development and for providing the basis for strategies of prevention or early diagnosis. The use of animal model systems provides a means by which stages of carcinogenesis can be dissected at the molecular level. One such model system, the induction of tumours in mouse skin, has a number of useful properties. First, tumours can be induced by a wide variety of chemical compounds and also by physical stimuli such as X-rays or UV light. Secondly, many of the currently accepted concepts of multistage carcinogenesis have been developed using the mouse skin model (Boutwell, 1974; Hecker et al., 1982). Hence, a wealth of detailed biological information exists relating to this particular system. Thirdly, the development of malignant skin carcinomas is preceded by the appearance of multiple benign papillomas. These premalignant lesions are histologically distinct and provide adequate material for the study of progressive changes which occur at different stages of tumour development.

Some of the important features of the mouse skin model of carcinogenesis may be summarized as follows. Treatment of mouse skin with a low dose of carcinogen results in the "initiation" of a small number of cells. With no further treatment, these cells do not give rise to tumours, but remain "dormant" in the skin. Repeated

application of tumour promoting agents leads to skin hyperplasia
followed with 6 - 10 weeks by the appearance of benign papillomas.
Some of these benign lesions seem to regress spontaneously while
others are capable of progression, either with or without further
promoter treatment, to malignant carcinomas.

The molecular events associated with the progression to
malignancy are unclear. However, recent experiments on RNA tumour
viruses and transfection of tumour-derived DNA into mouse NIH/3T3
fibroblast recipient cells have implicated a number of genes which
may be involved in various stages of tumour development (reviewed
by Bishop, 1983). The oncogenes of the RNA tumour viruses are
derived from normal cellular genes which have been termed proto-
oncogenes. These proto-oncogenes may be mutated, or activated, in
non-virus-infected cells such that the DNA of a significant
proportion of tumours is able to cause morphological transformation
of the recipient NIH/3T3 cells. Proto-oncogenes derived from normal
cells do not, on their own, have this ability. The proportion of
randomly selected human tumours with active transforming genes is
around 10-20% (Pulciani et al., 1982; Santos et al., 1984; Fujita et
al., 1984) but this figure can be much higher in certain animal model
systems (Sukumar et al., 1983; Balmain et al., 1984; Guerrero et al.,
1984). In the vast majority of cases, the activated proto-oncogenes
detected in the NIH/3T3 transformation system are members of the ras
gene family, related to the oncogenes of the Harvey and Kirsten
Murine Sarcoma Viruses (Cooper, 1982; Bishop, 1983). A limited
number of other non-ras oncogenes have also been described which can
transform NIH/3T3 cells (Goubin et al., 1983; Diamond et al., 1983;
Lane et al., 1984; Schechter et al., 1984; Cooper et al., 1984b).

Activated ras genes have been identified in tumours and cell
lines of a wide variety of cell types as detailed for human cells
in Table 1 and for animals cells in Table 2. The activation of the
c-H-ras gene seems to be largely confined to cells of epithelial
origin, with the exception of two melanoma cell lines and the mouse
myeloid tumour line WEHI 274. In contrast, c-K-ras and particularly
N-ras are activated in cells of fibroblastic, neuroblastic and
haematopoietic lineages. Molecular cloning and sequencing of ras
genes has identified two regions of the coding sequence where single
base mutations generate transforming alleles (Table 3). These regions
cover codons 12 and 61 of the genes. In vitro mutagenesis of cloned
ras sequences has shown that mutations which specify amino acid
changes at codons 13, 59 or 63 also activate the c-H-ras gene (Fasano
et al., 1984), but these mutants have not yet been identified in
natural tumours. A limited range of amino acid changes have been
noted for naturally occurring codon 12 mutations but Seeburg et al.
(1984) have shown by in vitro mutagenesis that any amino acid
substitution, except for proline, at codon 12 produces a transforming
allele of c-H-ras. The morphological phenotype of the transformed
cells can depend upon the particular amino acid substitution. It is

Table 1.

| Tumour type | Isolate number[2] | | ras gene[3] activated | Reference |
|---|---|---|---|---|
| CARCINOMA: | | | | |
|     Bladder | EJ/T24 | (C) | H | Der et al. (1982) |
| | | | | Santos et al. (1982) |
| | | | | Parada et al. (1982) |
| | J82 | (C) | H | Der et al. (1982) |
| | JBT44 | (T) | H | Fujita et al. (1984) |
| | A1698 | (C) | K | Pulciani et al. (1982) |
|     Renal Pelvic | JPT26 | (T) | H | Fujita et al. (1984) |
|     Lung | Hs242 | (C) | H | Yuasa et al. (1983) |
| | Lx-1 | (C) | K | Der et al. (1982) |
| | | | | McCoy et al. (1983) |
| | A427 | (C) | K | Pulciani et al. (1982) |
| | Calu-1 | (C) | K | Shimizu et al. (1983a,c) |
| | SK-LU-1 | (C) | K | Shimizu et al. (1983c) |
| | A2182 | (C) | K | Pulciani et al. (1982) |
| | PR310 | (C) | K | Nakano et al. (1984) |
| | A549 | (C) | K | McCoy et al. (1983) |
| | PR371 | (C) | K | Nakano et al. (1984) |
| | Lu65 | (C) | K | Taya et al. (1984) |
| | 1615 | (T) | K | Pulciani et al. (1982) |
| | LC-10 | (T) | K | Santos et al. (1984) |
| | SW1271 | (C) | N | Yuasa et al. (1984) |
|     Colon | SW480 | (C) | K | McCoy et al. (1983) |
| | Adenocarc. | (T) | K | McCoy et al. (1983) |
| | SK-CO-1 | (C) | K | Shimizu et al. (1983c) |
| | A2233 | (C) | K | Pulciani et al. (1982) |
|     Pancreas | A1165 | (C) | K | Cooper et al. (1984a) |
| | 1189 | (T) | K | Pulciani et al. (1982) |
|     Liver | HEP G2 | (C) | N | Notario et al. (1984) |
| | 2193 | (T) | N | Notario et al. (1984) |
|     Gall Bladder | A1604 | (C) | K | Pulciani et al. (1982) |
|     Ovary | OVCA-1 | (C) | K | Feig et al. (1984) |
|   Teratocarcinoma | PA1 | (C) | N | Cooper et al. (1984a) |

Table 2.

| Tumour Type | Isolate number | ras gene activated | Reference |
|---|---|---|---|
| **CARCINOSARCOMA:** | | | |
| Mammary | HS578T    (C) | H | Kraus et al. (1984) |
| **SARCOMA:** | | | |
| Fibrosarcoma | HT1080 (C) | N | Hall et al. (1983) |
| Rhabdomyosarcoma | RD      (C) | N | Hall et al. (1983) |
|  | 1085    (T) | K | Pulciani et al. (1982) |
| MELANOMA | SK2     (C) | H | Sekiya et al. (1984) |
|  | SK-MEL-146(C) | H | Albino et al. (1984) |
|  | SK-MEL-93 (C) | N | Albino et al. (1984) |
|  | SK-MEL-119(C) | N | Albino et al. (1984) |
|  | SK-MEL-147(C) | N | Albino et al. (1984) |
| NEUROBLASTOMA | SK-N-SH (C) | N | Shimizu et al. (1983b,c) |
| **LEUKAEMIA:** | | | |
| Acute lymphocytic (immature T cell) | RPMI8402 (C) | N | Souyri & Fleissner (1983) |
| (intermediate T cell) | T-ALL-1  (C) | N | Souyri & Fleissner (1983) |
| " | p12      (C) | N | Souyri & Fleissner (1983) |
| " | CCRF-CEM (C) | K | Eva et al. (1983) |
| " | MOLT-3   (C) | N | Eva et al. (1983) |
| " | MOLT-4   (C) | N | Eva et al. (1983) |
| Chronic myelocytic | PAC      (C) | N | Murray et al. (1983) |
|  | Marrow cells    (T) | N | Gambke et al. (1984) |
| Promyelocytic | HL60     (C) | N | Murray et al. (1983) |
| **LYMPHOMA:** | | | |
| Burkitts | AWRamos  (C) | N | Murray et al. (1983) |

1. Table only shows examples published before 31.12.84.
2. (C) denotes tumour-derived cell line, (T) denotes primary tumour material used as source of transforming DNA.
3. H: c-H-ras1 gene, K: c-K-ras2 gene, N: N-ras gene.

possible that the naturally occurring transforming alleles which have
been detected in the NIH/3T3 assay have high level transforming
activity.  A range of other transforming ras alleles may exist in
other tumours which are involved in the development of these tumours
but do not possess sufficient transforming activity to be detectable
by transfection into NIH/3T3 cells.  Thus ras activiation may occur in
a much higher proportion of human tumours than is presently
appreciated but it may be necessary to develop alternative and more
sensitive assay systems in order to detect more weakly transforming
genes.

We have demonstrated activation of the c-H-ras gene in the mouse
skin model for chemical carcinogenesis (Balmain and Pragnell, 1983;
Balmain et al., 1984).  In this system the activation of the gene
seems to occur at a relatively early stage of tumour progression since
benign papillomas taken after about 10 - 15 weeks of promoter
treatment have the same transforming activity as invasive carcinomas.
We have now further characterised the nature of the transforming
activity of c-H-ras in epidermal tumour progression.


RESULTS

Expression of the c-H-ras Gene in Epidermal Tumours

While the activation of ras genes in an increasing number of
tumour DNA isolates has been shown to be due to point mutations as
outlined above (Tables 1,2,3), other activating mechanisms have been
demonstrated for a variety of other proto-oncogenes.  For example,
aberrant regulation of the normal gene leading to an accumulation of
mRNA, possibly at an inappropriate stage of the cell cycle, may
produce an activated phenotype.  In support of this possibility, the
transfection of an in vitro construct of a normal H-ras allele with an
enhancer element can lead to the appearance of transformed recipient
cells (Chang et al., 1982).  To determine whether there is elevated
expression of the c-H-ras gene in epidermal tumours, RNA prepared from
a series of such tumours, as well as normal and hyperplastic
epidermis, was hybridized by Northern blotting to an H-ras specific
probe.  Figure 1 shows that the level of the 1.4kb c-H-ras specific
transcript is elevated in several individual Sencar strain papillomas,
in pooled small papillomas from NMRI mice and, to a lesser extent, in
a Sencar carcinoma.  This blot also appears to show a small increase
in c-H-ras transcripts in epidermis stimulated to proliferate by a
single dose of the promoting agent TPA.  However, upon rehybridizing
the blot with a probe specific for the ubiquitous highly abundant,
cytoplasmic 7S RNA (Balmain et al., 1982), it is demonstrated that the
sample from hyperplastic epidermis contains slightly more RNA than the
control epidermis lane (Fig. 1B, lanes b and a respectively).
Similarly the papilloma RNA in lane e hybridises more strongly than
the control with the 7S probe, hence the c-H-ras transcript level of

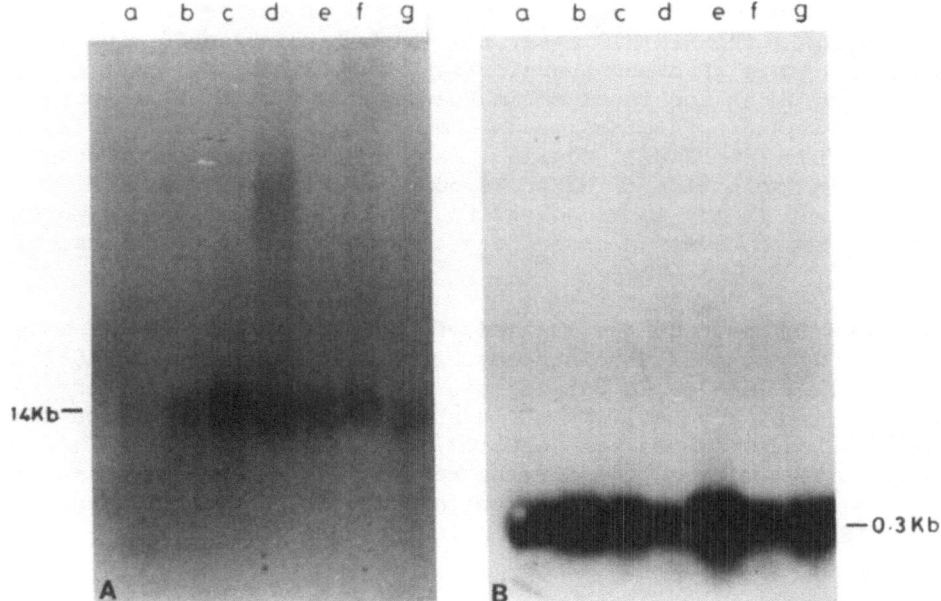

Fig. 1A   Northern blot analysis of c-H-ras transcripts in primary
          tumours.  Total cellular RNA was isolated as previously
          described (Balmain et al., 1984) from the following sources;
          a, normal epidermis;  b, TPA-treated epidermis (48hr after
          single treatment); c,d,e, individual papillomas from Sencar
          mice; f, pooled small papillomas from NMRI mice; g, Sencar
          carcinoma.  The blot was prepared and hybridised to a v-H-
          ras fragment (Ellis et al., 1980) using standard techniques
          (Maniatis et al., 1982).
       B  Comparison of RNA levels.  The blot used in panel A was
          stripped of probe by washing in water at 70°C and rehybrid-
          ised with the probe pA6 (Balmain et al., 1982) which carries
          sequences homologous to the ubiquitous 7S RNA species.

this tumour is slightly overestimated in Fig. 1.  The remaining tumour
RNAs hybridise to an equal or lesser extent to the 7S probe than the
control epidermal RNA, indicating a true increase in the relative
concentration of c-H-ras transcripts in these tumours.  We conclude
that there is a relatively small and variable increase in c-H-ras
transcript levels in primary tumours and that this effect is not due
simply to an increase in the proportion of proliferating cells within
the tumours, since no such increase was observed in the RNA of
hyperplastic epidermis.

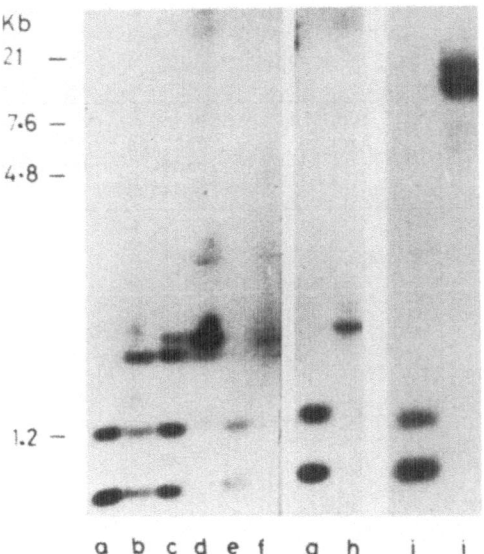

Fig. 2   Differential methylation of the c-H-ras locus in cells
         derived from different mouse tissues.   Sources of DNA;
         lanes a and b, normal epidermis, lanes c and d, brain;
         lanes e and f, F46 Friend erythroleukaemia cells;   lanes
         g and h, N18 neuroblastoma, lanes i and j, NIH/3T3 cells.
         The DNAs in lanes, a, c, e, g and i are digested with
         MspI, DNAs in lanes b,d,f,h and j digested with HpaII.


## The c-H-ras Locus is Undermethylated in Epidermal Cells

Numerous studies have implicated changes in DNA methylation -
notably.the presence or absence of 5-methylcytosine residues - in the
control of gene expression (reviewed by Razin and Riggs, 1980;
Felsenfeld and McGhee, 1982; Doerfler, 1983; Riggs and Jones, 1983).
Difference in the extent of DNA methylation have been observed in
comparisons of normal and tumour cells, both in general terms and at
specific sites around a variety of individual genes (Lapeyre and
Becker, 1979; Feinberg and Vogelstein, 1983a,b; Riggs and Jones, 1983;
Vedel et al., 1983).   It was of considerable interest to characterise
c-H-ras with respect to DNA methylation in view of the transcriptional
changes noted above, and also since the transforming abulity of the
c-H-ras gene is reproducibly activated in epidermal tumours.   In
addition, c-H-ras activation generally appears to be confined to
epithelial cell types (Table 1) and we wished to determine whether
there was a similar pattern of tissue specificity in DNA methylation
around the c-H-ras locus.   The methylation state of the locus was
assayed using the isoschizomeric restriction enzymes MspI, which
cleaves DNA even if the internal cytosine of the CCGG recognition

Table 3.

| Tumour type and origin[1] | | Inducing Agent | No. of Positive Trans- formants | ras gene involved[2] | Reference |
|---|---|---|---|---|---|
| **MOUSE** | | | | | |
| Epidermal carcinoma | (T) | DMBA+TPA | 4/6 | H | Balmain & Pragnell (1983) Balmain et al. (1984) |
| Epidermal papilloma | (T) | DMBA+TPA | 7/8 | H | " |
| Thymoma | (T) | γ-irradiation | 4/7 | K | Guerrero et al. (1984a) |
| Thymoma | (T) | NMU | 5/6 | N | " |
| Fibrosarcoma | (T) | MCA | 2/4 | K | Eva & Aaronson (1983) |
| Fibrosarcoma FS6M1 | (C) | BP | 1/1 | K | Vousden & Marshall (1984) |
| Lymphoma (T-cell) L5178Y-ES | (C) | MCA | 1/1 | K | " |
| Macrophage tumour P388D1 | (C) | MCA | 1/1 | K | " |
| Lewis Lung Carcinoma LLC | (C) | Spont. | 1/1 | N | " |
| Myeloid tumour WEHI 274 | (C) | Ableson MuLV | 1/1 | H | " |
| Fibroblast C3H/10T1/2 | | MCA | 10/10 | K | Parada & Weinberg (1983) |
| **RAT** | | | | | |
| Mammary carcinoma | (T) | NMU | 9/9 | H | Sukumar et al. (1983) |
| **GUINEA PIG** | | | | | |
| Foetal cells | (C) | MCA | 1/1 | R | Sukumar et al. (1984) |
| | | BP | 1/1 | R | " |
| | | MNNG | 2/2 | R | " |
| | | DENA | 1/1 | R | " |

1. (T) denotes primary tumour material, (C) denotes tumour-derived cell line.
2. H:  c-H-ras1 gene, K: c-K-ras2 gene; N: N-ras gene; R: ras-related.

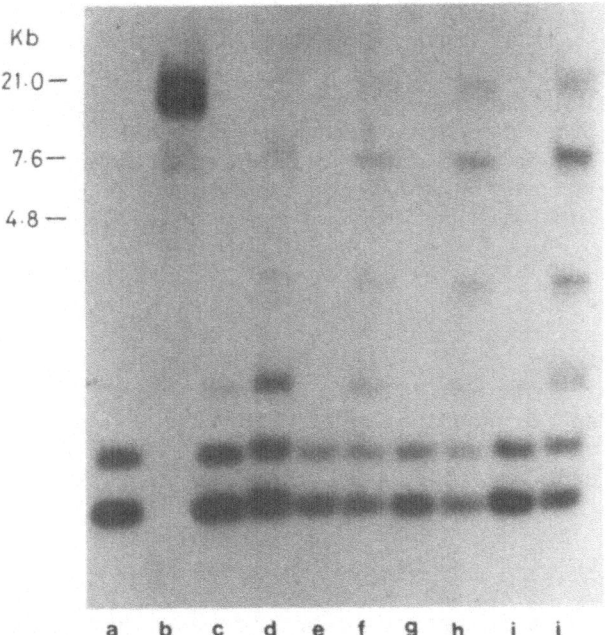

Fig. 3   Methylation levels at HpaII sites around the c-H-ras locus
         in normal and neoplastic epidermis.  Sources of DNA:  lanes
         a and b, NIH/3T3 cells;  lanes c and d, normal epidermis;
         lanes e and f, TPA-treated epidermis;  lanes g and h, pooled
         NMRI papillomas;  lanes i and j, representative NMRI carcinoma.
         The DNA samples in lanes, a, c, e, g and i are digested with
         MspI, those in lanes b, d, f, h, and j with HpaII.


sequence is methylated, and HpaII which is sensitive to methylation at
this site and will only cleave the unmethylated DNA sequence.  MspI or
HpaII digested DNAs of normal epidermis, brain, Friend erythro-
leukaemia, neuroblastoma and NIH/3T3 cells were Southern blotted and
probed for c-H-ras sequences.  Figure 2 shows that in all the MspI
digests the H-ras probe hybridises to two low molecular weight
fragments indicating that there are CCGG sequences close to the
c-H-ras gene.  Additional bands present in the MspI digest of brain
DNA (lane c) result from partial digestion of this sample.  The HpaII
digest of epidermal DNA (lane b) has a high proportion of the c-H-ras
gene copies in the low molecular weight fragments suggesting that the
majority of c-H-ras copies are unmethylated.  In contrast, in the
HpaII digest of NIH/3T3 DNA, virtually all of the hybridisation is to
fragments of 15-20kb (lane j) suggesting that a region of at least
15kb around the c-H-ras gene is highly methylated in this cell line.
In brain, Friend and neuroblastoma cell DNAs (Fig. 2, lanes d, f and h
respectively), the c-H-ras HpaII fragments are all of higher molecular

weight than the corresponding MspI fragments indicating that the CCGG
sequences closest to the c-H-ras gene are methylated but that the
region of heavy methylation does not extend as far into flanking
sequences as is the case in NIH/3T3 cell DNA.  It is clear that the
methylation status of the c-H-ras locus varies in different tissue
types, ranging between the highly methylated state in NIH/3T3 fibroblasts and the largely unmethylated form in epidermis, with intermediate levels in brain and hematopoietic cell lineages.

     Since the c-H-ras locus is undermethylated in normal epidermis,
it was of interest to determine whether this state persists in
epidermal tumours, or indeed whether there is further demethylation
during epidermal tumour progression.  DNA samples from normal and
hyperplastic epidermis, papillomas and carcinomas were therefore
digested with MspI or HpaII, Southern blotted and probed for H-ras
sequences.  Figure 3 shows that there was no substantial difference in
methylation around the c-H-ras locus in the various stages of tumour
progression and that the locus remains essentially unmethylated.

Genomic Map of the c-H-ras Locus

     Activation of a number of other oncogenes may be achieved by
chromosome rearrangement or insertion of a retrovirus element close
to the gene (reviewed by Yunis, 1983; Muller and Verma, 1984).  Since
the expression of the c-H-ras gene appears to be altered in epidermal
tumours, there was a possibility of this type of mechanism activating
c-H-ras in the epidermal tumours.  The region around the c-H-ras gene
was mapped with a number of restriction enzymes by Southern blotting
of double digested NIH/3T3 DNA and deduction of overlapping fragment
sizes.  The results of the mapping are summarised in Figure 4.
Mapping of this region is obviously limited to restriction fragments
which contain sequences homologous to the H-ras probe and thus only
the pair of sites closest to the gene are mapped for any restriction
enzyme.  Three XhoI sites are shown, the site marked 'X' being
methylated in NIH/3T3 cells but not always methylated in epidermal DNA
(Ramsden et al., 1985).  The c-H-ras gene must extend further than the
region indicated in Fig. 4 since BamHI and HindIII inactivate the
transforming ability of the gene (Vousden and Marshall, 1984) and the
H-ras-specific probe used (BS9, Ellis et al., 1980) does not carry
sequences homologous to exon 4 or the cellular gene.  Comparison of
single and double restriction digest fragments using papilloma and
carcinoma DNAs indicate no differences to the map in Fig. 4.  This
suggests that no insertions, deletions or re- arrangements have
occured, at least in the 23 kb of sequence around the c-H-ras gene
defined by the two EcoRI sites.  Activation of c-H-ras in epidermal
tumours is therefore unlikely to be caused by this type of mechanism.

The c-H-ras Gene Product is Altered in Epidermal Tumours

     In all cases so far examined in detail, ras gene activation is

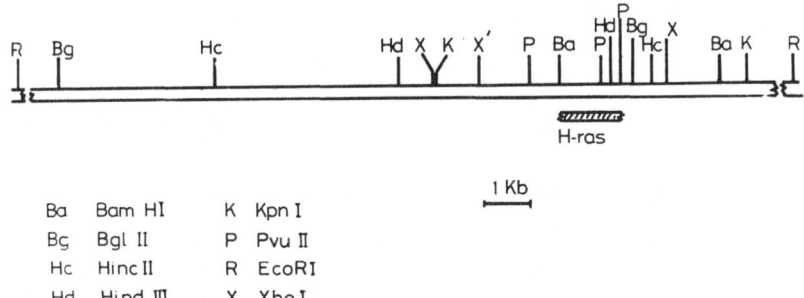

Fig. 4    Restriction map of the mouse c-H-ras locus derived by
blotting genomic DNA and hybridisation to a v-H-ras probe.
NIH/3T3 DNA was used to position the restriction sites.  The
XhoI site indicated 'X' is methylated in NIH/3T3 cells and
was mapped using PaeR71.  The position of this site was also
confirmed by digesting carcinoma DNA with XhoI.  The region
denoted H-ras is the minimum area which consistently hybridises
to the v-H-ras probe.

achieved by point mutation within the coding region (Table 3).  This
has been shown by cloning and sequencing of the normal and
transforming alleles of the gene.  One other method which can identify
altered ras gene product relies on the observations that the majority
of mutations at codons 12 or 61 of the ras gene give rise to a
product, the p21 protein, which exhibits an altered mobility on SDS-
polyacrylamide gel electrophoresis due to conformational changes in
the protein (for example Seeburg et al., 1984).  Normal or altered ras
genes can then be demonstrated by using p21-specific antisera to
immunoprecipitate in vivo labelled proteins.

NIH/3T3 cells transformed by papilloma or carcinoma were selected
and grown in Tissue Culture in the presence of $^{35}$S- methionine.
Cellular proteins were extracted and precipitated using either pre-
immune serum or the monoclonal antibody YA6-172, which is specific for
the Harvey type p21 (Furth et al., 1982).  Immunoprecipitates were
then electrophoresed through 30cm long 12% polyacrylamide gels and
labelled proteins visualised by fluorography.  Figure 5 shows the
ability of this technique to resolve different species of p21 protein.
NIH/3T3 cells express a low level of normal Harvey p21 (lane 6) which
is also immunoprecipitated from transformants (lane 1-5).  Four
variant forms of Harvey p21 are also resolved in Fig. 5.  Lane 5 shows
a slowly migrating Harvey p21 expressed in an NIH/3T3 transformant

Table 4.

| Gene | Codon | Sequence | Amino Acid | Source[1,2] | Reference |
|------|-------|----------|-----------|-------------|-----------|
| c-H-ras | 12 | GGC | Gly | Normal human | |
| | 12 | GTC | Val | T24/EJ | Reddy et al. (1982) Tabin et al. (1982) Taparowsky et al. (1982) |
| | 12 | GAC | Asp | 134-51 HS578T | Santos et al. (1983) Kraus et al. (1984) |
| | 12 | GGA | Gly | Normal rat | Sukumar et al. (1983) |
| | 12 | GAA | Glu | Rat mammary carcinoma | " |
| v-Has | 12 | AGA | Arg | Harvey Sarcoma Virus Rasheed Sarcoma Virus | Dhar et al. (1982) Rasheed et al. (1983) |
| V-Bas | 12 | AAA | Lys | Balb-c Sarcoma Virus | Reddy et al. (1985) |
| c-H-ras | 61 | CAG | Glu | Normal human | |
| | 61 | CTG | Leu | Hs242 SK2 | Yuasa et al. (1983) Sekiya et al. (1984) |
| c-K-ras | 12 | GGT | Gly | Normal human | |
| | 12 | TGT | Cys | Calu 1 PR371 Lu-65 | Shimizu et al. (1983a) Capon et al. (1983) Nakano et al. (1984) Taya et al. (1984) |
| | 12 | GTT | Val | SW480 | Capon et al. (1983) |
| | 12 | CGT | Arg | A2182 A1698 LC-10 | Santos et al. (1984) " " |
| | 12 | GGT | Gly | Normal mouse | Guerrero et al. (1984b) |
| | 12 | GAT | Asp | Mouse lymphoma | " |
| v-K-ras | 12 | AGT | Ser | Kirsten Sarcoma virus | Tsuchida et al. (1982) |
| c-K-ras | 61 | CAA | Gln | Normal human | |
| | 61 | CAT | His | PR310 | Yamamoto & Perucho (1984) |

Table 5.

| Gene | Codon | Sequence | Amino Acid | Source[1,2] | Reference |
|------|-------|----------|------------|-------------|-----------|
| N-ras | 12 | GGT | Gly | Normal human | |
| | 12 | GAT | Asp | PA1 | Tainsky et al. (1984) |
| | 61 | CAA | Gln | Normal human | |
| | 61 | AAA | Lys | HT1080 SK-N-SH | Brown et al. (1984) Taparowsky et al. (1983) |
| | 61 | CGA | Arg | SW1271 | Yuasa et al. (1984) |
| | 61 | CAC or CAT | His | RD301 | Bos et al. (1984) |

1.  Further details of tumour type in Table 1.
2.  Synthetic mutant constructs not included.
    (see Fasano et al., 1984; Seeburg et al., 1984)

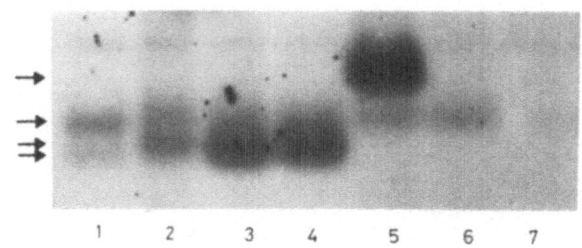

Fig. 5   Fluorograph of ras p21 proteins immunoprecipitated from
         NIH/3T3 transformants using the Harvey-specific monoclonal
         YA6-172 (Furth et al., 1982).   The $^{35}$S-labelled p21s were
         from transformants induced by the following epidermal tumour
         DNAs: 1, papilloma 4 (a mixture of 10 pooled NMRI papillomas);
         2, papilloma 3; 3, papilloma 2; 4, carcinoma 2; 5, carcinoma
         1; 6, untransformed NIH/3T3 cells; 7, NIH/3T3 cells with pre-
         immune serum.   The arrows indicate the migration of Harvey
         p21 variant proteins.

induced by carcinoma DNA.   This migration is very similar to that of
the Harvey p21 of the T24 cell line which has a codon 12 mutation
(data not shown).   Transformed NIH/3T3 foci induced by a single
papilloma DNA and a second carcinoma DNA (lanes 3 and 4 respectively)
have identical rapidly migrating Harvey p21s.   This form of Harvey p21
was also detected in two other papilloma DNA-induced foci (data not
shown).   Single examples of two further Harvey p21 variants are also
shown.   Lane 2 shows the p21 derived from a papilloma DNA-induced
focus which has a greater mobility than the normal Harvey p21 but
migrates slightly more slowly than the form shown in lanes 3 and 4.
Lane 1 shows p21 derived from a NIH/3T3 transformant induced by the
DNA of a pool of 10 small papillomas which appears to have two variant
forms present.   The upper band appears to migrate marginally faster
than the normal Harvey p21.   While the lower band has the same
mobility as the common variant shown in lanes 3 and 4.


DISCUSSION

     The activation of transforming ability in the c-H-ras gene is a
molecular event which occurs reproducibly during the induction of
epidermal tumours by chemical carcinogens.   This activation is
complete by the time benign papillomas develop (Balmain et al., 1984)
and is therefore an early event in epidermal tumorigenesis.   This
contrasts with evidence from other systems suggesting that ras gene
activation is a late event associated with the development of
malignancy;   for example the detection of transforming ras genes from
late, but not early, passage carcinogen-treated guinea pig cells
(Sukumar et al., 1984) and in a metastatic variant of a T-cell

are pre-malignant lesions they can be autonomous and rapidly proliferate to substantial size.  Tumour cells with similar properties but located in tissues such as dermis, brain or bone marrow could have much more serious consequences for the host since they may not be contained within the normal geographical boundaries imposed by epithelial tissue organisation (Cairns, 1975).  In other words, the number of events required to generate a skin papilloma, formally classified as benign, may be similar to that required for a fibro-sarcoma or leukaemia, either of which could kill the host animal.  In support of this interpretation, analysis of age-incidence curves for different human cancers has suggested that the total number of events required for carcinoma formation may be greater than for many other types of tumour (Peto, 1977).

The mechanism by which the c-H-ras gene is activated in epidermal tumours is not entirely clear.  However, we have shown that 4 variant forms of the Harvey p21 are detectable in a series of NIH/3T3 trans-formants induced by papilloma or carcinoma DNA.  One of these variants has a reduced mobility on SDS-polyacrylamide gel electrophoresis. This appears to be a common property of Harvey p21s with alterations of amino acid residue 12 (see for example Seeburg et al. (1984).  The other p21 variants we have detected exhibit increased mobility on electrophoresis, suggesting that these represent codon 61 mutants by analogy with published examples (Shimizu et al., 1983c; Yuasa et al., 1983; Fasano et al., 1984).  All of the epidermal tumours in our study were initiated by treatment with the same carcinogen, dimethyl-benzanthracene (DMBA).  The data are consistent with the ability of DMBA to form bulky adducts  with deoxyadenosine or deoxyguanosine residues, leading to the induction of a variety of point mutations (Singer and Kusmierek, 1982; Dipple et al., 1983).  These observations may provide evidence for the direct interaction between DMBA and the c-H-ras gene being a crucial event in the initiation of carcino-genesis.  This suggestion has previously been put forward by Sukumar et al. (1983) to explain the consistent induction of rat mammary carcinomas by nitrosomethylurea (NMU).  In this system, all 39 carcinomas analysed have an identical G to A transition affecting codon 12 of the c-H-ras gene (Zarbl et al., 1985).  This particular mutation is predicted by the ability of NMU to methylate the 0-6 position of deoxyguanosine residues leading to mispairing during replication and transition mutations (Margison and O'Connor, 1978). Obviously, more detailed analysis of large numbers of activated ras genes in tumours induced by defined carcinogens is required to confirm or refute the suggestion of direct carcinogen-ras gene interaction.

The available evidence presently does not preclude the possibility that other changes occur at the c-H-ras locus during chemical carcinogenesis which have either a predisposing or modulating influence upon the activation of the transforming potential of the gene.  Such influences may give a molecular basis for the intriguing observation that c-H-ras activation occurs in a much narrower category

of cell types than does the activation of either c-K-ras or N-ras.
Lane et al. (1982) and Sukumar et al. (1983) have suggested that there
may be specificity in the activation of particular proto-oncogenes
dependent upon either the tissue of origin or differentiation state of
the original target cell.  The activation of c-H-ras in NMU-induced
rat mammary carcinomas only occurs if the carcinogen is administered
during a restricted period of the juvenile animals' maturation
(Sukumar et al., 1983).  This is thought to reflect a modulating
influence exerted by the hormonal state of the animal.  Apart from
hormones, a number of other mechanisms are known to influence gene
expression and may also have a role in the apparent tissue-specific
activation of c-H-ras.  There is an increase in the levels of c-H-ras
transcripts in some epidermal tumours, suggesting that the expression
of the gene is modulated in this model system.  The increased
transcript level is not accompanied by chromosomal rearrangement or
insertion of DNA elements close to the gene and it is not clear what
role, if any, this phenomenon has in the aetiology of epidermal
tumours.  There does not appear to be a simple correlation between the
degree of expression of the c-H-ras gene and the overall DNA
methylation levels around the locus.  For example, although under-
methylated at CCGG sequences in normal epidermis, c-H-ras expression
is at a similar low level to the expression in NIH/3T3 cells where the
locus is highly methylated.  However, the level of methylation at the
c-H-ras locus does appear to exhibit a tissue specificity similar to
the specificity of c-H-ras activation.  The c-H-ras gene is under-
methylated and capable of frequent activation in epidermis, but is
highly methylated in fibroblastic cells where carcinogen-induced
transformation is associated with c-K-ras activation (Eva and
Aaronson, 1983; Parada and Weinberg, 1983).  It is plausible that in
fibroblast or other cell types, c-H-ras activation may not occur since
in addition to mutational events, demethylation steps are required to
allow the effective expression of the c-H-ras transforming ability.
It is also possible that demethylation of c-H-ras in epidermal DNA
renders the gene more easily accessible to carcinogenic agents.  This
effect may be mediated by differential protein binding to c-H-ras in
different cell types in association with the DNA methylation levels.
Obviously the elucidation of such possibilities requires much greater
insight into the role c-H-ras plays in the cell, the mechanisms by
which expression of the gene is regulated and also the mechanism of
activation by carcinogen treatment.  As a preliminary step we have
identified and isolated a genomic clone containing the normal mouse
c-H-ras gene.  This clone was identified in a library (provided by Dr
R. Krumlauf, Fox Chase Cancer Center, Philadelphia) of partial Sau3AI
digested genomic DNA ligated into the $\lambda$ phage vector Charon 30,
packaged in vitro and propagated in E.coli.  Subcloning, restriction
mapping and sequencing of this clone should provide a sound basis for
a characterisation of the c-H-ras locus leading towards an
understanding of the regulation and activation of the gene.

ACKNOWLEDGEMENTS

     The Beatson Institute is supported by the Cancer Research
Campaign.  M.Q. was supported by an EMBO Long Term Fellowship and a
grant from Imperial Chemical Industries PLC.  We thank G. Cole and J.
Smith for excellent technical assistance.

REFERENCES

Albino, A.P., Le Strange, R., Oliff, A.I., Furth, M.E. and Old, L.J.,
     1984, Transforming ras genes form human melanoma: a manifestation
     of tumour heterogeneity? Nature 308:69.
Balmain, A., Krumlauf, R., Vass, J.K. and Birnie, G.D., 1982, Cloning
     and characterisation of the abundant cytoplasmic 7SRNA from mouse
     cells. Nucl. Acids Res., 10:4259.
Balmain, A. and Pragnell, I.B., 1983, Mouse skin carcinomas induced in
     vivo by chemical carcinogens have a transforming Harvey-ras
     oncogene, Nature, 303:72.
Balmain, A., Ramsden, M., Boweden, G.T. and Smith, J., 1984,
     Activation of the mouse cellular Harvey-ras gene in chemically
     induced benighn skin papillomas, Nature, 307:658.
Bishop, J.M., 1983, Cellular oncogenes and retroviruses, Ann. Rev.
     Biochem., 52:301.
Bos, J.L., Verlaan-de Vries, M., Jansen, A.M., Veeneman, G.H., van
     Boom, J.H., and van der Eb, A.J., 1984, Three different mutations
     in codon 61 of the human N-ras gene detected by synthetic
     oligonucleotide hybridization, Nucl. Acids Res., 12:9155.
Boutwell, R.K., 1974, The function and mechanism of promoters of
     carcinogeness, CRC Crit. Rev. Toxicol. 2:419.
Brown, R., Marshall, C.J., Pennie, S.G. and Hall, A., 1984, Mechanism
     of activation of an N-ras gene in the human fibrosarcoma cell
     line HT1080, EMBO J., 3:1321.
Cairns, J., 1975, Mutation selection and the natural history of
     cancer, Nature, 255:197
Capon, D.J., Seeburg, P.H., McGrath, J.P., Hayflick, J.S., Edman,U.,
     Levinson, A.D. and Goeddel, D.V., 1983, Activation of Ki-ras 2
     gene in human colon and lung carcinomas by two different point
     mutations, Nature, 304:507.
Chang, E.M., Furth, M.E., Scolnick, E.M., and Lowy, D.R., 1982,
     Tumorigenic transformation of mammalian cells induced by a normal
     human gene homologous to the oncogene of Harvey murine sarcoma
     virus, Nature 297:479
Cooper, C.S., Blair, D.G., Oskarsson, M.K., Tainsky, M.A., Eader, L.A.
     and Vande Woude, G.F., 1984a, Characterisation of human
     transforming genes from chemically transformed, teratocarcinoma
     and pancreatic carcinoma cell lines, Cancer Res., 44:1.
Cooper, C.S., Park, M., Blair, D.G., Tainsky, M.A., Huebner, K.,
     Croce, C.M., and Vande Woude, G.F., 1984b, Molecular cloning of a
     new transforming gene from a chemically transformed human cell
     line, Nature, 311:29.

Cooper, G.M., 1982, Cellular transforming genes, Science 218:801 Der,
    C.J., Krontiris, T.G. and Cooper, G.M., 1982, Transforming genes
    of human bladder and lung carcinoma cell lines are homologous to
    the ras genes of Harvey and Kirsten sarcoma viruses, Proc. Natl.
    Acad. Sci. USA, 79:3637.

Dhar, R., Ellis, R.W., Shih, T.Y., Oroszlan, S., Shapiro, B., Maizel,
    J., Lowy, D., and Scolnick, E., 1982, Nucleotide sequence of the
    p21 transforming protein of Harvey Murine Sarcoma Virus, Science,
    217:934.

Diamond, A., Cooper, G.M., Ritz, J. and Lane, M.A., 1983,
    Identification of molecular cloning of the human Blym
    transforming gene activated in Burkitt's lymphoma, Nature 305:
    112.

Dipple, A., Sawicki, J.T., Moschel, R.C. and Bigger, A.H., 1983, 7,
    12-Dimethylbenz(a)anthracene-DNA interactions in mouse embryo
    cell cultures and mouse skins, in: "Extrahepatic Drug Metabolism
    and Chemical Carcinogenesis". Rydstrom, J.,
    Montelins, J. and Bengtsson, eds., Elsevier Science Publishers
    B.V. Amsterdam.

Doerfler, W., 1983, DNA methylation and gene activity, Ann. Rev.
    Biochem. 52:93.

Ellis, R.W., DeFeo, D., Maryak, J.M., Young, H.A., Shih, T.Y., Chang,
    E.H., Lowy, D.R. and Scolnick, E.M., 1980, Dual evolutionary
    origin for the rat genetic sequences of Harvey Murine Sarcoma
    Virus, J. Virol., 36:408.

Eva, A. and Aaaronson, S.A., 1983, Frequent activation of c-kis as a
    transforming gene in fibrosarcomas induced by methylcholanthrene,
    Science, 220:955.

Eva, A., Tronick, S.R., Gol, R.A., Pierce, J.H. and Aaronson, S.A.,
    1983, Transforming genes of human hematopoietic tumours: frequent
    detection of ras-related oncogenes whose activation appears to be
    independent of tumour phenotype, Proc. Natl.Acad. Sci. USA,80:
    4926.

Fasano, O., Aldrich, T., Tamanoi, F., Taparowsky, E., Furth, M., and
    Wigler, M., 1984, Analysis of the transforming potential of the
    human H-ras gene by random mutagenesis, Proc. Natl.Acad. Sci.,
    USA, 81:4008.

Feig, L.A., Bast, R.C., Knapp, R.C. and Cooper, G.M., 1984, Somatic
    activation of ras  gene in a human ovarian carcinoma, Science
    223:698.

Feinberg, A.P. and Vogelstein, B., 1983a, Hypomethylation
    distinguishes genes from some human cancers from their normal
    counterparts, Nature 301:89.

Feinberg, A.P. and Vogelstein, B., 1983b, Hypomethylation of ras
    oncogenes in primary human cancers, Biochem. Biophys. Res.
    Commun. 111:47.

Felsenfeld, G. and McGhee, J., 1982, Methylation and gene control,
    Nature, 206:602.

Fujita, J., Yoshida, O., Yuasa, Y., Rhim, J.S., Hatanaka, M. and

Aaronson, S.A., 1984, Ha-ras oncogenes are activated by somatic
    alteration in human urinary tract tumours, Nature, 309:464.
Furth, M.E., Davis, L.J., Fleurdelys, B. and Scolnick, E.M., 1982,
    Monoclonal antibodies to the p21 products of the transforming
    gene of Harvey murine sarcoma virus and of the cellular ras gene
    family, J. Virol.,  43:294.
Gambke, C., Signer, E. and Moroni, C., 1984, Activation of N-ras gene
    in bone marrow cells from a patient with acute myeloblastic
    leukaemia, Nature, 307:476.
Goubin, G., Goldman, D.S., Luce, J., Neiman, P.E. and Cooper, G.M.
    1983, Molecular clo  g and nucleotide sequence of a transforming
    gene detected by transfection of chicken B-cell lymphoma DNA,
    Nature 302:114.
Guerrero, I., Calzada,   , Mayer, A. and Pellicer, A., 1984a, A
    molecular approach to leukemogenesis: mouse lymphomas contain an
    activated c-ras oncogene, Proc. Natl. Acad. Sci. USA, 81:202.
Guerrero, I., Villasante, A., Corces, V. and Pellicer, A., 1984b,
    Activation of a c-K-ras oncogene by somatic mutation in mouse
    lymphomas induced by gamma radiation, Science, 225:1159.
Hall, A., Marshall, C.J., Spurr, N.K. and Weiss, R.A., 1983, Identifi-
    cation of transforming gene in two human sarcoma cell lines as a
    new member of the ras gene family located on chromosome 1, Nature
    303:396.
Hecker, E., Fusenig, N.E., Kunz, W., Marks, F. and Theilmann, H.W.
    (eds.) 1982, "Carcinogenesis - a Comprehensive Survey" Vol 7,
    Raven Press, New York.
Kraus, M.H., Yuasa, Y. and Aaronson, S.A., 1984, A position 12-
    activated H-ras oncogene in all HS578T mammary carcinosarcoma
    cells but not normal mammary cells of the same patient, Proc.
    Natl. Acad. Sci. USA 81:5384.
Lane, M.A., Sainten, A. and Cooper, G.M., 1982, Stage-specific trans-
    forming genes of human and mouse B- and T-lymphocyte neoplasms,
    Cell 28:873
Lane, M.A., Sainten, A., Doherty, K.M. and Cooper, G.M., 1984,
    Isolation and characterisation of a stage-specific transforming
    gene, Tlym-I from T cell lymphomas, Proc. Natl. Acad.Sci. USA,
    81:2227.
Lapeyre, J.M. and Becker, F.F., 1979, 5-methylcytosine content of
    nuclear DNA during chemical hepatocarcinogenesis and in carcinoma
    which result, Biochim. Biophys. Res. Commun. 87:698.
Maniatis, T., Fritsch, E.F. and Sambrook, J., 1982, "Molecular Cloning
    (a laboratory manual)", Cold Spring Harbor Lab., New York.
Margison, G.P. and O'Connor, P.J., 1978, Nucleic acid modifications by
    N-nitroso compounds, in: "Chemical Carcinogens and DNA" Vol. 1,
    Grover, ed., CRC Press, Florida.
McCoy, M.S., Toole, J.J., Cunningham, J.M., Chang, E.H., Lowy, D.R.
    and Weinberg, R.A., 1983, Characterisation of a human colon/lung
    carcinoma oncogene, Nature 302:79.
Muller, R. and Verma, I.M., 1984, Expression of cellular oncogenes.
    Curr. Topics Microbiol. Immunol., 112:73.

Murray, M.J., Cunningham, J.M., Parada, L.F., Dautry, F., Lebowitz, P., and Weinberg, R.A., 1983, The HL-60 transforming sequence: A ras oncogene co-existing with altered myc genes in hematopoietic tumours, Cell 33:749.

Nakano, H., Yamamoto, F., Neville, C., Evans, D., Mizuno, T. and Perucho, M., 1984, Isolation of transforming sequences of two human lung carcinomas:  structural and functional analysis of the activated c-K-ras oncogenes, Proc. Natl. Acad. Sci. USA, 81:71

Notario, V., Sukumar, S., Santos, E., and Barbacid, M., 1984, A common mechanism for the malignant activation of ras oncogenes in human neoplasia and in chemically induced animal tumours, in: "Cancer Cells 2/ Oncogenes and Viral Genes," Vande Woude, G.F., Levine, A.J., Topp, W.C. and Watson, J.D., eds., Cold Spring Harbor Lab., New York.

Parada, L.F., Tabin, C.J., Shih, C. and Weinberg, R.A., 1982, Human EJ bladder carcinoma oncogene is homologue of Harvey sarcoma virus ras gene, Nature, 297:474.

Parada, L.F. and Weinberg, R.A., 1983, Presence of a Kirsten murine sarcoma virus ras oncogene in cells transformed by 3-methyl-cholanthrene, Mol. Cell. Biol. 3:2298.

Peto, R., 1977, Epidemiology, multistage models and short term mutagenicity tests, in: "Origins of Human Cancer", Hiatt et al eds., Cold Spring Harbor Lab., New York.

Pulciani, S., Santos, E., Lauver, A.V., Long, L.K., Aaronson, S.A. and Barbacid, M., 1982, Oncogenes in solid human tumours, Nature, 300:539.

Ramsden, M., Cole, G., Smith, J. and Balmain, A., 1985, Differential methylation of the c-H-ras gene in normal mouse cells and during skin tumour progression, EMBO J., (in press).

Rasheed, S., Norman, G.L. and Heidecker, G., 1983, Nucleotide sequence of the Rasheed rat sarcoma virus oncogene:  new mutations, Science, 221:155.

Razin, A. and Riggs, A.D., 1980, DNA methylation and gene function, Science, 210:604.

Reddy, E.P., Reynolds, R.K., Santos, E. and Barbacid, M., 1982, A point mutation is responsible for the acquisition of transforming properties by the T24 human bladder carcinoma oncogene. Nature, 300:149.

Reddy, E.P., Lipman, D., Andersen, P.R., Tronick, S.R. and Aaronson S.A., 1985, Nucleotide sequence analysis of the BALB/c murine sarcoma virus transforming gene, J. Virol. 53: 984.

Riggs, A.D. and Jones, P.A., 1983, 5-methylcytosine, gene regulation and cancer, Adv. Cancer Res., 40:1

Santos, E., Tronick, S.R., Aaronson, S.A., Pulciani, S., and Barbacid, M., 1982, T24 human bladder carcinoma oncogene is an activated form of the normal human homologue of BALB- and Harvey-MSV transforming genes, Nature, 298:343.

Santos, E., Reddy, E.P., Pulciani, S., Feldmann, R.J. and Barbacid, M., 1983, Spontaneous activation of a human proto-oncogene, Proc. Natl. Acad. Sci. USA, 80:4679.

Santos, E., Martin-Zanca, D., Reddy, E.P., Pierotti, M.A., DellaPosta, G. and Barbacid, M., 1984, Malignant activation of a K-ras oncogene in lung carcinoma but not in normal tissue of the same patient, Science, 223:661.

Schechter, A.L., Stern, D.F., Vaidyanathan, L., Decker, S.J., Drebin, J.A., Greene, M.I. and Weinbert, R.A., 1984, The neu oncogene: an erb-B-related gene encoding a 185,000-Mr tumour antigen, Nature, 312:513.

Seeburg, P.H., Colby, W.W., Capon, D.J., Goeddel, D.V. and Levinson, A.D., 1984, Biological properties of human c-Ha-ras 1 genes mutated at codon 12, Nature, 312:71.

Sekiya, T., Fushimi, M., Hori, H., Hirohashi, S., Nishimura, S. and Sugimura, T., 1984, Molecular cloning and the total nucleotide sequence of the human c-Ha-ras-1 gene activated in a melanoma from a Japanese patient, Proc. Natl. Acad. Sci. USA, 81:4771.

Shimizu, K., Birnbaum, D., Ruley, M.A., Fasano, O., Suard, Y., Edlund, L., Taparowsky, E., Goldfarb, M. and Wigler, M., 1983a, Structure of the Ki-ras gene of the human lung carcinoma cell line Calu-1, Nature, 304:497.

Shimizu, K., Goldfarb, M., Perucho, M. and Wigler, M., 1983b, Isolation and preliminary characterisation of the transforming gene of a human neuroblastoma cell line. Proc. Natl. Acad.Sci. USA, 80:383.

Shimizu, K., Goldfarb, M., Suard, Y., Perucho, M., Li, Y., Kamata, T., Feramisco, J., Stavnezer, E., Fogh, J. and Wigler, M.H., 1983c, Three human transforming genes are related to the viral ras oncogenes, Proc. Natl. Acad. Sci. USA, 80:2112.

Singer, B. and Kusmierek, J.T., 1982, Chemical mutagenesis, Ann. Rev. Biochem. 51:655.

Souyri, M. and Fleissner, E., 1983, Identification by transfection of transforming sequences in DNA of human T-cell leukaemia, Proc. Natl. Acad. Sci. USA 80:6676.

Sukumar, S., Notario, V., Martin-Zanca, D. and Barbacid, M., 1983, Induction of mammary carcinomas in rats by nitroso-methylurea involves malignant activation of H-ras-1 locus by single point mutations, Nature, 306:658.

Sukumar, S., Pulciani, S., Doniger, J., DiPaolo, J.A., Evans, C.H., Zbar, B. and Barbacid, M., 1984, A transforming ras gene in tumorigenic Guinea Pig cell lines initiated by diverse chemical carcinogens, Science, 223:1197.

Tabin, C.J., Bradley, S.M., Bargmann, C.I., Weinberg, R.A., Papageorge, A.G., Scolnick, E.M., Dhar, R., Lowy, D.R., and Chang, E.H., 1982, Mechanism of activation of a human oncogene Nature, 300:143.

Tainsky, M.A., Cooper, C.S., Giovanella, B.C. and Vande Woude, G.F. 1984, An activated ras gene: detected in late but not early passage human PA1 teratocarcinoma cells, Science 225:643.

Taparowsky, E., Suard, Y., Fasano, O., Shimizu, K., Goldfarb, M. and Wigler, M., 1982, Activation of the T24 bladder carcinoma transforming gene is linked to a single amino acid change, Nature, 300:762.

Taparowsky, E., Shimizu, K., Goldfarb, M. and Wigler, M., 1983,
    Structure and activation of the human N-ras gene, Cell 34:581.
Taya, Y., Hosogai, K., Hirohashi, S., Shimosato, Y., Tsuchiya, R.
    Tsuchida, N., Fushimi, M., Sekiya, T. and Nishimura, S., 1984, A
    novel combination of K-ras and myc amplification accompanied by
    point mutational activation of K-ras in a human lung cancer,
    EMBO J., 3:2943.
Tsuchida, N., Ryder, T., and Ohtsubo, E., 1982, Nucleotide sequence of
    the oncogene encoding the p21 transforming protein of Kirsten
    Murine Sarcoma Virus, Science, 217:937.
Vedel, M., Gomez-Carcia, M., Sala, M. and Sala-Trepat, J.M., 1983,
    Changes in methylation pattern of albumin and  -fetoprotein genes
    in developing rat liver neoplasia, Nucleic Acids Res., 11:4335.
Vousden, K.H. and Marshall, C.J., 1984, Three different activated ras
    genes in mouse tumours; evidence for oncogene activation during
    progression of a mouse lymphoma, EMBO J., 3:913.
Yamamoto, F. and Perucho, M., 1984, Activation of a human c-K-ras
    oncogene, Nucl. Acids Res., 12:8873.
Yuasa, Y., Srivastava, S.K., Dunn, C.Y., Rhim, J.S., Reddy, E.P., and
    Aaronson, S.A., 1983, Acquisition of transforming properties by
    alternative point mutations within c-bas/has human proto-
    oncogene, Nature, 303:775.
Yuasa, Y., Gol, R.A., Chang, A., Chiu, I.M., Reddy, E.P., Tronick,
    S.R. and Aaronson, S.A., 1984, Mechanism of activation of an
    N-ras oncogene of SW-1271 human lung carcinoma cells, Proc. Natl.
    Acad. Sci. USA 81:3670.
Yunis, J.J., 1983, The chromosomal basis of human neoplasia, Science,
    221:227.
Zarbl, H., Sukumar, S., Arthur, A.V., Martin-Zanca, D. and Barbacid,
    M., 1985, Kirect mutagenesis of Ha-ras-1 oncogenes by N-nitroso
    -N-methylurea during initiation of mammary carcinogenesis in
    rats, Nature, 315:382.

# THE INTERACTIONS OF HERPES SIMPLEX VIRUS WITH DIFFERENTIATED CELLS

N.J. Maitland

Department of Pathology
University of Bristol
The Medical School
University Walk, Bristol BS8 1TD

Herpes simplex virus is a large, DNA tumour virus whose most common clinical symptoms are the "cold sores" in both facial and genital sites. The biochemical and physical properties of HSV have been extensively reviewed elsewhere (1,2) and this review will concentrate on the genetic properties of the virus and how virus gene expression might be related to the interactions of HSV with different host cells during its three distinct types of reaction with these hosts viz.

(i)   Productive infection
(ii)  Latent infection
(iii) Non-permissive infection

Gene expression during each of the three life cycles will be briefly reviewed but before this is possible it will be essential to describe the genome structure of HSV (reviewed in 3).

## HERPES SIMPLEX VIRUS GENOME STRUCTURE

Genetic analysis of HSV has proved both a complex and frustrating exercise, firstly because of the sheer size of the viral DNA (150 kilobases) and the recognition as long ago as 1976 that even a plaque purified stock of HSV exhibited considerable heterogeneity.

First indications of the genetic complexity came from the classical genetic studies of recombination frequencies between different plaque morphology markers and unknown temperature sensitive mutants. Predicted recombination frequencies were often wildly inaccurate and indicative of a non linear arrangement of the viral genes.

Secondly, the DNA reassociation studies of Sheldrick and Berthelot (4) showed that, if denatured HSV was allowed to reanneal and was inspected under the electron microscope, dumbell shaped molecules were seen. As shown in figure 1 these dumbells revealed the presence of inverted repetitions at the ends and in the centre of the genome. Sheldrick and Berthelot speculated that the terminal repetitions would allow the formation of 4 possible isomers, each with identical termini.

This speculation was rapidly confirmed by the initial restriction endonuclease cleavage analyses of HSV DNA (5,6). Results of these studies suggested that each population of HSV DNA consisted of equimolar proportions of each of the isomers, since DNA fragments present in submolar yield were detected after electrophoretic separation of the fragment mixtures as shown in figure 2. Recent studies have suggested that the 4 isomers may not be present in exactly equimolar proportions, but nevertheless it is generally true that "molar" fragments derive from the long and the short unique regions of the HSV genome while "half molar" fragments derive from the ends of the molecule and "quarter molar" fragments from the 'joint' between the long and short segments.

The effects of the presence of 4 isomers in a genetic recombination experiment are briefly summarized in figure 3 i.e. recombination frequencies between markers within each unique region will follow the normal pattern whereas recombination between markers in the different unique regions will be the average of the two possibilities. A further consequence of the presence of the inverted repeats which flank the unique regions is the partially diploid nature of the HSV genome.


PRODUCTIVE INFECTION BY HSV

Herpes simplex virus has a remarkably large host cell range, with respect to productive or lytic infection. Indeed, a major problem in studies of viral latency and transformation has been the prevention of viral replication. The productive cycle is complex and is subject to a number of subtle controls of gene expression. Reviews of the details of messenger RNAs and proteins synthesised have been published elsewhere (7), but for the purposes of this discussion I shall confine myself to what is known about switching between the 3 phases of the infectious cycle. The three phases of the productive cycle are as follows.

**a. Reassociation of Single Stranded HSV DNA**

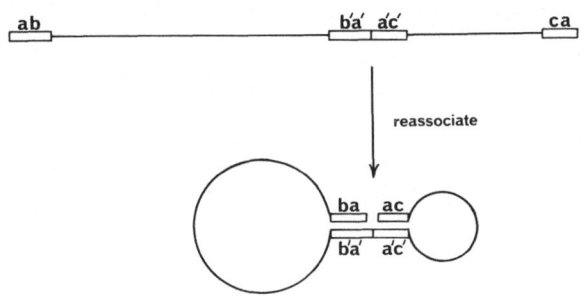

**b.  HSV  Genome  Structure**

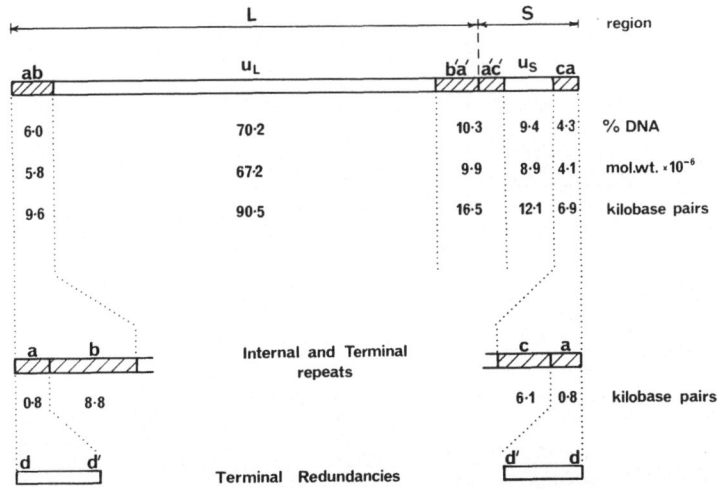

Fig. 1   Structure of the Herpes Simplex Virus Genome.
         (a) Illustrates the formation of "dumbell" structures on
         reannealing of single stranded HSV DNA.

(i)  Immediate Early (IE) phase, which has been defined as containing those viral genes which require no prior protein synthesis after viral

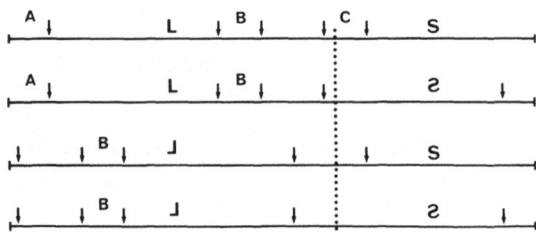

**a. Normal DNA population**

3 FRAGMENTS A, B, C, present in equimolar yields

i.e $\dfrac{\text{yield A}}{\text{mol.wt. A}} = \dfrac{\text{yield B}}{\text{mol.wt. B}}$

**b. HSV DNA population**

3 FRAGMENTS A, B, C.

A located at end of molecule – present in 50% of molecules

B located in centre of molecule (in unique region) – present in 100% of molecules

C located across "joint" region – present in 25% of molecules

i.e $\dfrac{\text{yield A}}{\text{mol.wt. A}} : \dfrac{\text{yield B}}{\text{mol.wt. B}} : \dfrac{\text{yield C}}{\text{mol.wt. C}} = 2 : 4 : 1$

Figure 2.  Consequences of restriction endonuclease cleavage of normal DNA (a) and HSV DNA (b) populations.

infection i.e. genes expressed in cells which had been treated with cycloheximide before infection.  There are relatively few of these functions on the HSV genome (8) and they tend to be clustered in the

Linkage experiment between markers A,B,C, on HSV genome (all values refer to map units)

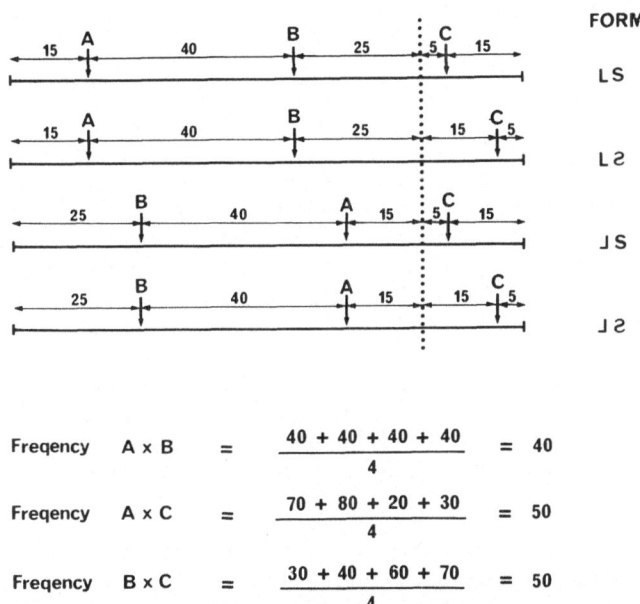

$$\text{Freqency} \quad A \times B \quad = \quad \frac{40 + 40 + 40 + 40}{4} \quad = \quad 40$$

$$\text{Freqency} \quad A \times C \quad = \quad \frac{70 + 80 + 20 + 30}{4} \quad = \quad 50$$

$$\text{Freqency} \quad B \times C \quad = \quad \frac{30 + 40 + 60 + 70}{4} \quad = \quad 50$$

Figure  3. Genetic consequences of the 4 HSV isomers in a recombination experiment.

repeat regions.   The IE functions must play a central role in the initiation of the infectious cycle and are the first step in the viral strategy of turning the cell into a virus 'factory'.   IE gene products are non-structural as far as virus architecture is concerned, and their enzymatic functions, if any, are still unknown.  At least two IE functions are present in 2 copies (8,9) but if both copies are non-functional the effect would be to produce a non-viable virus.  This serves to emphasise the important control functions of the IE genes.

(ii) Delayed Early (DE) genes are defined as genes expressed in the absence of viral DNA replication i.e. genes expressed in cells treated with inhibitors of DNA replication, such as cytosine arabinoside. These genes are more numerous than the IE genes and have been mapped (7) throughout the small and large unique regions of the viral genome. Many of their functions are now known and include several enzymes of

DNA synthesis, whose properties are quite different from their cellular analogues. Expression of the delayed early genes is critically dependent on prior synthesis of IE gene products.

(iii) Late genes are defined as all functions which are expressed after the onset of viral DNA replication. These genes normally encode viral structural proteins, from the capsid and viral envelope.

STRUCTURE AND EXPRESSION OF HERPES SIMPLEX VIRUS GENES

Increasing sequence data from the HSV genome have confirmed many of the original results of HSV gene structure which suggested that the genome of 150 kilobase pairs (kbp) encoded more than 50 polypeptides (7,10). Most of the HSV genes are unspliced, excepting two immediate early genes with common 5' termini which are transcribed from the short repetitive regions into the short unique region. Differential splicing of these two mRNA's (IE RNA's 1 and 12) ensures the production of two unique proteins (i.e. IE 68K and IE 12K) since the 5' RNA termini are not translated (11). All other HSV genes sequenced to date are unspliced. Transcription takes place from both strands of the HSV DNA and most genes mapped to date are non-overlapping apart from the IE 12K protein and a 33K late protein encoded in the short unique region (7,11).

Sequence data also indicates that the normal consensus sequences for transcription are utilised in HSV1 (11, 12) but, probably due to the extremely high G + C content of HSV, there is distinct codon usage bias towards G and C in the "wobble" 3rd base position of the codons (12).

Putative cis acting control sequences have also been identified and their functions tested using transient expression sequences (13). For example, a transcriptional enhancer sequence has been identified, in close proximity to the 5' end of the IE 175K protein (14). The latter gene appears to be of critical importance for the control of the complex cascade of HSV gene expression. Genetic evidence has indicated that mutations in the IE175K protein prevent expression of all other HSV genes (15). The features of IE control identified to date are threefold (16):

(i) The presence of the 5' transcriptional enhancer sequence,
(ii) A repetitive "alpha control" sequence located at 175 nucleotides 5' to the start of the protein coding sequence and
(iii) A binding site for a virion protein (Vmw64/65) within the alpha control regions of IE175K. It has been shown that merely transfecting HSV1IE175K genes (which have been cloned into a bacterial plasmid) into susceptible cells does not in itself lead to a gross increase in other IE gene products. However, when these transfected cells are co-infected with HSV2 the level of HSV1 IE gene product synthesis was

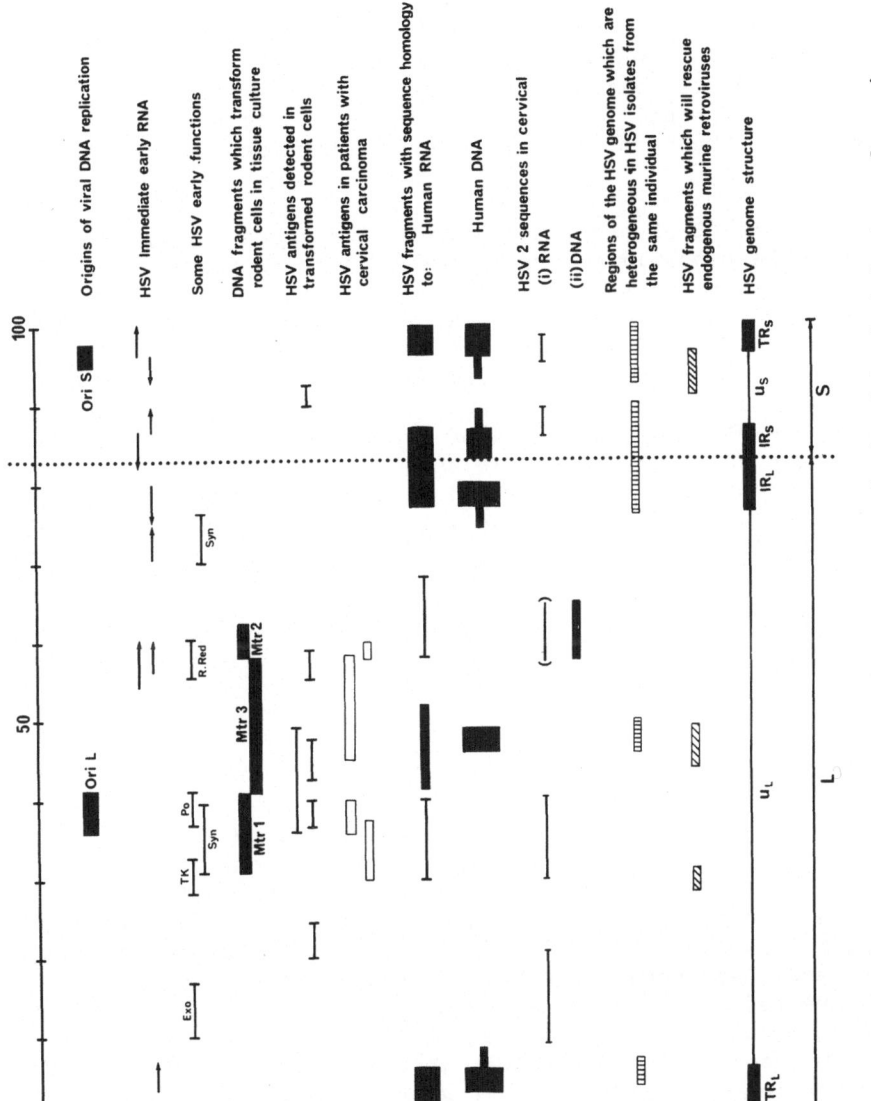

Fig. 4  Herpes simplex virus gene products detected in transformed
and tumour cells.
Data compiled from the references cited in the text.

greatly stimulated (S. Faber and K. Wilcox, personal communication). Thus, there must be a combination of the cis and transacting control features which ensures both preferential expression of HSV IE genes in the infected cell and fine control of gene expression if required.  In addition, further levels of control of gene expression have been proposed, including stability of mRNA and mRNA transport from nucleus to cytoplasm (3).  Since the latter controls were suggested by experiments involving recombinant virus, rather than transient expression of isolated viral genes cloned in bacterial plasmids, these controls may be of equal importance in vivo to that effected by transcriptional enhancers (S. Silver and B. Roizman, personal communication).

Further control of the expression of HSV genes during the infectious cycle probably occurs by the binding of transacting IE products to (initially) DE control sites and later to L control sites, which have been tentatively identified up to 900 bp 5' to the start of DE and L genes.  The presence of an active HSV origin of replication with viral DNA synthesis is not sufficient to activate late genes, IE and DE products are an absolute requirement (17, 18).  However, IE 175 is also capable of transactivation of genes from different viruses (19).  In these cases no nucleotide sequence homology was observed in the cis located control sequences and it has been suggested that the regulatory effects of IE175 operate via a secondary interaction with a cellular gene (12, 19).

LATENT INFECTION WITH HERPES SIMPLEX VIRUS

Considerable clinical and experimental evidence exists to demonstrate the ability of HSV to persist as a latent or inapparent infection (20, 21).  It is without the scope of this article to discuss this in detail but the reader is referred to several recent reviews on the subject (22, 23).  The study of HSV latency at the molecular level has proved extremely difficult since:
(i) there are few, if any, reliable in vitro latency systems which employ the correct differentiated cells (24),
(ii) latency itself implies a silent infection and detection of very few virus particles or genes in a large cell mass is an almost impossible task,
(iii) in the detection of latent infection, the most common experimental assay is for virus reactivation.
It is clearly very difficult to decide whether a particular virus is incapable of entering, maintaining or reactivating from the latent state.

It has been demonstrated, however, by cell culture and electron microscopy that the most common site of latency lies in sensory ganglia (25), probably within the neurones.  Evidence of virus has also been detected in the central nervous system of animals and man (26) and other sites of virus persistence have been noted (reviewed in 23) although the neurons are now generally accepted as the principal site of true latency, as opposed to persistence of a low grade productive infection e.g. in guinea pig skin or mouse footpad (27).

The influence of viral gene expression on experimental HSV latency in the mouse has been investigated, principally using conditional lethal HSV mutants (27).  While there is an incipient fault with experiments in vivo using temperature sensitive virus mutants in that the temperature of the experimental animal is extremely variable these experiments indicated that certain viral genes are absolutely required to induce latency (within the limits of the reactivation assay for latency induction).  For example synthesis of active IE175K protein is an absolute requirement, particularly since this gene product has been detected in latently infected cells (28).  Given the central role of IE175K in the induction of the productive infectious cycle, this is not surprising. The presence of IE175K in the latently infected tissues however does suggest either that this protein is not the only trigger for productive infection or that absolute levels of IE 175K in latency are not sufficiently high to induce a productive infection.

The status of other HSV genes with respect to latency is more controversial.  A number of workers have reported that an active viral TK is required to induce latency (29), while others have shown that TK-virus is quite capable of inducing latency (30).  This controversy remains to be resolved but possible causes of the discrepancy include:

(i)   leaky TK-mutants e.g. point mutations which revert to TK+,
(ii)  the presence of an active portion of the TK gene (31), and
(iii) the influence of the reactivation system on the final result.

Since TK-HSV grows poorly in non-dividing cells (32) it is likely to reactivate better in growing cells.  Again the weakness of the experiments lies in using reactivation as an assay for induction of latency.  Recently mutations within the HSV genome which greatly increase and decrease viral neurovirulence have been mapped (33,34). These results also imply a positive role for viral genes in the interaction of HSV with neurons.  The ability of these mutant viruses to induce and maintain latency has not yet been reported but they should provide useful tools for future study of the influence of viral gene expression on the latent state.

To overcome these experimental difficulties the use of molecular and in situ hybridization to detect the presence and expression of HSV genes during latency has recently been exploited.  In situ hybrid-

isation of HSV DNA to frozen sections of human tissue identified
transcription of a number of regions of the HSV genome in latently
infected neuronal tissue (35).  In addition HSV genetic information
was detected in the central nervous system (CNS) of humans and in the
brain stems of mice in an experimental latency system (36,37).  It has
also been demonstrated (38) that the terminal fragments of virus
isolated after several cycles of latency/reactivation in vivo show
changes in molecular weight as detected by restriction endonuclease
cleavage.  The most striking feature of the latter results was the
relative absence of fragments from the termini of HSV when the brain
stem DNA was digested by restriction endonucleases (37).  This
suggests that in brain stem the virus genomes (which are present in
high copy numbers of greater than 100 molecules per cell), exist as
endless concatamers, circles or perhaps even integrated in tandem into
the host cell chromosomes.  Much work remains to be done in this
intriguing system.

What mechanism could be proposed for the induction maintenance
and reactivation of latent HSV in neurons, bearing in mind that all
three states occur within the same cell?  Under the non-permissive
conditions the virus genome assumes the "endless" state as outlined
above.  Latency is therefore established.  Whether the contribution of
the neuron is active (synthesis of a repressor protein, for example),
or passive (lack of cellular replicative functions in the non-dividing
neuron) remains to be determined.

The physical stimuli for reactivation of latent HSV have been
well documented (23) and include physical trauma and exposure to
sunlight.  Immunological deficiency may not be a critical factor in
primary reactivation and is perhaps of more importance in limiting the
spread and severity of recrudescent HSV in humans.  A fuller
assessment of the importance of immune mechanisms in HSV latency is
reviewed in (22).  It has recently been shown that HSV infection
induces the synthesis of heat shock or stress proteins in the infected
cells (39).  Could it be that this primitive reaction to stress is the
trigger for virus reactivation from latency?  These stress proteins
are absent from resting cells such as neurons and have wide ranging
effects on cellular transcription after their stimulation by heat
shock.

Thus the molecular nature of the interactions between HSV and a
single differentiated cell, the neuron, during in vivo and
experimental latency are poorly understood.  Perhaps with improvements
in the culture of neuronal tissues and development of micro-cloning
techniques more information will be forthcoming on this important
clinical problem.  Since currently available vaccination and
chemotherapy regimes can limit the severity and spread of primary and
recurrent disease, understanding of viral latency leading to its
prevention is the best available route to the elimination of HSV from
the general population.

NON PERMISSIVE INTERACTIONS

## 1.    Cell Transformation In Vitro By HSV

Transformation of mainly rodent fibroblasts in culture by HSV has been demonstrated many times since the pioneering experiments of Duff and Rapp (40). However, when compared to in vitro transformation by other DNA tumour viruses such as adenoviruses and polyomaviruses there are several important differences.

For in vitro transformation to occur it is necessary to have a non-permissive system, in which no viral replication occurs. While it is possible to achieve this by choosing appropriate cell types for the smaller DNA tumour viruses, this is not possible with HSV which will replicate to some extent in almost every cell type. To achieve non-permissivity it is therefore necessary to use virus which has been treated with chemicals or radiation (41) or maintenance of cells infected with wild type or temperature sensitive mutant viruses at elevated temperatures (42,43). In addition, introduction of fragmented viral DNA into cells has also proved most effective (44,45) and by using particular cloned DNA fragments the "transformation regions" of HSV have been identified (46) (figure 4). Unlike SV40 and human adenoviruses, however, no single transforming region has been identified on HSV1 (Mtr1) and HSV2 (Mtr 2 and 3) whereas all other gene assignments have up till now proved to be colinear (7,12) for these two closely related viruses. In HSV2 the two separate regions have been identified by different transformation assay systems and it has been suggested that one region is responsible for induction of anchorage independence (46), which enables transformants to grow in semi-solid support medium, while the other region carries an immortalizing function (47), which confers unlimited growth potential on the transformed cells. For the HSV1 transforming region, both anchorage independence and morphological changes were observed in the transformed cells (46). However, in all cases the transformed cells were tumorigenic when injected into appropriate host animals.

By comparison with the smaller DNA tumour viruses, e.g. SV40, the efficiency of transformation by HSV is considerably lower, using the same host cells and the morphology of the HSV transformed cells more resembles that of spontaneous transformants than that of "true" viral transformants (48). In addition it has recently been shown that the minimal HSV2 DNA fragment required for trans- formation, although it includes a protein coding region has no start of 5' signal sequence present (46). Therefore to express HSV functions the transforming DNA would have to insert into the host DNA after a cellular start codon and in perfect phase for reading the genetic code.

## 2.    Maintenance of the Transformed State

Faced with the conflicting evidence for the involvement of HSV

gene expression in establishment of the transformed state, it is
perhaps not surprising that the experiments designed to detect the
presence and expression of HSV genes within transformed cells have
also produced results which are difficult to reconcile in terms of an
HSV "tumour" antigen.

The experimental results summarised in figure 4 indicate that
many independent researchers, using independently derived antisera
have detected evidence of HSV antigens in HSV transformed cells.
However there appears to be no consensus about the antigens present
and they are often present in abnormal cellular locations, i.e. not at
the same position as intracellular site as in productive infections.
Some of the cell lines showed cell cycle specific expression of HSV
antigens (49) and it remains possible that these viral antigens are
either cellular antigens which are induced after HSV infection or
cellular antigen present only in specific differentiated cells which
cross-react with an antibody against an HSV antigen.  The strongest
candidates for the HSV tumour antigen are the VP143 (DNA binding
protein) (50), and the 38,000mol wt protein (51) encoded by the HSV2
"transforming" region, however.

Detection of viral nucleic acid sequences in transformed cells
has also proved difficult, particularly in cells transformed by
treatment with HSV DNA fragments (52).  In cells transformed by u.v.
inactivated virus however, particularly the 333-8-9 lines and sublines
(53) some clues to the role of HSV in cellular transformation may be
found.  Several investigators were able to demonstrate the presence of
HSV DNA sequences in early passage (post-transformation) 333-8-9 cells
(54,55), but after extensive passage progressively less HSV DNA was
detectable, while the cells themselves became cytogenetically unstable
and, if anything more tumourgenic.

An interesting but indirect demonstration of the presence of HSV
sequences has also been possible by using HSV transformed rat cells to
complement HSV temperature sensitive mutants to permit growth at non-
permissive temperatures (56).  However, similar experiments with
polyoma virus host mutants (57) have shown that viral mutations, even
in tumour antigens, can be complemented by functions present in
specific differentiated cell types, previously not exposed to virus.

When cells transformed by fragments of HSV2 DNA were tested for
the presence and expression of HSV genes no single HSV2 tumour antigen
was detected (46) while only transient expression of HSV1 glycoprotein
gB was expressed in cells transformed by an HSV1 DNA fragment encoding
the gene for gB (58,59).

Therefore at present it is not yet certain whether an HSV tumour
antigen exists, although present and consistent failure to isolate
such a tumour antigen argues against its existence.

## 3.    Herpes Simplex Virus Mutagenesis

As a result of the anomalous behaviour of HSV in comparison to the other DNA tumour viruses zur Hausen (60) and others have proposed that HSV transformation is not mediated by a tumour antigen but occurs by a mutagenic or "hit and run" mechanism.  A growing amount of evidence exists for the mutagenic potential of inactivated HSV (61), the virus appears, in several assays, to be at least as mutagenic as a number of known chemical carcinogens (62).  Unfortunately the molecular basis of this mutagenesis is uncertain i.e. the HSV genes responsible and the effect on the host cell genes are unknown. However the capacity of HSV to induce chromosome breaks has been known for many years (63) and a fuller understanding of HSV induced mutagenesis will be of critical importance.  Our own results (N. Maitland and C. Lynas, unpublished) indicate that in one particular assay viz. mutagenesis of hypoxanthin-guanine phosphoribosyl transferase (HGPRT), independently derived mutant cell clones all possess different lesions in the HGPRT gene.  In addition permanent HGPRT-cell lines have proved difficult to isolate, although small colonies of HGPRT-cells are readily obtained.  Since transfection of HSV DNA into these cells produces multiple chromosomal breaks we presently attribute the low frequency of stable cell line isolation to random mutagenesis by HSV of many cell genes, in addition to the HGPRT gene.  We have further investigated the effects of HSV infection on the expression of HGPRT gene as mRNA (figure 5).  While RNA accumulation experiments using the indicated metabolic inhibitors to block HSV replication indicated that the primary effect of HSV infection was to repress HGPRT transcription, measurements of steady state levels of HGPRT mRNA through a time course of infection with no drugs present indicated no decrease in transcription of the gene (data not shown).  Therefore the primary effect is probably on transport, half-life or translation of cell genes in HSV infected cells.  This result suggests that the HGPRT gene remains transcriptionally active and therefore more available to mutagenic agents than silent genes in condensed chromatin (Maitland et al., manuscript in preparation).

## 4.    Herpes Simplex Virus and Human Cancer

Considerable sero-epidemiological evidence has accumulated over the last 15 years to implicate HSV2 as an aetiological agent in human carcinoma of the cervix (54,65).  However, as shown in figure 4 no consensus about HSV antigens present both in the serum of cancer patients and in the cancer cells themselves has been reached (64).  Similarly attempts to detect HSV nucleic acid sequences in carcinoma tissue biopsies have proved largely unsuccessful (65) until the advent of cloned fragments of HSV for use as radioactive hybridization probes.  By in situ hybridisation increased binding of HSV2 DNA probes, compared to controls was observed on carcinoma cells (66,67), when probed for viral RNA.  However, most of this hybridization was probably due to homology between the cellular RNA and HSV DNA

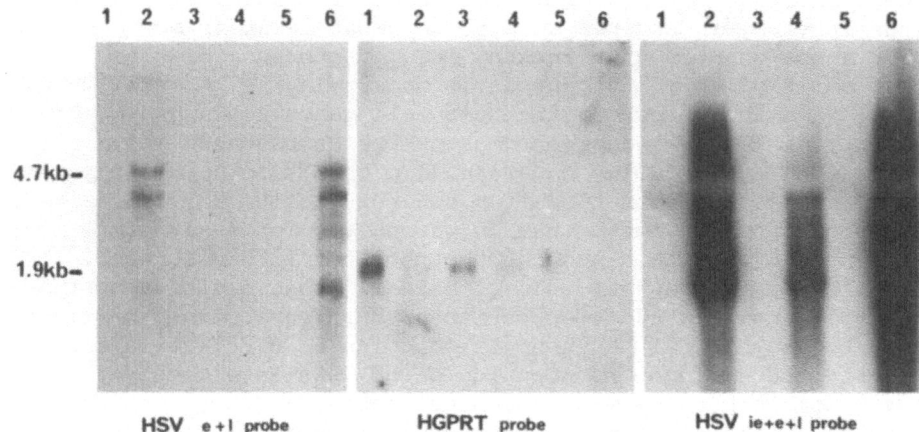

Fig. 5   The effect of HSV infection on HGPRT gene expression in
         human tissue culture cells.

         Total cell RNA was extracted from human cells grown in media
         supplemented as shown.   Addition of cycloheximide ensures
         production of IE RNA only.   Cytosine arabinoside allows
         production of DE RNA only over a six hour accumulation period.
         The effectiveness of the inhibitors was assayed by their effects
         on viral DNA synthesis, i.e. no HSV1 DNA was synthesised in the
         presence of either inhibitor.   Ten micrograms of total cell RNA
         was separated on a formaldehyde/agarose gel, transferred to
         "genescreen" membrane and hybridized with a radioactive cDNA
         probe for the murine HGPRT gene (kindly supplied by Dr T. Caskey,
         University of Houston, Texas, USA) and various cloned DNA
         fragments from the HSV1 genome, as described in Maitland and
         Lynas (manuscript in preparation).   The resulting autoradiograph
         was exposed for 72 hours.

                                                          (continued)

Probe type used is given below each autoradiograph.  All probes
were of the same specific activity.  Tracks 1,3,5 were mock-
infected cells while tracks 2,4,6 were infected with 10-50 plaque
forming units/cell of HSV1.  Tracks 1,2 contained RNA extracted
from cells treated with 50 micrograms/ml of cytosine arabinoside
at 30 minutes post infection to allow only synthesis of immediate
and delayed early RNA's.  Tracks 3,4 contained RNA extracted from
cells treated with 50 micrograms/ml of cycloheximide at 1 hour
pre-infection and cytosine arabinoside at 30 minutes post
infection to allow only synthesis of immediate early RNA's.
Tracks 5,6 contained RNA from untreated cells maintained (as were
all the other cultures) for 6-8 hours at 37oC after infection.
HSV DNA and gross cytopathic effects were detected in the cells
from track 6 indicating the presence of late viral gene products.
The progress of the viral infection may be followed by observing
the e+1 probe hybridization to tracks 2,4 and 6.  Track 2 (IE+DE)
contains 2 major RNA's, while track 4 (IE only) contains no
hybridizing RNA and track 6 (mainly DE+L) contains the same 2
major species as track 2 but several additions.  The apparent
effect of HSV infection on HGPRT mRNA levels is to deplete the
levels per cell as the synthesis of HSV mRNA increases.

(Maitland et al., manuscript submitted).  This cellular RNA which
cross hybridizes with HSV2 DNA is largely non-polyadenylated, of high
G + C content and partially repetitive, including ribosomal genes.
However by hybrid selection of mRNA from human placenta using a cloned
HSV2 DNA fragment and subsequent in vitro translation of the selected
mRNA in a rabbit reticulocyte lysate system (figure 6) it is apparent
that at least one cell messenger RNA will hybridize to HSV2 DNA from
the short terminal repeat region.  In addition DNA sequence homology
has been reported between the 5' untranslated sequence of a cellular
oncogene (Ha-ras) and a similar sequence from HSV1 (A. Puga et al.,

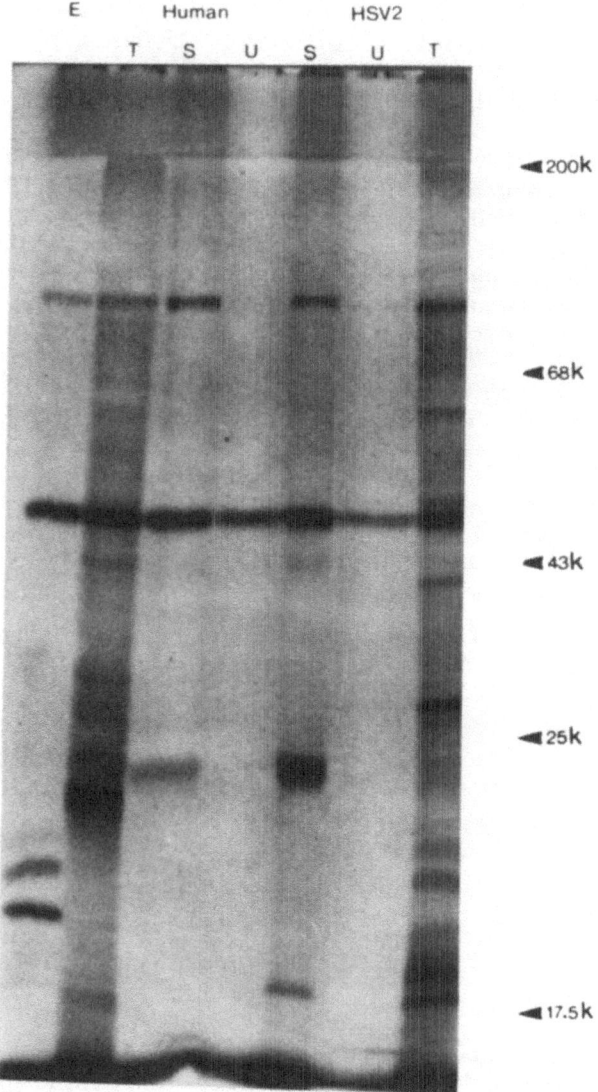

Figure 6.  In vitro translation of human mRNA selected by
     hybridization to a joint region fragment from HSV2 DNA.

     Ten micrograms of poly A+ RNA from human tissue culture cells,
     either infected or mock-infected with HSV2 virus was hybridized
                                                         (continued)

under standard conditions (2xSSC, 45% formamide at 50° C for 16
hours) to a cloned fragment of HSV2 DNA from the "joint" region
of the molecule, which had been immobilized on nitrocellulose
filters.  The filters were then washed for 4 hours in 2xSSC, 45%
formamide at 45 C and 1 hour at 64 C in 1xSSC before the RNA was
eluted by incubation of the filter at 80 C in double distilled
water.  The eluted RNA was then translated in vitro using a
rabbit reticulocyte lysate, purchased from Amersham, and used
according to the maker's instructions, with a supplement of 35S
methionine.  The resultant proteins were separated by
electrophoresis in a 10% SDS-polyacrylamide gel, fluorographed
and exposed for 5 days to Kodak XAR-5 X-ray film.
In addition to the expected HSV2 specific products at 18K and 43K
a protein of molecular weight 23K was observed in the hybrid
-selected tracks (designated S) for both uninfected (human) and
infected (HSV2) polyA+ RNA.  Control tracks of total, unselected
polyA+ RNA (designated T), the endogenous reaction with no RNA
added to the lysate (designated E) and the reaction with polyA-
RNA selected with the HSV2 DNA clone (designated U) are also
shown.

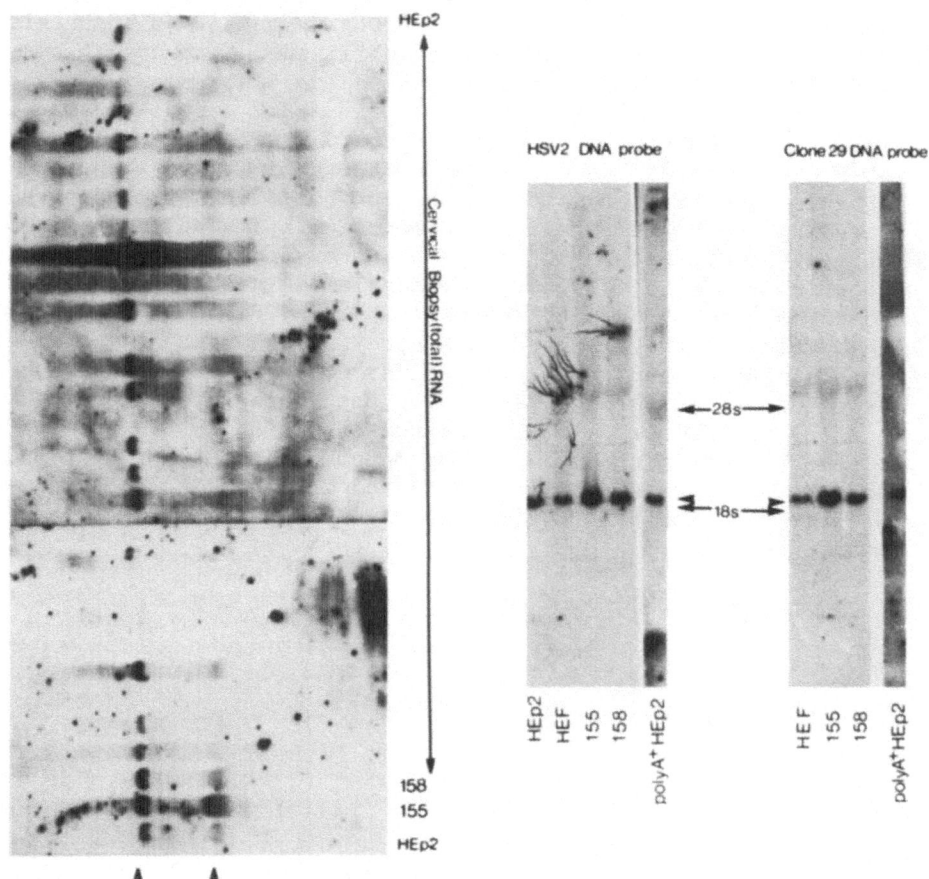

Figure 7.   Hybridization of HSV2 DNA to RNA extracted from human
            cervical neoplasias.
        Extracted total cell RNA was separated by electrophoresis in
        formaldehyde/agarose gels, transferred to 'Genescreen' membrane,
        and hybridized with a 32-P labelled total HSV2 DNA probe (taken
        from Maitland et al., submitted).
        (a) Principal hybridization was to an RNA which co-migrated with
        18S ribosomal RNA although this may be a doublet of two RNA's
        (see below).  In addition the two tracks 155 and 158
        RNA extracted from cervical cell cultures.  Note the presence of
        extra RNA species hybridizing to HSV at about 26S molecular
        weight (arrowed).
        (b) Shows similar results obtained when total HSV2 and a cloned
        HSV2 DNA fragment were used as probes on RNA extracted from
        cultures of cervical epithelium, and human tissue culture cell
        line HEp2.  The cervical cultures consisted of islets of
        epithelium in fibroblasts and the degree of hybridization to the
        18S RNA correlated with the epithelial content of the cultures.

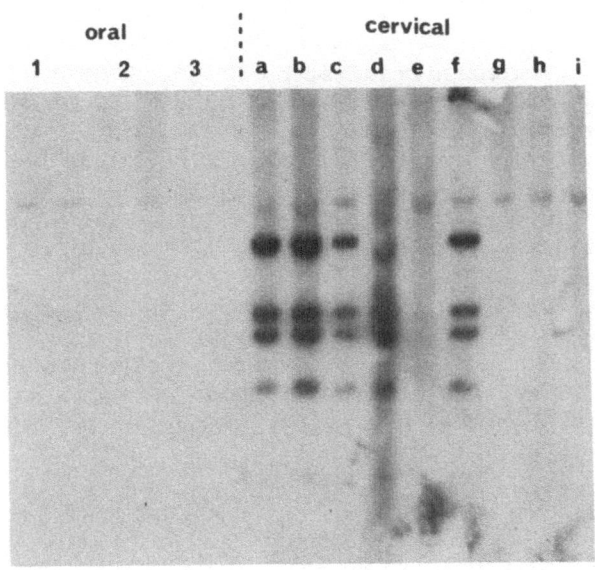

$^{32}$P HPV 16 Probe

Figure 8.  Detection of human papillomavirus type 16 DNA in PstI
   digests of DNA extracted from human cervical biopsies.

Ten micrograms of total cell DNA from human tissue were digested
with PstI, separated by electrophoresis in 0.8% agarose gels,
transferred to 'Genescreen' membranes, and hybridised with a 32-P
labelled HPV16 DNA probe, excised from pBR322 plasmid (clone
kindly supplied by Professor H. zur Hausen, German Cancer
Research Centre, Heidelberg).  Tracks 1, 2, 3 contain 10
micrograms of DNA extracted from oral carcinoma biopsies (kindly
supplied by Professor C. Scully and Dr S. Prime, University of
Bristol), while tracks a,b,c,d,f contained 10 micrograms of
cervical tumour DNA and tracks e,g,h,i contained 10 micrograms of
DNA from histologically normal cervical biopsies (supplied by Dr
C. Meanwell, University of Birmingham).
After 72 hours' exposure of the autoradiographs hybridisation was
seen only in tracks containing DNA from tumour biopsies and not
in tracks containing DNA extracted from normal tissues.

personal communication). This result is in agreement with our own
demonstration that HSV2 DNA probes will hybridiize more to RNA from
carcinoma than to normal human RNA (figure 7) since increased
expression as mRNA of this oncogene has been associated with human
neoplasms (68).

In addition, recent hybridization of the HSV2 _in vitro_
transforming DNA fragment (BgIII"n") to carcinoma DNA has produced a
small percentage of positive results, (69,70) indicating retention of
HSV2 DNA. However virus specific mRNA has not been detected and the
tumour type was generally adenocarcinoma which had been used as a
negative control in previous experiments, since sero-epidemiology had
linked HSV2 to squamous cell carcinoma.

In view of recent positive results for the presence and
expression of human papilloma virus (HPV) DNA in cervical carcinoma
tissue, (70, 71 and figure 8), it is more likely that HPV is the
reason for the "infectious" nature of human cervical carcinoma,
although the role of HSV as a possible co-carcinogen or mutagen should
still not be eliminated (60).


CONCLUSIONS

Herpes Simplex Virus is a genetically complex DNA virus with a
large natural host range for productive infection, probably because it
encodes many of the enzymes required for DNA replication in its own
genome. In contrast to other DNA tumour viruses, which activate most
cell genes early in infection, most cell functions are repressed in
HSV-infected cells, quite soon after infection and two HSV "shut-off"
functions have been genetically mapped, although their biochemical
nature is unknown. The results reported in this article suggest that,
for one particular DNA synthetic enzyme (HGPRT), the viral effect on
host gene expression is not at the level of transcription, but cn mRNA
processing and stability. Thus the selective utilization of cellular
genes during HSV production infection may be achieved by prolonging
the life of "useful" mRNA while degrading other mRNA's. What is still
unclear however is the means by which HSV subverts the cellular gene
control mechanisms to promote expression of its own immediate-early
genes, although a concentration of transcription enhancer sequences
around the IE genes may be part of the answer. This would in turn be
followed by a cascade type enhancement of early and late gene
expression, which may also involve a cellular gene in the cascade.
Infection of neurons superimposes a second level of control on the HSV
gene expression sequence. In these cells the virus remains non-
productive for long periods, but can replicate quite adequately when
particular stimuli are applied. These intracellular controls must be
cellular and may include heat-shock functions since heat shock
proteins have been detected early in productive HSV infection. Heat
shock or stress is an efficient method for the reactivation of latent

HSV from neurons, however the heat shock response is also induced by viral productive infection and whether the activation of these cellular genes is the cause or effect of HSV reactivation from the latent state remains to be determined while the elements of cellular control of viral replication can be recognized in viral latency, the degree to which cell factors affect virus induced transformation is unknown. To produce cell transformation with a DNA tumour virus a non-permissive state must be achieved. With HSV the virus itself has been mutated to prevent replication and to achieve in vitro transformation. In vivo, populations of replication defective viruses can be produced by high multiplicity of infection passage of wild-type virus but no evidence has been produced to demonstrate an increased transformation frequency with these defectives. In addition the defective viruses do not contain the Mtr regions of the HSV genome, but consist of reiterations of the origins of viral DNA replication. The effect of the differentiated cell type may also be important in vivo for the induction of a non-permissive state, however it has been shown that HSV will replicate quite normally in cultured squamous cell epithelium, the presumed target cell for the induction of squamous cell carcinoma. The interactions between different cell types in vivo may therefore be required to produce a non-permissive state for both latency and cell transformation and our present ideas of "one cell-one result" for viral infection could be a gross oversimplification, based as they are on in vitro studies of the HSV infectious cycle.

It is therefore of increasing importance to understand both the cellular and viral aspects of HSV infections in order to understand fully the mechanisms behind the virus's capacity to interact in three different ways with its host.


## ACKNOWLEDGEMENTS

I wish to thank the Cancer Research Campaign for their continuing support of the research into the viral aetiology of human cancer, firstly in the Institute of Animal Genetics, University of Edinburgh with a grant to Dr K.W. Jones (in whose laboratory much of this work was done) and latterly in the Department of Pathology, University of Bristol. I also wish to acknowledge the support of the Nuffield Foundation for the award of research funds to new science lecturers in support of the HGPRT mutagenesis project. Technical assistance of Anne Purves and Caroline Lynas and help with illustrations by Cliff Jeal and Dave Neale were also very much appreciated. My thanks are also due to Jane McRill for helping to type and organize the manuscript.


## REFERENCES

1.    J. Tooze, "DNA Tumour Viruses", Cold Spring Harbor Laboratory, (1980).

2.    B. Roizman, "The family Herpesviridae:  general description,
        Taxomonmy and classification", in: "The Herpesviruses,"
        vol. 1, pp1-23 B. Roizman et al., eds., Plenum Press, New
        York and London (1982).
3.    B. Roizman, The structure and isomerziation of herpes simplex
        virus genomes, Cell, 16: 481-494, (1979)
4.    P. Sheldrick and B. Berthelot, Inverted repetitions in the
        chromosome of herpes simplex virus.  Cold Spring Harbor
        Symposia and Quantative Biology 39: 667-679 (1974).
5.    G.S. Hayward, N. Frenkel and B. Roizman, Anatomy of herpes
        simplex virus DNA.   Strain differences and heterogeneity
        of the location of restriction endonuclease cleavage sites.
        Proc. Natl. Acad. Sci. (USA) 72: 1768-1772.
6.    N.M. Wilkie, Physical maps for herpes simplex virus type 1 DNA
        for restriction endonucleases Hind III, Hpa and Xbad.
        J. Virol., 20: 222-233.
7.    E.K. Wagner, Transcription patterns in HSV infections in:
        "Advances in Viral Oncology Vol. 3: 239-270, G. Klein, ed.,
        Raven Press, New York (1983)
8.    J.B. Clements, J.J. McLaughlan and D.J. McGeogh, Orientation of
        the herpes simplex type 1 immediate-early mRNA7s. Nucleic
        Acids Res., 7: 77-91 (1979).
9.    M.-J. Murchie and D.J. McGeogh, DNA sequence analysis of an
        immediate early gene region of the herpes simplex virus
        type 1 genome (map co-ordinates 0.959 to 0.978), J. Ger.
        Virol., 62: 1-15 (1982).
10.   D.J. McGeogh, The nature of animal virus genetic material, in:
        "The Microbe 1981", Part 1, Viruses, 36th Symposium of the
        Society for General Microbiology, pp75-107, B.W.J. Mahy and
        J.R. Pattison eds., Cambridge Univ. Press, Cambridge
        (1984).
11.   D.J. McGeogh, A. Dolan, S. Donald and F.J. Rixon, Sequence
        determination and genetic content of the short unique
        region in the genome of herpes simplex virus type 1. J.
        Mol. Biol., 181: 1-13 (1985).
12.   R.W. Honess, Herpes simplex and the herpes complex diverse
        observations and a unifying hypothesis - The Eight Fleming
        Lecture.  J. Gen. Virol., 65: 2077-2107, (1984).
13.   J. Banerji, S. Rusconi and W. Schaffner, Expression of a  -
        globin gene is enhanced by remote SV40 sequences, Cell, 27:
        299-308.
14.   J.C. Lang, D.A. Spandidos and N.M. Wilkie, Transcriptional
        regulation of a herpes simplex virus immediate early gene
        is mediated through an enhancer type sequence, E.M.B.O.
        Journal, 3: 389-395 (1984).
15.   C.M. Preston, Control of herpes simplex virus type 1 mRNA
        synthesis in cells infected with wild-type virus or the
        temperature sensitive mutant tsK, J. Virol., 29: 275-285
        (1979).

16.  C.M. Preston, M.G. Cordingley and N.D. Stow, Analysis of DNA
     sequences which regulate the transcription of a herpes
     simplex virus immediate early gene, J. Virol., 50: 708-716,
     (1984).
17.  R.D. Everett, DNA sequence elements required for regulated
     expression of the HSV1 glycoprotein D gene lie within 83bp
     of the RNA cap sites. Nucl. Acids. Res., 11:6647-6666
     (1983).
18.  R.M. Sandri-Goldin, A.L. Goldin, L.E. Holland, J.C. Glorioso and
     M. Levine, Expression of herpes simplex virus b and x genes
     integrated in mammalian cells and their induction by an a
     gene product. Mol. Cell Biol., 3:2028-2044.
19.  L.T. Feldman, M.J. Imperiale and J.R. Nevins, Activation of early
     adenovirus transcription by the herpes virus immediate
     early gene-evidence for a common cellular control factor,
     Proc. Natl. Acad. Sci. (USA) 79: 4952-4956, (1982).
20.  F.M. Burnet and S.W. Williams, Herpes simplex: a new point of
     view, Med. J. Aust., 1: 637-647, (1939).
21.  P. Wildy, H.J. Field and A.A. Nash, Classical Herpes latency
     revisited, in: "Symposium 33, Society for General
     Microbiology," pp133-149, B.W.J. Mahy, A.C. Minson and G.K.
     Darby, eds., Cambridge University Press, London
22.  W.A. Blyth and T.J. Hill, Establishment, maintenance and control
     of herpes simplex virus (HSV) latency, in: "Immunology of
     Herpes Simplex Virus Infection," B.T. Rouse and C. Lopez,
     eds., CRC Press, Inc., Boca Raton, Florida, USA (1984).
23.  T.J. Hill, Herpes simplex virus latency, in: "The Herpes
     Viruses," B.Roizman, ed., Plenum Press, New York and London
     (1985).
24.  B. Wigdahl, A.C. Scheck, R.J. Zigler, E. de Clercq and F. Rapp
     Analysis of the herpes simplex virus genome during in vitro
     latency in human diploid fibroblasts and rat sensory
     neurons, J. Virol., 49: 205-213 (1984).
25.  J.L. McLennan and G. Darby, Herpes simplex virus latency:  The
     cellular location of virus in dorsal root ganglia and the
     fate of the infected cell following virus activation J.
     Gen. Virol., 51: 233-243.
26.  D.A. Galloway, C.M. Fenoglio, M. Shevchuck and J.K. McDougall
     Detection of herpes simplex RNA in sensory ganglia.
     Virology 95: 265-268 (1979).
27.  S.A. Al-Saadi, G.B. Clements and J.H. Subak-Sharpe, Viral genes
     modify herpes simplex virus latency both in mouse footpad
     and sensory ganglia, J. Gen. Virol., 64: 1175-1179, (1984).
28.  M.T. Green, R.J. Courtney and E.G. Dunkel, Detection of an
     immediate early herpes simplex virus type 1 polypeptide in
     trigeminal ganglia from latently infected animals, Infect.
     Immun., 34: 987-999, (1981).
29.  R.B. Tenser, S. Ressel, and M.E. Dunstan, Herpes simplex virus
     thymidine kinase expression in trigeminal infection:
     correlation of enzyme activity with ganglion virus titre

and evidence of in vitro complementation, Virology, 112: 328-341 (1981).

30. H.J. Field and P. Wildy, The pathogenicity of thymidine kinase -deficient mutants of herpes simplex virus in mice, J. Hyg., 81: 267-277 (1978).

31. M.E. Halpern and J.R. Smiley, Effects of deletions on expression of the herpes simplex virus thymidine kinase gene from the intact viral genome:  the amino terminus of the enzyme is dispensible for catalytic activity. J. Virol., 50: 733-758 (1984).

32. A.T. Jamieson, G.A. Gentry and J.H. Subak-Sharpe, Introduction of both thymidine kinase and deoxycytidine kinase and deoxycytidine kinase activity by herpes viruses. J. Gen. Virol., 24: 465-480 (1974).

33. R.L. Thompson and J.G. Stevens, Biological characterization of a herpes simplex virus intertypic recombinant which is completely and specifically non-neuro-virulent. Virology 131: 171-179 (1983).

34. R.L. Thompson, E.K. Wagner and J.G. Stevens, Physical location of a herpes simplex virus type-1 gene function(s) specifically associated with a 10 million-fold increase in HSV neurovirulence, Virology, 131: 180-192 (1983).

35. D.A. Galloway, C.M. Fenoglio and J.K. McDougall, Limited transcription of the herpes simplex virus genome when latent in human sensory ganglia, J. Virol., 41: 686-691 (1982)

36. N.W. Fraser, W.C. Lawrence, Z. Wroblewska, D.K. Gilden and H. Koprowski, Herpes Simplex type 1 DNA in human brain tissue, Proc. Natl. Acad. Sci. USA 78: 6461-6465, (1981)

37. L. Rock and N.W. Fraser, Detection of HSV-1 in central nervous system of latently infected mice, Nature, 302: 523-525, (1983)

38. N.J. Maitland, I.W. Smith, J.F. Peutherer, D.H.H. Robertson and K.W. Jones, Restriction endonuclease analysis of DNA frcm genital isolates of herpes simplex virus type 2. Inf. and Immun., 38: 834-842, (1982).

39. N.B. La Thangue, K. Shriver, C. Dawson and W.L. Chan, Herpes simplex virus infection causes the accumulation of heat shock protein, EMBO Journal, 3: 267-277, (1984).

40. R. Duff and F. Rapp, Properties of hamster embryo fibroblasts transformed in vitro after exposure to ultraviolet irradiated herpes simplex virus type 2, J. Virol., 8: 469-477 (1971).

41. F. Rapp, J.H. Li and M. Jerkofsky, Transformation of mammalian cells by DNA containing viruses following photodynamic inactivation, Virology, 55: 339-346 (1973).

42. G. Darai and K. Munk, Human embryonic lung cells abortively infected with herpes virus hominis type 2 show some properties of cell transformation, Nature New Biol., 241: 268-269 (1973).

43.  J.C.M. MacNab, Transformation of rat embryo cells by temperature
        sensitive mutants of herpes simplex virus, J. Gen. Virol.,
        24: 143-153 (1974).
44.  N.J. Maitland, The transformation of mammalian cells in tissue
        culture with fragments of herpes simplex virus type 2 DNA.
        PhD. Thesis, University of Birmingham, (1977).
45.  G.B. Reyes, R. LaFemina, S.D. Hayward and G.S. Hayward,
        Morphological transformation by DNA fragments of human
        herpes viruses:  Evidence for two distinct transforming
        regions in herpes simplex virus type 1 and 2 and lack of
        correlation with biochemical transfer of the thymidine
        kinase gene, Cold Spring Harbor. Symp. Quant. Biol. 44:
        629-641, (1979).
46.  D.A. Galloway and J.K. McDougall, The oncogenic potential of
        herpes simplex viruses:  evidence for a 'hit-and-run'
        mechanism, Nature (London), 302: 211-214, (1983).
47.  R.J. Jariwalla, L. Aurelian and P.O.P. Ts'O, Tumorigenic
        transformation induced by a specific fragment of DNA from
        herpes simplex virus type 2. Proc. Natl. Acad. Sci. USA,
        77: 2279-2883 (1980).
48.  B. Hampar, A.L. Boyd, J.G. Derge, M. Zweig, L. Eader and S.D.
        Showalter, Comparison of properties of mouse cells
        transformed spontaneously by ultraviolet light irradiated
        herpes simplex virus or by simiam virus 40. Cancer Res.,
        40: 2213-2222, (1980).
49.  J.G. Lewis, L.S. Kucera, R.Eberle and R.J. Courtney, Detection of
        herpes simplex virus type 2 glycoproteins expressed in
        virus-transformed rat cells, J. Virol., 42: 275-282,(1982).
50.  V.L. Flannery, R.J. Courtney and P.A. Schaffer, Expression of an
        early nonstructural antigen of herpes simplex virus in
        cells transformed in vitro by herpes simplex virus,
        J. Virol, 21: 284-291 (1977).
51.  J.J. Docherty, J.H. Subak-Sharpe and C.M. Preston, Identification
        of a virus-specific polypeptide associated with
        transforming fragment (BgIII-N) of herpes simplex type 2
        DNA, J. Virol., 40: 126-132.
52.  D.A. Galloway, C.D. Copple and J.K. McDougall, Analysis of viral
        DNA sequences in hamster cells transformed by herpes
        simplex virus type 2, Proc. Natl. Acad. Sci. USA, 77:
        880-884 (1980).
53.  R. Duff and F. Rapp, Properties of hamster embryo fibroblasts
        transformed in vitro after exposure to ultraviolet-
        irradiated herpes simplex virus type 2, J. Virol., 18: 885
        -893, (1976).
54.  M. Park, D.M. Lonsdale, M.C. Timbury, J.H. Subak-Sharpe and J.C.
        M. MacNab, Genetic retrieval of viral genome sequences from
        hepes simplex virus transformed cells, Nature (London),
        285: 412-415, (1980).
55.  T.L. Benjamin and E. Goldman, Indirect complementation of a non-
        transforming mutant of polyoma virus, Cold Spring Harbor

Symp. Quant. Biol., 39: 41-52 (1975).

56. A. Camacho and P.G. Spear, Transformation of hamster embryo fibroblasts by a specific fragment of the herpes simplex virus genome, Cell 15: 993-1002 (1978).

57. P.G. Spear, Transformation of cultured cells by human herpes viruses, Int. Rev. Exp. Pathol., 25: 327-360, Academic Press, (1983).

58. H. zur Hausen, Human genital cancer - synergism between two virus infections or synergism between a virus infection and initiating events, Lancet pp1370-1372, (1982).

59. J.R. Schlehofer and H. zur Hausen, Induction of mutations within the host cell genome by partially inactivated herpes simplex virus type 1, Virology, 122: 471-475, (1982).

60. J.R. Schlehofer, L. Gissman, B. Matz and H. zur Hausen, Herpes simplex viurs-induced amplification of SV40 sequences in transformed Chinese hamster embryo cells, Int. J. Cancer 32: 99-103 (1983).

61. B. Hampar and S.A. Ellison, Chromosomal aberrations induced by an animal virus, Nature (London), 192: 145-147, (1961).

62. F. Rapp, Viral aetiology of cervical cancer, International Cancer Research Data Bank Program of the National Cancer Institute (Publ., by the U.S. Dept. of Health and Human Services), (1982).

63. H. zur Hausen, Herpes simplex virus in human genital cancer, Int. Rev. Exp. Pathol., 25: 307-326 (1983).

64. N.J. Maitland, J.H. Kinross, A. Busuttil, S.M. Ludgate, G.E. Smart and K.W. Jones, The detection of DNA tumour virus-specific RNA sequences in abnormal human cervical biopsies by in situ hybridisation, J. Gen. Virol., 55: 122-137, (1981).

65. J.K. McDougall, C.P. Crum, C.M. Fenoglio, L.C. Goldstein and D.A. Galloway, Herpesvirus specific RNA and protein in carcinoma of the uterine cervix. Proc. Natl. Acad. Sci.USA 79: 3853-3857, (1982).

66. D.J. Slamon, J.B. de Kernion, I.M. Verma and M.J. Kline, Expression of cellular oncogenes in human malignancies, Science, 224: 256-262, (1984).

67. M. Park, H.C. Kitchner, and J.C.m. MacNab, Detection of herpes simplex virus type 2 DNA restriction fragments in human cervical carcinoma tissue, E.M.B.O. Journal, 2: 1029-1034, (1983).

68. S.S. Prakash, W.C. Reeves, G.R. Sisson, M. Brenes, J. Godoy, R.C. de Britton, and W.E. Rawls, Herpes simplex virus type 2 and human papilloma virus type 16 in cervicitis, dysplasia and invasive cervical carcinoma, Int. J. Cancer, 35: 51-57 (1985).

69. M. Boshart, L. Gissman, H. Ikenberg, A. Kleinheinz, W. Scheurlen and H. zur Hausen, A new type of papilloma-virus DNA, its presence in genital cancer biopsies and in cell lines derived from cervical cancer, E.M.B.O. Journal, 3:1151-1157 (1984).

# TRANSFORMATION OF HUMAN CELLS BY VIRAL AND CELLULAR ONCOGENES

Philip J. Byrd and Phillip H. Gallimore

Cancer Research Campaign Laboratories
Department of Cancer Studies
University of Birmingham
Birmingham, B15 2TJ, U.K.

## INTRODUCTION

Human adenoviruses have been widely used in studies on the expression of genes in eukaryotic cells and in studies of experimentally produced cancer (for reviews see Flint, 1982; Branton et al., 1985; Gallimore et al., 1985a). The oncogenic potential of these viruses was identified by the ability of certain serotypes to induce tumours following injection of newborn rodents. Human adenoviruses have been assigned to three subgroups on the basis of their tumourigenicity, with subgroup A viruses being highly oncogenic and viruses of subgroups B and C being weakly and non-oncogenic respectively. Although these viruses exhibit a spectrum of tumourigenicity, virions or viral DNA of all serotypes tested have the ability to morphologically transform non-permissive or semipermissive mammalian cells in vitro. The use of defined subgenomic adenovirus DNA fragments in in vitro transformation experiments, coupled with analysis of the tumourigenic potential of cell lines established from transformed foci, facilitate investigations into the roles of viral genes in malignant transformation.

The RNA tumour viruses or retroviruses are divided into two groups according to whether they do or do not contain transforming genes (Bishop and Varmus, 1982). The oncogenes of retroviruses represent cellular genes that have been transduced by reverse transcription. Consequently the viral oncogenes contain no introns and may differ from their cellular counterparts at many sites in the coding sequence or may be incomplete versions of the cellular proto-oncogenes (Bishop, 1983). While retroviral transduction is a specialised mode of activating the transforming potential of proto-oncogenes they can also be activated by chromosomal translocation,

131

by amplification and by point mutation (Bishop, 1983). Identification of dominant activated proto-oncogenes in human tumours has been accomplished by transfection of murine NIH 3T3 cells; DNA from 10-20% of human tumours has been found to induce foci of morphologically transformed cells (Fujita et al., 1984). The cellular proto-oncogenes most commonly identified in this way belong to the ras family i.e. genes with homology to Harvey murine sarcoma virus (Ha-MSV) and Kirsten murine sarcoma virus (Ki-MSV; Fujita et al., 1984). So far the activated ras genes isolated from human tumours have been found to have single amino acid alterations either at position 12 or 61 in these 21000 m.w. proteins (Santos et al., 1984). Since murine NIH 3T3 cells are immortal and exhibit a relatively high level of spontaneous transformation it has been impossible to determine the roles of proto-oncogenes in the multistage route to cancer.

In this study we determined the ability of segments of the adenovirus transforming region to effect transformation of primary human embryo retinal (HER) cells. We also investigated whether a cloned activated human proto-oncogene i.e. the N-ras proto-oncogene (Hall et al., 1983) has transforming activity in human cells either alone or in combination with adenovirus genes.

MATERIALS AND METHODS

Retinas were dissected out of the eyes of aborted human foetuses (14-20 weeks old) and disrupted by gentle pipetting. The cells from each retina were plated out in ten 5 cm tissue culture dishes and grown in RPMI 1640 medium containing 20% foetal calf serum (FCS). After 8 to 10 days incubation at 37°C the cultures had normally grown to ∿70% confluency and were composed of a variety of neuroblastic, glial and fibroblastic cells. At this point the cultures were transfected (Graham and Van der Eb, 1973) with cloned adenovirus genes and/or cloned N-ras proto-oncogene. Ten micrograms of each cloned sequence were transfected onto each dish of cells; single DNA clones were mixed with 10 μg pAT153 for comparison with dishes that were cotransfected with two different plasmids. The medium was removed from each dish and the DNA added in 0.5 ml Hepes buffered saline (Hebs) pH 7.1 containing 125 mM CaCl$_2$. After five minutes at room temperature 4.5 ml of growth medium containing 10% FCS was added and the cultures were incubated for 4 hours at 37°C. The growth medium was then removed and each dish was treated with 10% glycerol in Hebs for 1 minute followed by multiple washes in serum free medium. Cultures were incubated at 37°C and carefully observed for up to 12 weeks for the appearance of transformed foci.

Adenovirus type 12 (Ad 12) transforming region segments were cloned in this laboratory (Byrd et al., 1982b); Ad 5 clones were provided by Dr. L. Babiss (Department of Microbiology, Columbia University, U.S.A.) and the Ad 2 E1A clone was the gift of Dr. N. Stow (MRC Institute of Virology, Glasgow).  The activated N-ras proto-oncogene clone was provided by Dr. A. Hall (Chester Beatty Laboratories, Institute of Cancer Research, London).

Southern (1975) blotting analysis was performed according to Maniatis et al. (1982).

RESULTS

The adenovirus genome is a linear double stranded DNA molecule of 34-36 Kbp.  A detailed transcription map of the genome has been constructed (Gingeras et al., 1982) and analysis of virion trans- formed rodent cells has identified early region 1 (E1) located within the left end 11-12% of the viral genome as the transforming region.  The E1 region is divided into two transcriptional units E1A and E1B which together encode at least four tumour (T) antigens; Figure 1 shows the organisation of the E1 region for Ad 12 but the general structure is the same for all serotypes.

In a study of the ability of cloned Ad 12 E1 segments to trans- form baby rat kidney (BRK) cells we found that the specific trans- forming activities decreased in the order E1A + E1B: E1A + 5'E1B: E1A alone (Gallimore et al., 1984; 1985b).  Attempts to reproduce these results in human skin fibroblasts (embryonic and adult) and human embryo kidney cells were largely unsuccessful but four Ad 12 E1A + E1B transformed HEK cell lines were established from six extremely rare transformed foci (Whittaker et al., 1984).

Since Albert et al. (1968) had shown that Ad 12 could transform hamster neural retinal cells in vitro and Mukai et al. (1980) had shown that Ad 12 induced retinoblastoma like tumours following intra-ocular injection of newborn rodents and baboons, we investi- gated whether HER cells were susceptible to transformation by the adenovirus E1 region.  The complete Ad 12 E1 region was found to transform HER cells reproducibly and the efficiency of transformation (0.093 transformants/µg plasmid; Table 1) was only 4 to 5 fold lower than that on BRK cells (Gallimore et al., 1984; 1985b); by comparison the specific transforming activity of the cloned Ad 12 E1 region in HEK cells was more than two orders of magnitude lower than in HER cells (Whittaker et al., 1984; Gallimore and Byrd, unpublished observations).  The transforming efficiency of the cloned Ad 12 E1A region in HER cells was 19-fold lower than the complete E1 region and approximately 2-fold lower than the cloned Ad 12 E1A + 5' E1B segment (Table 1).  Although the same relative transforming activi- ties were found on BRK cells, a major difference between the two transformation systems was in the ease of establishment of cell lines from cells transformed by cloned segments representing E1A alone or

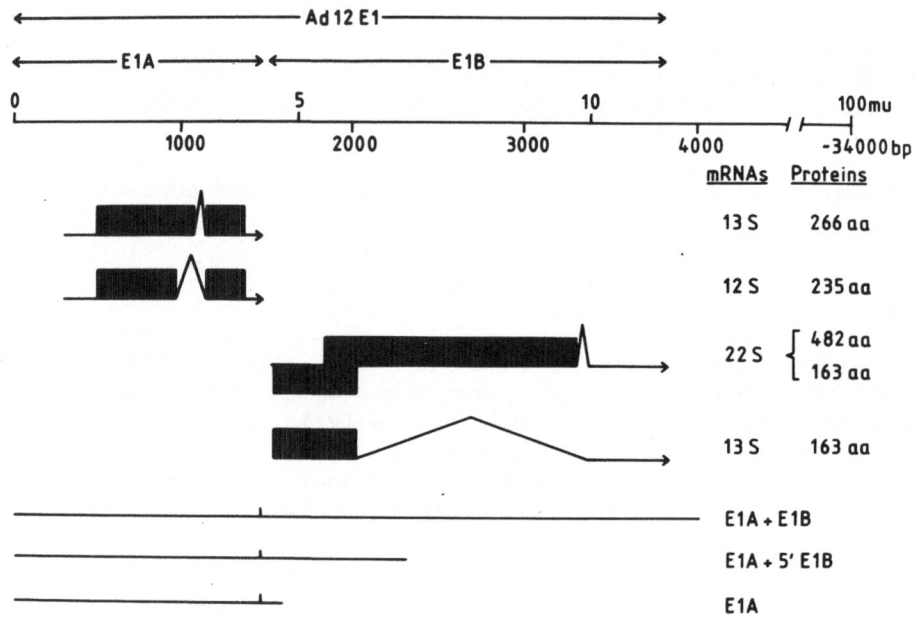

Figure 1.    Organisation of the Ad 12 E1 transforming region.  By
             convention the map of the human adenovirus genome is
             divided into 100 equal map units (m.u.).  The Ad 12 E1
             region is within the left end 3809 bp or ∿11.2 m.u.
             Both E1A and E1B are transcribed in the rightward
             direction.  The major mRNA species are shown as single
             headed arrows; carets denote splicing.  The protein
             coding sequences of these mRNAs are shown as filled
             boxes.  The sizes of the mRNAs and the number of amino
             acids (a.a.) in each protein are shown.  The 22S E1B
             mRNA species has the potential to code for the 482 a.a.
             and the 163 a.a. proteins.  The cloned Ad 12 E1 segments
             used in this study are shown at the bottom.  These plas-
             mids have been referred to previously as pAsc 2 (E1A +
             E1B), pAsc 6.8 (E1A + 5'E1B) and pAsc 4.7 (E1A; Byrd
             et al., 1982b).

E1A + 5' E1B.  The rat cell foci generated by these cloned segments
could be established into continuous cell lines with a high success
rate, although several attempts at isolation were required before
vigorous cell growth was obtained from the majority of E1A trans-

Table 1. Transformation of HER cells by cloned segments of the human adenovirus E1 region and by the activated human N-ras proto-oncogene in combination with adenovirus E1A.

| | No. transformants/ No. 5 cm dishes | Transformants/ μg plasmid | Transforming activities relative to Ad 2 E1A[c] |
|---|---|---|---|
| Ad 5 E1A + E1B | 785/50 | 1.640 | 568.5 |
| Ad 12 E1A + E1B | 77/77 | 0.093 | 27.2 |
| Ad 12 E1A + 5' E1B | 14[a]/66 | 0.012 | 2.3 |
| Ad 12 E1A | 7[b]/50 | 0.012 | 1.4 |
| Ad 2 E1A | 2[a]/38 | 0.006 | 1.0 |
| Ad 2 E1A + N-ras | 53/29 | 0.183 | 31.0 |
| N-ras | 0/30 | 0.000 | 0.0 |

a All abortive transformants.
b All but one were abortive transformants.
c In calculating the relative transforming activities, the values in the second column were adjusted to take into account the sizes of the plasmids; the number of molecules per microgram is determined by the size of the plasmid.

This table was compiled from the results of 26 experiments.

formants (Gallimore et al., 1985b).  In contrast all but one of the
HER cell foci generated by these plasmids aborted before or soon
after isolation.  The exception, an Ad 12 E1A transformant, grew so
slowly that nine months elapsed from the time of isolation before a
single confluent 9 cm dish of cells was obtained.  The only viral
genes contained and expressed in this cell line are those from E1A
(Byrd and Gallimore, manuscript in preparation).

We extended our analysis to include cloned E1 segments of the
non-oncogenic subgroup C viruses Ad 2 and Ad 5, to determine whether
the inability of the E1A region to transform HER cells was unique
to Ad 12.  As shown in Table 1 the complete Ad 5 E1 region induced
foci of small epithelioid transformed cells (Figure 2) at a
frequency >20-fold higher than that for Ad 12; the difference in the
transforming activities of the Ad 12 and Ad 5 E1 regions on BRK
cells is of the same order (Bernards et al., 1982).  However, the
increased transforming activity of the Ad 5 E1A + E1B sequences
was not reflected in comparisons of the E1A plasmids (Table 1; the
Ad 2 E1A used in these experiments is >90% homologous to the Ad 5
E1A and the properties of the E1 region of these viruses are identical).

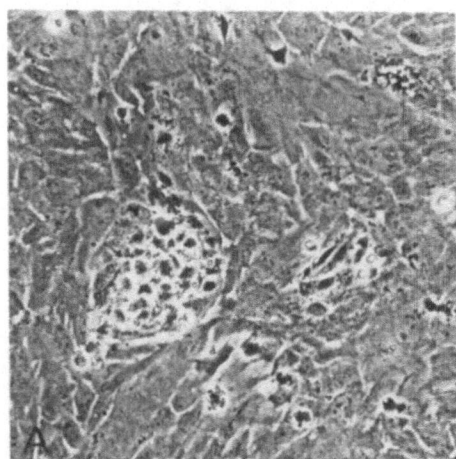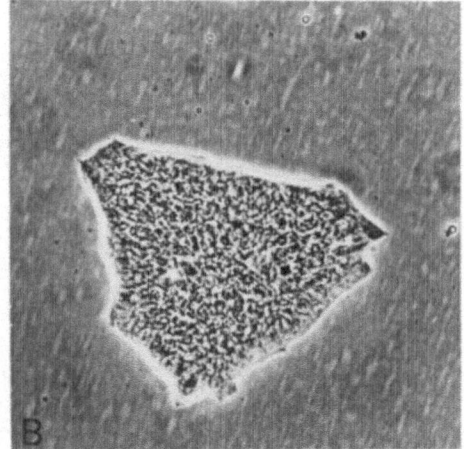

Figure 2.   The morphologies of normal and Ad 5 transformed HER
            cells.
            A.   Normal primary HER cells, 14 days after plating the
            disrupted retina.
            B.   A colony of Ad 5 E1A + E1B transformed HER cells.
            The tight packing of the cells and the well defined
            border of the colony are characteristic of Ad 5 trans-
            formants.
            Magnification X225.

The rare transformation of HER cells by the adenovirus E1A region, together with the reduction in expression of E1A or E1B proteins in a minority of complete E1 transformed cell lines at high passage levels (Grand, Byrd and Gallimore, unpublished observations), led us to investigate whether viral and cellular genes could cooperate to initiate and maintain transformation. In these experiments we used the activated N-ras human proto-oncogene. As shown in Table 1 we were unable to detect any transforming activity for the N-ras gene alone. However, when primary HER cells were cotransfected with N-ras and Ad 2 E1A, transformed foci were produced at an efficiency approximately 20-fold lower than that of the complete Ad 5 E1 region but >30-fold higher than the E1A region alone. Additionally, whereas both Ad 2 E1A foci we identified ultimately aborted several N-ras + Ad 2 E1A transformed cell lines were isolated. These transformants were very difficult to grow and although we were successful in every case, for some foci it was necessary to passage them with all the cells in their dishes before established lines were recovered. The growth of some of these transformants was found to be very slow and marked by periods of crisis (Byrd and Gallimore, manuscript in preparation).

To show that the N-ras + Ad 2 E1A transformants contained exogenously added copies of the N-ras gene, Southern blotting analysis was performed (Figure 3). When DNA from the cell line HER E1A/N-ras A2 was digested with EcoRI a band equivalent to a segment of the endogenous N-ras proto-oncogene was found (compare track 1 with track 2). The same enzyme releases a 12.3 Kbp fragment from the cloned N-ras proto-oncogene (track 3) and a band corresponding to a fragment of this size was found in EcoRI digested HER E1A/N-ras A2 cell DNA. Three other bands containing N-ras exon 1 sequences were evident and exogenously added N-ras sequences were present at the level of between five and ten copies per cell.


DISCUSSION

In the study reported here we investigated the ability of adenovirus E1 genes and the human N-ras proto-oncogene to transform HER cells. The complete adenovirus E1 region transformed HER cells reproducibly with the Ad 5 E1 region being more efficient than that of Ad 12. Although we have been able to transform BRK cells with the Ad 12 E1A region alone at a much reduced frequency compared to the complete Ad 12 E1, transformation of HER cells by E1A was an exceptionally rare event and was not serotype dependent. The human N-ras proto-oncogene was found to be incapable of eliciting transformation unless cotransfected with the adenovirus E1A. Sager et al. (1983) found that early passage human skin fibroblasts were resistant to transformation induced by exogenously added cloned activated human Ha-ras proto-oncogene. In primary baby rat kidney cells Ruley (1983) found that the activated human Ha-ras proto-

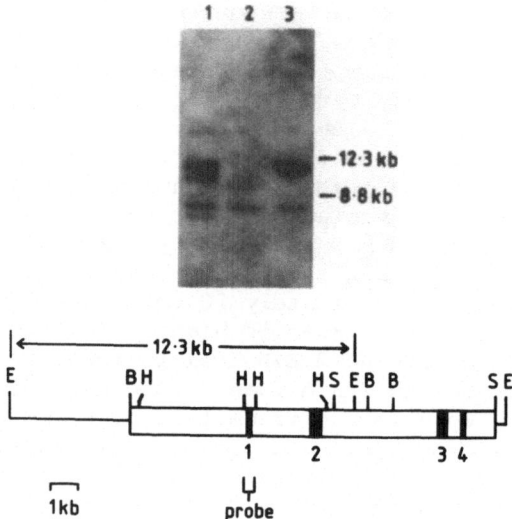

Figure 3.    Southern hybridisation analysis of an HER E1A/N-ras
             transformant.
             The diagram shows the structure of the cloned activated
             human N-ras proto-oncogene (Brown et al., 1984) desig-
             nated pN-ras (HT); the plasmid is shown linearised
             through the EcoRI site in the sequences of the vector.
             The four exons of N-ras are shown as filled boxes, non-
             coding sequences as open boxes and plasmid sequences a
             single line.  A 12.3 Kb fragment containing exon 1 is
             released from pN-ras (HT) by EcoRI digestion while the
             same enzyme releases an 8.8 Kb exon 1 fragment from
             genomic DNA.  The sites for the restriction enzymes
             BamHI (B), EcoRI (E), HindIII (H) and SstI (S) are shown.
                Ten microgram samples of DNA were cut to completion
             with EcoRI and the fragments were separated by electro-
             phoresis on a 1% agarose gel.  Following transfer to a
             nitrocellulose filter the DNA was probed with a $^{32}$P-
             labelled 300 bp DNA fragment that spans N-ras exon 1.
             Track 1, HER E1A/N-ras A2; track 2, normal HER cell DNA;
             track 3, normal HER cell DNA containing ∿5 copies/cell
             of pN-ras (HT).

oncogene required the co-operation of other oncogenes such as
adenovirus E1A for morphological transformation in vitro.  However,
Land et al. (1983) were able to demonstrate morphological transformation of secondary rat embryo fibroblasts with the activated
human Ha-ras proto-oncogene but the transformants had very limited

replicative capacity, were not tumourigenic in nude mice and required
other co-operating oncogenes for expression of the complete transformed phenotype.  Similarly Newbold and Overell (1983) found that
the Ha-ras proto-oncogene could only fully transform Syrian hamster
dermal fibroblasts if they had been previously 'immortalised' by
carcinogens.  Contrary to the results reported here and the published work described above Spandidos and Wilkie (1984) found that
increasing the expression of the human Ha-ras proto-oncogene with
transcriptional enhancers endowed the normal gene with the ability
to immortalise primary rodent cells and endowed the activated gene
with the ability to malignantly transform the same cells; this
applied to Chinese and Syrian hamster cells and cells from a variety
of rat tissues.  At the present time it is unclear how elevated
expression of a single oncogene can effect malignant transformation
when the genesis of cancer is thought to involve multiple stages.
It is presumed that activation and enhanced expression of the
proto-oncogene count as different stages in the route to cancer
(Spandidos and Wilkie, 1984; Marshall, 1984), but it seems likely
that other cellular genetic alterations may facilitate the transformation by single oncogenes.  Whether single transcriptionally
enhanced, activated proto-oncogenes can induce malignant transformation in vitro of genetically more stable human cells such as
HER cells is unknown but under evaluation.

At this point we do not know why HER cells are so susceptible
to morphological transformation by adenovirus genes and cellular
proto-oncogenes in combination with E1A.  The simple explanation
that they transfect more readily than other cell types seems
unlikely because we know that SV40 virus transforms human skin
fibroblasts, HEK cells and HER cells efficiently (Whittaker et al.,
1984; Gallimore and Byrd, manuscript in preparation) and adenovirus
E1 genes are fully expressed in HEK cells.

There is no evidence that adenoviruses could be aetiological
agents of human retinoblastoma and indeed the genetic lesions
underlying this cancer seem to involve regulatory genes (see
Murphree and Benedict, 1984 for a recent review).  Interestingly,
one or more products of the E1A region are known to be transacting transcriptional activators and it could be that the viral
proteins compete against regulatory factors, attempting inappro-
priately to induce or maintain the expression of genes involved in
cell proliferation.

The cell of origin of retinoblastoma is still a subject of
debate but a recent report suggests that it derives from a primitive
bi- or multipotential neuroectodermal cell (Kyritsis et al., 1984).
Some of our Ad 12 transformed HER cell lines produce retinoblastoma-
like tumours when injected intracerebrally into athymic nude mice
(Byrd et al., 1982a; Byrd and Gallimore, manuscript in preparation),
suggesting that the cell type which is susceptible to transformation

in vitro is the same as that which generates retinoblastoma in humans. The transformation system described here should therefore be of great value in studies of carcinogenesis and cellular differentiation.

## REFERENCES

Albert, D.M., Rabson, A.S., and Dalton, A.J., 1968, In vitro neoplastic transformation of uveal and retinal tissue by oncogenic DNA viruses, Invest. Ophthalmol., 7:357.

Bernards, R., Houweling, A., Schrier, P.I., Bos, J.L. and Van der Eb, A.J., 1982, Characterization of cells transformed by Ad 5/Ad 12 hybrid early region 1 plasmids, Virology, 120:422.

Bishop, J.M., 1983, Cellular oncogenes and retroviruses, Ann. Rev. Biochem., 52:301.

Bishop, J.M., and Varmus, H.E., 1982, Functions and origins of retroviral transforming genes, in: "The Molecular Biology of Tumor Viruses, Part III RNA Tumour Viruses", R.A. Weiss, N. Teich, H.E. Varmus, and J.M. Coffin, eds., Cold Spring Harbor Laboratory, Cold Spring Harbor, New York, pp. 999-1108.

Branton, P.E., Bayley, S.T., and Graham, F.L., 1985, Transformation by human adenoviruses, Biochimica et Biophysica Acta., in press.

Brown, R., Marshall, C.J., Pennie, S.G., and Hall, A., 1984, Mechanism of activation of an N-ras gene in the human fibrosarcoma cell line HT1080, The EMBO Journal, 3:1321.

Byrd, P.J., Brown, K.W., and Gallimore, P.H., 1982a, Malignant transformation of human embryo retinoblasts by cloned adenovirus 12 DNA, Nature, 298:69.

Byrd, P.J., Chia, W., Rigby, P.W.J., and Gallimore, P.H., 1982b, Cloning of DNA fragments from the left end of the adenovirus type 12 genome: transformation by cloned early region 1, J. Gen. Virol., 60:279.

Flint, S.J., 1982, Expression of adenoviral genetic information in productively infected cells, Biochimica Et Biophysica Acta., 651:175.

Fujita, J., Yoshida, O., Yuasa, Y., Rhim, J.S., Hatanaka, M., and Aaronson, S.A., 1984, Ha-ras oncogenes are activated by somatic alterations in human urinary tract tumours, Nature, 309:464.

Gallimore, P.H., Byrd, P.J., Grand, R., Whittaker, J., Breiding, D., and Williams, J., 1984, An examination of the transforming and tumour-inducing capacity of a number of adenovirus type 12 early-region 1, host-range mutants and cells transformed by subgenomic fragments of Ad 12 E1 region, in: "Cancer Cells 2; Oncogenes and viral genes", G.F. Vande Woude, A.J. Levine, W.C. Topp and J.D. Watson, eds., Cold Spring Harbor Laboratory, Cold Spring Harbor, New York, pp. 519-526.

Gallimore, P.H., Byrd, P.J., and Grand, R.J.A., 1985a, Adenovirus

genes involved in transformation.  What determines the oncogenic
phenotype?  The Society for General Microbiology 37th Symposium,
"Viruses and Cancer", P.W.J. Rigby and N.M. Wilkie, eds., in
press, Cambridge University Press, Cambridge.

Gallimore, P.H., Byrd, P.J., Whittaker, J.L., and Grand, R.J.A.,
1985b, The properties of rat cells transformed by DNA plasmids
containing adenovirus type 12 E1 DNA or specific fragments of
the E1 region: A comparison of transforming frequencies,
Cancer Res., in press.

Gingeras, T.R., Sciaky, D., Gelinas, R.E., Bing-Dong, J., Yen,
C.E., Kelly, M.M., Bullock, P.A., Parsons, B.L., O'Neill,
K.E. and Roberts, R.J., 1982, Nucleotide sequences from the
adenovirus 2 genome, J. Biol. Chem., 257:13475.

Graham, F.L., and Van der Eb, A.J., 1973, A new technique for the
assay of infectivity of human adenovirus 5 DNA, Virology,
52:456.

Hall, A., Marshall, C.J., Spurr, N.K., and Weiss, R.A., 1983,
Identification of transforming gene in two human sarcoma cell
lines as a new member of the ras gene family located on
chromosome 1, Nature, 303:396.

Kyritsis, A.P., Tsokos, M., Triche, T.J., and Chader, G.J., 1984,
Retinoblastoma-origin from a primitive neuro-ectodermal cell?
Nature, 307:471.

Land, H., Parada, L.F., and Weinberg, R.A., 1983, Tumorigenic
conversion of primary embryo fibroblasts requires at least
two cooperating oncogenes, Nature, 304:596.

Maniatis, T., Fritsch, E.F., and Sambrook, J., 1982, Molecular
Cloning: A Laboratory Manual, Cold Spring Harbor Laboratory,
Cold Spring Harbor, New York.

Marshall, C., 1984, Functions of ras oncogenes, Nature, 310:448.

Mukai, N., Kalter, S.S., Cummins, L.B., Matthews, V.A., Nishida, T.
and Nakajima, T., 1980, Retinal tumour induced in the baboon
by human adenovirus 12, Science, 210:1023.

Murphree, A.L., and Benedict, W.F., 1984, Retinoblastoma: Clues to
human oncogenesis, Science, 223:1028.

Newbold, R.F., and Overell, R.W., 1983, Fibroblast immortality is
a prerequisite for transformation by EJ c-Ha-ras oncogene,
Nature, 304:648.

Ruley, H.E., 1983, Adenovirus early region 1A enables viral and
cellular transforming genes to transform primary cells in
culture, Nature, 304:602.

Sager, R., Tanaka, K., Lau, C.C., Ebina, Y. and Anisowicz, A.,
1983, Resistance of human cells to tumourigenesis induced by
cloned transforming genes, Proc. Natl. Acad. Sci. USA, 80:7601.

Santos, E., Martin-Zanca, D., Reddy, E.P., Pierotti, M.A., Della
Porta, G., and Barbacid, M., 1984, Malignant activation of a
K-ras oncogene in lung carcinoma but not in normal tissue of
the same patient, Science, 223:661.

Southern, E.M., 1975, Detection of specific sequences among DNA
fragments separated by gel electrophoresis, J. Mol. Biol.,
98:503.

Spandidos, D.A., and Wilkie, N.M., 1984, Malignant transformation
    of early passage rodent cells by a single mutated human
    oncogene, Nature, 310:469.
Whittaker, J.L., Byrd, P.J., Grand, R.J.A., and Gallimore, P.H.,
    1984, Isolation and characterization of four adenovirus type
    12-transformed human embryo kidney cell lines, Mol. Cell.
    Biol., 4:110.

# TISSUE-SPECIFIC EXPRESSION OF CLONED CHICKEN CRYSTALLIN GENES IN MAMMALIAN CELLS

H. Kondoh, S. Hayashi, K. Okazaki, K. Yasuda
and T. S. Okada

Institute for Biophysics, Faculty of Science
University of Kyoto, Kyoto 606, Japan

Crystallins are a group of soluble proteins specific to vertebrate lenses (Clayton, 1974; Piatigorsky, 1984). We have cloned a continuous stretch of a chicken δ-crystallin gene on a bacterial plasmid vector (Kondoh et al., 1983). The gene is approximately 9 kb long, consists of 17 exons (Ohno et al., 1985), and is associated with 5' and 3' flanking DNA sequences of 2.2 kb and 0.5 kb long, respectively.

We attempted to reintroduce the cloned δ-crystallin gene into nuclei of mammalian cells, mouse cells in particular, to see whether any tissue-specific gene expression took place. The choice of mouse cells took advantage of the fact that δ-crystallin is found only in avians and reptilians and is replaced in other vertebrates by completely different γ-crystallin. Thus, expression of chicken δ-crystallin gene in mouse cells should be detectable in a high sensitivity.

We prepared primary cultures of various tissues of mouse, mainly from fetuses in order to get differentiated cell populations. Lens epithelial cultures were usually prepared from mice just after weaning, but we found no age-dependent difference in the result using animals from the day 14 of gestation to one year old.

Introduction of the δ-crystallin genes to mouse cells was accomplished by direct microinjection into nuclei using the Injectoscope (Olympus). We could inject from 1 to 500 copies of the δ-crystallin gene per nucleus by adjusting the DNA concentration and by assuming an injection volume of $10^{-14}$ l per nucleus. Successful nuclear injection was established by recovery of the injected DNA copies after 2 days from nuclei of injected cultures, as revealed by Southern blot analysis (Hayashi et al., 1985). The δ-crystallin sequences were found almost exclusively in the Hirt's supernatant fraction, indicating that the large majority of the injected DNA remained unintegrated from the mouse chromosome at least for two days. The same analysis revealed no substantial difference in the stability of the injected DNA between nuclei of different tissues.

Among the mouse tissues, lens epithelial cells were, of course, the first choice of interest. We found that the chicken δ-crystallin gene was expressed in the mouse lens epithelial cells as efficiently as in the homologous chick cells (Fig. 1) (Kondoh et al., 1983). Synthesis of δ-crystallin took place in the initial 2-3 days after the gene injection. The δ-crystallin polypeptide synthesized in the mouse lens epithelium had the native molecular weight (50,000) and antigenicity.

When injected into nuclei of other non-lens tissues, the expression of the δ-crystallin  gene was inefficient, and was 1-5% of the level when compared with that in lens epithelium. This cell type preference in the high-level expression indicated that the exogenous δ-crystallin gene was regulated almost normally in the xenogenic environment. Considering the absence of the δ-crystallin gene in mouse, the observations suggested that there are crystallin-specific or lens-specific regulatory mechanisms for gene expression. It was also indicated that there are built-in regulatory signals in the δ-crystallin and associated DNA sequences for the tissue-specific regulatory mechanisms. The presence of crystallin- or lens-specific regulatory mechanisms

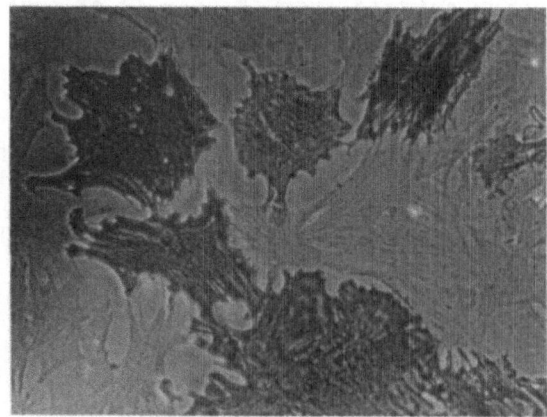

Fig. 1.   Expression of chicken δ-crystallin in mouse lens epithelial cells in culture. Two days after injection of the gene, the culture was stained immunochemically for δ-crystallin.  Only injected cells are stained.

was supported by the study of one other class of crystallin, α-crystallin.  Chicken α-crystallin gene has also been cloned (Okazaki et al., 1985).  We modified the chicken α-crystallin gene so as to distinguish the exogenous genes's expression from the endogenous mouse α-crystallin.  This was accomplished by constructing a chimeric gene using the 5' half and the upstream sequences of the chicken α-crystallin gene and the 3' half of the δ-crystallin gene shown to be neutral in the tissue preference. This chimeric gene, αδ, was used in place of the chicken α-crystallin gene, and the expression was assessed using δ-specific immunochemical methods.  The αδ gene also was expressed strictly in the lens-specific manner, demonstrating that chicken crystallin genes are correctly regulated by the mouse systems (Okazaki., 1985).

When the promoter region of the δ-crystallin gene was replaced by the transcriptional signals of Moloney murine leukaemia virus LTR, the expression of the gene, Mo-δ, was no longer lens-specific, and we observed an almost constant level of expression in various cell types (Kondoh and Okada, 1986).  This observation indicated that the region which confers lens-specificity to the δ-crystallin gene probably resides in the promoter region.  We thus carried out deletion analysis of the promoter region of the δ-crystallin gene to localize the regulatory signals in the DNA sequences.  The analyses indicated that the lens-specific high level expression depends on the region 50-80 bp upstream of the transcriptional initiation site (cap site), while non-specific, low-level expression depends on the region 80-100 bp upstream from the cap site (Hayashi et al., 1985).  This difference in the dependence of the upstream sequences indicated that transcriptional regulation of the crystallin genes in lens and non-lens cells are basically different.

With this information, we reinvestigated various mouse tissues for their potency of expression of the exogenous δ-cystallin gene. The gene expression was assessed by comparing with a co-injected, non-specific Mo-δ gene.  We found that among a number of mouse tissues in fresh primary culture, not only lens but also epidermal cells supported a high-level expression of the δ-crystallin gene (Kondoh and Okada, 1986).  The expression in epidermis required the same 50-80 bp upstream region as in the lens cells.  These two cell types are closely related in that both originate from embryonic ectoderm, and the lens is separated from epidermis only after induction by an optic cup.  In addition, retinal cells in long term culture acquired the capacity to express the exogenous δ-crystallin gene at a high level, in the course of transdifferentiation into lens, but before expressing the lens phenotype (Kondoh and Okada, 1986). However, we never observed such lens-like expression in any other tissues in various culture conditions. We thus conclude that the high-level expression of the exogenous δ-crystallin gene reflects a differentiated state of the cells which is very close to the lens and such cells share crucial regulatory mechanisms with the lens cells.

In conclusion, we observed regulated expression of cloned chicken crystallin genes after introduction to mouse cells by nuclear injection. Taking advantage of this gene transfer system, we could localize the DNA sequences responsible for the tissue specificity of the δ-crystallin gene within the 80 bp region upstream from the transcriptional initiation site.

However, the expression of δ-crystallin in this experimental system deviates from the normal expression in the chicken in two respects. First, a low but significant level of the expression took place in virtually all cell types we examined. This appears to be due to the extrachromosomal localization of the injected DNA, since expression of this type was suppressed in stably transformed cell lines (Kondoh et al., 1984). Secondly, an efficient expression of δ-crystallin was not confined to authentic lens cells but also observed in other lens-related cells. This suggests multistep regulation of δ-crystallin expression. Probably, our experimental system succeeded in mimicking in large part the normal regulation but lacks the mechanism to confine the expressing tissue to lens. Unsuccessful regulation in the latter part may be due to the lack of the chromosomal effect or may be due to xenogenic combination of the gene and the recipient cells.

In any event, we feel it promising that the gene transfer experiments uncover clues to elucidate tissue specific gene regulation.


REFERENCES

Clayton, R.M., 1974, Comparative aspects of lens proteins, in: "The Eye," H. Davson and L.T. Graham, ed. Vol. 5, Academic Press, New York.
Hayashi, S., Kondoh, H., Yasuda, K., Soma, G., Ikawa, Y., and Okada, T.S., 1985, Tissue-specific regulation of a chicken δ-crystallin gene in mouse cells: involvement of the 5' end region, EMBO J., 4:2201.
Kondoh, H., Yasuda, K., and Okada, T.S., 1983, Tissue-specific expression of a cloned chick δ-crystallin gene in mouse cells, Nature, 301:440.
Kondoh, H., Takahashi, Y., and Okada, T.S., 1984, Differentiation-dependent expression of the chicken δ-crystallin gene introduced into mouse teratocarcinoma stem cells, EMBO J., 3:2009.

Kondoh, H., and Okada, T.S., 1986, Dual regulation of expression
    of exogenous δ-crystallin gene in mammalian cells: a
    search for molecular background of instability in
    differentiation, <u>Curr. Top. Dev. Biol.</u>, 20:153.
Ohno, M., Sakamoto, H., Yasuda, K., Okada, T.S., and Shimura, Y.,
    1985, Nucleotide sequence of a chicken δ-crystallin gene,
    <u>Nucl. Acids Res.</u>, 13:1593.
Okazaki, K., Yasuda, K., Kondoh, H., Okada, T.S., 1985, DNA
    sequences responsible for tissue-specific expression of a
    chicken α-crystallin gene in mouse lens cells, <u>EMBO J.</u>,
    4:2589.
Piatigorsky, J., 1984, δ-crystallin and their nucleic acids, <u>Mol.
    Cell. Biochem.</u>, 59:33.

THE EXPRESSION OF GENES INJECTED INTO OOCYTES AND EGGS OF

XENOPUS LAEVIS

J.G. Williams, M.M. Bendig, P.J. Mason and
J.A. Elkington

The Imperial Cancer Research Fund
Burtonhole Lane
Mill Hill
London NW7

The Xenopus laevis β1-globin gene was injected into oocytes
and unfertilized eggs of X.laevis. In oocytes the injected globin
gene was actively transcribed but the majority of the transcripts
were incorrectly initiated. Processing of Xenopus globin RNA in
oocytes was analyzed using a fusion gene containing the promoter of
the Herpes Thymidine Kinase gene and the coding and 3' non-coding
sequences from the β1 globin gene. The transcripts were spliced and
polyadenylated at the correct sites with a very high efficiency. In
unfertilized eggs the injected β1 globin gene was transcribed at a
low level but only from the correct start sites. In oocytes the
injected circular plasmid DNA containing the cloned globin genes
persisted but did not replicate. In contrast, DNA injected into
unfertilized eggs replicated up to 15-fold within a 22hr period.
Naked DNA injected into either oocytes or eggs is assembled into a
chromatin-like structure. The ability of the egg to selectively
transcribe the injected Xenopus globin gene from the correct
promoter sites may be related to differences in chromatin  structure
between the oocyte and the unfertilized egg.

INTRODUCTION

The availability of cloned genes and the ability to study their
expression after introduction into eukaryotic cells has resulted in
major insights being gained into gene function. The oocyte and the
unfertilized egg of X.leavis have been two favoured systems for the
analysis of gene expression and gene replication respectively. In
Xenopus the oocyte and the egg are related yet very different cells.
The oocyte is not active in DNA replication but, when the egg is

'activated', by fertilization or by pricking with a micropipette, rapid chromosomal replication begins. Oocytes are very active in RNA synthesis but, after maturation into eggs, very little RNA is synthesized and active transcription does not resume until fertilized eggs reach mid-blastula. Although very different in transcriptional activity and capacity to replicate their chromosomes both oocytes and eggs contain large amounts of the components, such as ribosomes, histones, and polymerases, which will be needed for rapid development of the early embryo (1). When purified DNA is injected into unfertilized eggs, it replicates semiconservatively (2,3,4) and this provides a model system for studying eucaryotic DNA replication (5). For transcriptional studies genes are usually injected into oocytes rather than unfertilized eggs because there is generally 10 to 20 times more transcription of the injected gene in oocytes (6). Few genes, however, are transcribed with sufficient fidelity to make oocyte injection a suitable functional assay. Thus oocytes do not accurately transcribe the rabbit β-globin genes (7) or the ovalbumin gene (8,9).

        Previous experiments, injecting the Xenopus β1-globin gene into fertilized eggs, showed that the injected gene was transcribed in developing embryos at a low level, but from the correct promoter (10,11). We have now analyzed the expression of the Xenopus β1 globin gene after injection into oocytes and unfertilized eggs. There are major differences between the transcripts produced in the two cell types. The oocyte yields predominantly incorrectly initiated transcripts while in the unfertilized egg the correct promoter is utilized. We also show that, although initiation of transcription in the oocyte occurs with very low fidelity, splicing and poly-adenylation of β1 globin gene transcripts are both accurate and efficient.

RESULTS

Transcription of Xenopus β1-Globin Genes Injected into Oocytes and Unfertilized Eggs of X.laevis

        The Xenopus major adult α- and β-globin genes were injected into oocytes or unfertilized eggs on the recombinant plasmid pXGαβ1 (Fig.1). Approximately 4ng per oocyte or egg was injected, an amount of DNA well below the saturating levels for transcription in oocytes (6) and for chromatin assembly in either oocytes (12) or eggs (13). After incubation, total RNA was extracted from the injected oocytes and eggs and analyzed by primer extension for transcripts of the Xenopus β1-globin gene. When hybridized to RNA from Xenopus adult erythroblasts the primer, which anneals within the first exon of the β1-globin gene, was extended to give two major fragments of 127 and 129 nucleotides in length (Fig.2). These are the sizes expected for correctly initiated transcripts of the X.laevis major adult β-globin gene, which displays heterogeneity in the start point of transcription (14). In RNA from injected oocytes, there

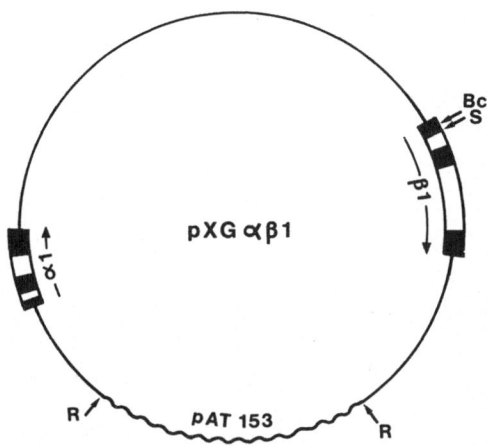

Fig.1.  The restriction map of recombinant plasmid pXGαβ1.  The
        plasmid pXGαβ1 contains the major adult α- and β-globin genes
        of <u>Xenopus</u> <u>laevis</u> on a 14.3Kb EcoRI fragment of genomic DNA.
        Wavy lines represent bacterial plasmid DNA sequences and
        straight lines represent <u>Xenopus</u> genomic DNA sequences. The
        α1- and β1-globin genes are shown as boxes with the filled-in
        portions corresponding to exons and with arrows showing the
        direction of transcription. The symbols used for restriction
        sites are: Bc - BclI, R - EcoRI and S - Sau96.

was an array of extended fragments ranging in size from just
slightly larger than the 52 nucleotide primer to over 500 nucleotides in length (Fig.2). Included within this array, there were
extended fragments of the size predicted for transcripts initiating
from the correct promoter. However these constituted only a minority
of the total extension products. In contrast to the complex pattern
of transcripts found in RNA from oocytes injected with the β1-globin
gene, RNA from unfertilized eggs injected with pXGαβ1 gave only two
major extended fragments which are identical to those observed with
adult erythroblast RNA (Fig.2). Thus in unfertilized eggs, the
injected <u>Xenopus</u> β1-globin gene is accurately transcribed from the
correct promoter but in oocytes the injected β1-globin gene is
inaccurately transcribed with the majority of the transcripts
initiating at incorrect start sites.

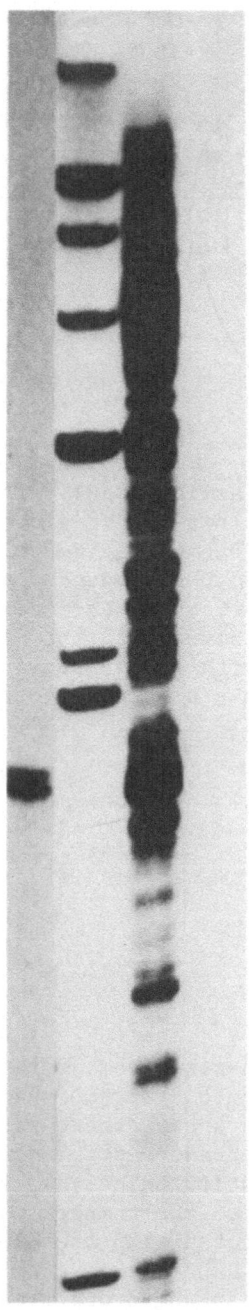

Fig.2. The detection of β1-globin
gene transcripts in
unfertilized eggs and
oocytes. Transcripts were
detected by primer extension
analysis (see Materials and
Methods). The positions of
the two extension products
from correctly initiated
β1-globin gene transcripts
are indicated on the left
of the figure. The sizes of
the pAT153/HinfI fragments
(lane 2) are listed on the
right. Lane 1 is an analysis
of RNA from unfertilized
eggs injected with 4ng of
pXGαβ1 DNA. Lane 3 is an
analysis of RNA from oocytes
injected with 4ng of pXGαβ1
DNA. Lane 4 is a control
using RNA from uninjected
oocytes.

The situation is complicated by the fact that, in oocytes, the ratio of correct versus incorrect transcription of the injected β1-globin gene varied with different batches of oocytes. There was variability from female to female in the total amount of correct transcripts per oocyte as well as variability in the ratio of correct to incorrect transcripts (data not shown). This variability in transcription of the injected genes did not arise from irreproducibility in the amount of DNA injected or from differences in the persistence of the injected DNA. While oocytes from different females vary in their relative ability to transcribe from the correct promoter of the injected β1-globin gene, eggs from different females displayed very little variability, the injected β-globin genes being in all cases transcribed at low levels and exclusively from the normal site of initiation.

The amount of correct transcription of the injected β1-globin gene in oocytes and eggs was estimated by comparing the intensity of the  bands corresponding to extended fragments from correctly initiated transcripts to the intensity of the bands observed with known amounts of control RNA (data not shown). There were from 1 to 20pg of correctly initiated transcripts per three oocytes injected, depending upon the batch of oocytes used, and this represents 0.005 to 0.1 correct transcripts per gene during the 20hr incubation period. Compared with the transcription of some other polymerase II-transcribed genes injected into oocytes, this is a very low level of correct transcription. With the Herpes Simplex Virus (HSV) thymidine kinase (tk) gene (15), a minimum of 3.0 specific transcripts are produced per gene copy per day, and Etkin and Maxson (16) estimated injected sea urchin histone genes to be transcribed at approximately 2.4 transcripts per gene copy per day. We estimate the rate of correct transcription of the β1-globin gene injected into unfertilized eggs to be approximately 2pg of correctly initiated transcripts in 22hr (0.01 transcripts per gene in 22hrs). This represents a low level of transcription which is within the range of correct transcription observed for the β1-globin gene injected into oocytes. Thus the principal difference between transcription of the β1-globin gene in eggs and that in oocytes is that oocytes produce a large number of β1-globin gene transcripts initiated from incorrect start sites in addition to the low level of correctly initiated transcripts.

In order to determine whether the incorrectly initiated transcripts in oocytes were the products of polymerase II or III, oocytes were coinjected with pXGαβ1 DNA and α-amanitin. A low level of α-amanitin (0.2ng/oocyte) abolished nearly all transcription of the β1-globin gene (data not shown) indicating that, in oocytes, polymerase II is responsible for both the incorrect and the correct transcription of the injected β1-globin gene.

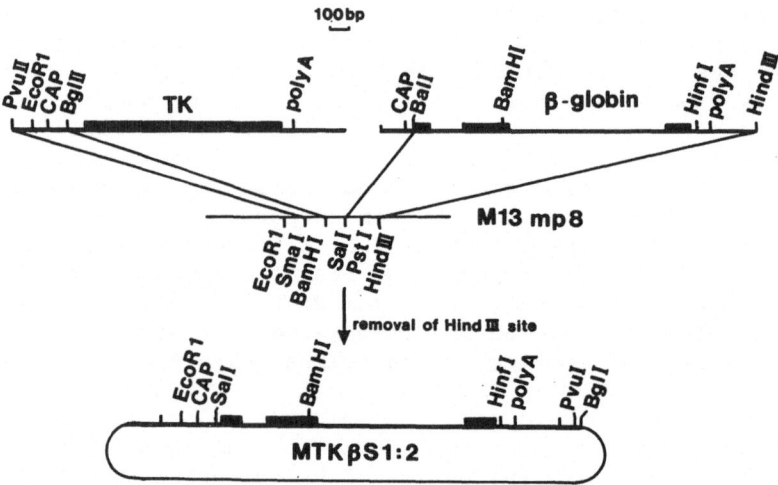

Fig.3.   Construction of a TK/β1-globin fusion gene.  The tk promoter
was fused to the Xenopus laevis β1 globin gene in the vector
M13mp8 to generate pMTK S1 as described in Materials and
Methods. Only those restriction enzyme cleavage sites used
in plasmid construction and in the preparation of S1
nuclease mapping probes are shown.

## Transcripts of a thymdine kinase/β-globin fusion gene are efficiently processed in Xenopus oocytes

The results presented above show that the oocyte yields
predominantly incorrectly initiated transcripts. In order to
determine whether this lack of fidelity extended to RNA processing,
we decided to produce uniformly initiated transcripts of the β1
globin gene in high concentration by construction of a fusion gene.
We joined the β1-globin gene to a promoter known to be active in
oocytes - that of the thymidine kinase (tk) gene from Herpes Simplex
Virus (17). The fusion gene (pMTKβS1:2, abbreviated to pS1:2 hence-
forth) was constructed using the single stranded bacteriophage
M13mp8 as vector (18). In the fusion gene, the bulk of the 5' non-
coding region is from the tk gene but the ATG initiation codon
derives from the Xenopus β1 globin gene (Figure 3).

The fusion gene was injected into germinal vesicles of Xenopus laevis oocytes. After incubation of the oocytes, total nucleic acid was extracted and nuclease S1 mapping was used to analyse the 5' end of the mRNA and splicing of the two introns (data not shown). The results show that the fusion gene is efficiently transcribed. About half of the mRNA molecules have the correct 5' end - the remainder initiating upstream of the tk cap site. The splice at the boundary between intron 1 and exon 2 is made correctly and both splice junctions in intron 2 are processed correctly (data not shown).

We estimate that each injected oocyte contains the equivalent of 0.5-2.5ng of β-globin RNA, i.e. between one tenth and one half of the concentration of tk transcripts found by McKnight et al. (15) after microinjection of a plasmid containing the intact tk gene.

The site of polyadenylation in the β1 globin mRNA has been deduced from the nucleotide sequence adjacent to a segment of the poly(A) tail contained within the cDNA clone pXG8D2 (19,20). The nucleotide sequence of the 3' proximal region of the  1 globin gene is known (14) and the site of polyadenylation is shown in Fig.4. We used a fragment from the β1 globin gene to show that transcripts were correctly polyadenylated and this experiment revealed the

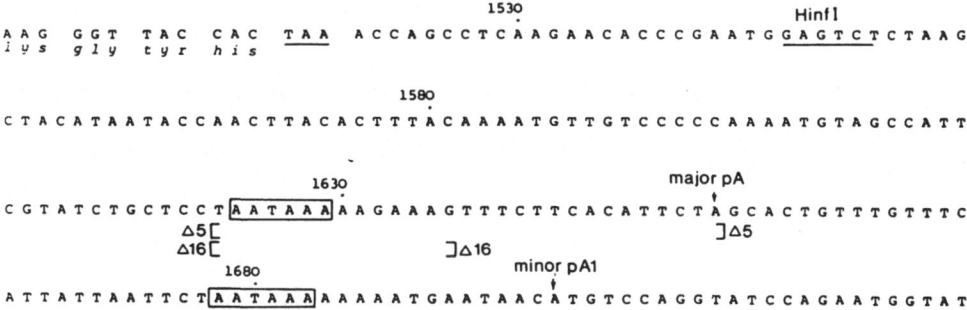

Fig.4.  The nucleotide sequence of the 3' end of the β1 globin gene of Xenopus laevis.  The three AATAAA sequences are boxed and the sites of polyadenylation indicated by the symbol pA. The minor site, pA1, was shown to be 14+1 bases downstream of the AATAAA hexanucleotide, by size determination of the appropriate fragment after S1 mapping and by comparison of the migration of the fragment with a sequencing ladder of the probe run on the same gel. The A residue is arrowed because the site of addition of the poly(A) tail is almost always an A in the genomic sequence. The three A residues at positions 1780-1782 were found to be C residues by Patient et al. (14), but the sequence was derived from the genomic clone λXGαβ103 which is allelic to λXGαβ1. We assume that this difference is a reflection of allelic polymorphism.

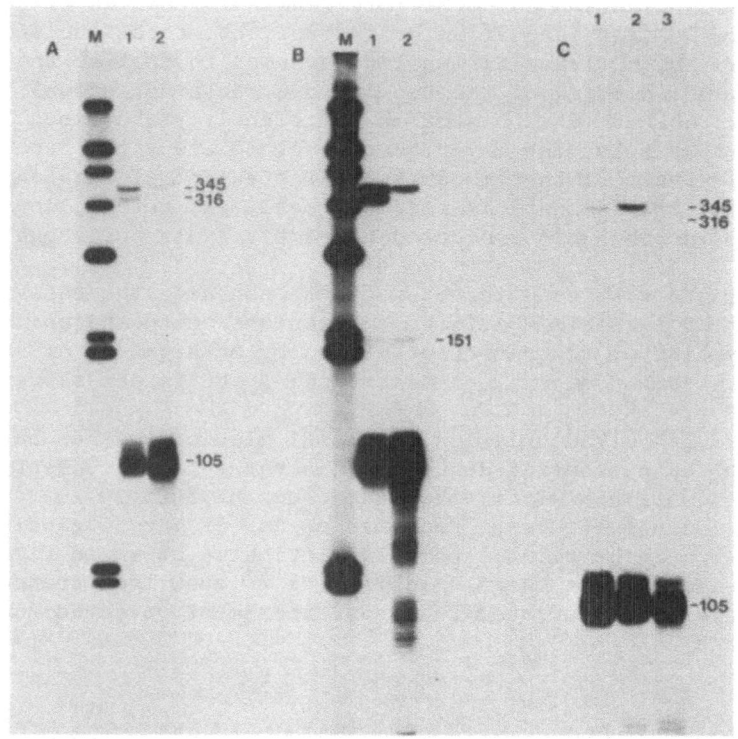

Fig.5.   Nuclease S1 mapping of the 3' end of β-globin RNA from adult
         reticulocytes and of RNA from oocytes injected with pS1:2.
         Nuclease mapping was carried out as described in Materials
         and Methods and the products of the reaction resolved on 7.5%
         denaturing polyacrylamide gels. Normally 2 oocyte equivalents
         of nucleic acid and 5-10ng of single stranded probe (a 345
         base HinfI/EcoRI fragment) were used per reaction. The probe
         was end labelled at the HinfI site (Fig.4) and the coding
         strand was purified by strand separation on a native
         acrylamide gel. This probe is only homologous to the
         injected DNA for a distance of 316 bases from the labelled
         end, hence a band of this size represents either
         "read-through" RNA or hybridization of the probe to the
         injected DNA.
              The RNAs analysed were:
         A and B. Lane 1) Total RNA from oocytes injected with
                              2ng/oocyte of single stranded pS1:2 DNA.
                    Lane 2) 400ng total cytoplasmic RNA from reticulo-
                              cytes of anaemic frogs.
         C. Lane 1) Total RNA from oocytes injected with 4ng/oocyte
                       of double stranded pS1:2 DNA (5ng probe).
            Lane 2) As 1) but with 10ng of probe.
            Lane 3) 250ng total cytoplasmic RNA from frog reticulocytes

Panels A and B are different exposures of the same gel.
This experiment shows the presence of major and minor
polyadenylation sites in adult β-globin RNA and in RNA from
injected oocytes. The band of 316 nucleotides seen in A1
and B1 is mainly due to hybridization of the probe with
residual single stranded DNA, as the band is much weaker
when double stranded DNA is injected (Panel C).
M. Molecular weight markers, a HinfI digest of pAT153.

existence of a minor downstream polyadenylation site which is present
in both reticulocyte RNA and in fusion gene transcripts.

Total cytoplasmic RNA, isolated from erythrocytes of anaemic
animals was used in S1 mapping with a single stranded probe from the
β1 globin gene (Figure 5). The major protected fragments were between
101 and 109 nucleotides in length, which is the approximate size
expected for an RNA processed at the polyadenylation site (19). There
was an additional minor band derived from a fragment of 151 nucleotides in length. We estimate that mRNA processed at this site, which
we term minor site 1, is approximately 100 fold less abundant than
the major species. This minor polyadenylation site lies $14\pm1$ nucleotides downstream from an AATAAA hexanucleotide (Fig.4). Analysis of
RNA extracted from oocytes injected with pS1:2 DNA showed a pattern
very similar to that observed with reticulocyte RNA with the major
and minor RNA species being present in a ratio approximately similar
to that observed with reticulocyte RNA (Fig.5). Chromatography on
oligo dT cellulose showed that both RNA species were polyadenylated
(data not shown).

Replication of the injected DNA

Oocytes and unfertilized eggs were injected with pXGαβ1 DNA
and total nucleic acids were extracted from samples taken
immediately after injection and after incubation for 20 to 22hrs
at 10°C. The amount of pXGαβ1 DNA present in the various samples
was determined by hybridization of $^{32}$P-labelled pAT153 DNA to
nitrocellulose blots of the samples separated on agarose gels
(data not shown). The relative amounts of pXGαβ1 DNA present in the
various samples was determined by liquid scintillation counting of
the appropriate areas of the radioactively labelled filters
(Table 1). The DNA did not replicate in oocytes during the 22hrs
incubation period but 35-50% of the injected DNA persisted 22hrs
after injection. In unfertilized eggs, there was extensive
replication of the DNA. Thus when 4ng was injected there was, within
22hrs, a greater than 6-fold increase in the amount of pXGαβ1 DNA
and when 24ng was injected there was a 1.5-fold increase (Table 1).
The majority of the newly replicated DNA in unfertilized eggs
comigrated with high molecular weight cell DNA (data not shown).
These results are similar to those found in fertilized Xenopus

Table 1.   The replication of pXGαβ1 DNA injected into <u>Xenopus</u>
           oocytes and eggs.

<u>pXGαβ1 DNA (cpm)</u>

Sample time (hrs)          0          22

<u>Oocytes</u>

4ng DNA injected        25,900      3,990

<u>Eggs</u>

4ng DNA injected        35,000     220,000


eggs where the injected DNA replicates and eventually comigrates
with chromosomal DNA (10,11,21,22).


DISCUSSION

    It is not immediately apparent why injected <u>Xenopus</u> globin
genes should be faithfully transcribed from the correct promoters in
unfertilized and fertilized eggs (10,11) and incorrectly transcribed
in oocytes. Eggs are less transcriptionally active than oocytes so
that a variety of genes, injected into unfertilized eggs, produce
10 to 20 times fewer hybridizable transcripts than when injected into
oocytes (6). Thus an overall lower level of transcription of the
injected globin genes in eggs was not surprising. The higher degree
of transcriptional fidelity in eggs was, however, unexpected.

    When DNA is injected into either oocytes or eggs it is
assembled into a chromatin-like structure (13,12,23). Differences in
the properties of chromatin assembled on injected DNA in <u>Xenopus</u>
oocytes and eggs have been observed previously (24). When DNA
containing the <u>Drosophila</u> histone gene repeat was injected into
<u>Xenopus</u> oocytes and eggs the DNA was shown by micrococcal nuclease
and DNaseI digestion to be assembled into chromatin with a 180bp
nucleosome periodicity in oocytes but in eggs the injected DNA
became resistant to both micrococcal nuclease and DNaseI digestion.
Further work from the same laboratory (25) has shown that a proportion of the DNA injected into oocytes adopts an unusual chromatin
conformation and that this 'dynamic' chromatin may be the transcriptionally active form for RNA-polymerase III. Possibly, this
torsionally strained chromatin may also permit the initiation of

transcription by RNA polymerase II in regions other than the
authentic globin gene promoter.

The other major conclusion to derive from this study concerns
the fidelity of RNA processing in oocytes. We have shown that
transcripts from a thymidine kinase/β-globin fusion gene are
accurately spliced and polyadenylated. Correct processing of mRNA
sequences in frog oocytes has been inferred previously from the
detection of the protein product (7,8) but accurate splicing and
polyadenylation by direct RNA analysis has only previously been
demonstrated in the case of oocytes injected with SV40 DNA (26). The
fusion between the tk gene promoter and the β1 globin gene was made
in the 5' non-coding region of both genes and approximately one half
of the stable transcripts initiate at the tk cap site. The remaining
transcripts initiate upstream of the tk promoter. The stable
transcripts we detect are correctly processed hence the 5' non-
coding sequences do not appear to influence RNA processing. When the
recombinant plasmid pS1:2 is transcribed in oocytes a low level of
transcripts are detected which extend to, or beyond, the HindIII
site that lies 210 bases downstream of the major polyadenylation
site. This implies that transcription proceeds beyond this HindIII
site and that there is no transcription termination in this region.
A similar conclusion has also been reached for several viral genes(27,
28) and for the mouse β-globin gene (29).


MATERIALS AND METHODS

Enzymes

Restriction enzymes, T4 DNA ligase, T4 polynucleotide kinase
and the Klenow fragment of DNA polymerase I were purchased from
either New England Biolabs, Inc. (Beverly, Mass.) or from Bethesda
Research Laboratories, Inc. (Gaithersburg, Md.) and were used
according to manufacturers recommendation.

DNA injected

Xenopus oocytes or unfertilized eggs were injected with pXGαβ1
plasmid DNA (Fig.1). This plasmid contains the X.laevis major adult
α- and β-globin genes (α1 and β1) which were originally cloned by
inserting a 14.3Kb EcoRI fragment of X.laevis genomic DNA into a
bacteriophage  vector (30). From λXGαβ1 the 14.3Kb EcoRI fragment
containing the globin genes was recloned into the EcoRI site of the
plasmid vector pAT153 (31). The DNAs used in construction of the
fusion gene were: pHSV106 (17) containing the herpes simplex virus
thymidine kinase (HSVtk) gene and pXG1C3 containing the β1 globin
gene from  XGαβ1 (30) in pAT153 (31) (Figure 4). The 250 base pair
PvuII/BglII fragment containing the HSVtk promoter derived from
plasmid pHSV106 was ligated into SmaI/HindIII cleaved M13mp8 to give

plasmid pMTK4. The BalI/HindIII fragment of pXG1C3 containing the
β-globin gene was purified and ligated into pMTK4 that had been
cleaved with SalI, the ends "filled in" with the Klenow enzyme and
then cleaved with HindIII. The resulting plasmid was designated
pMTKβS1 (abbreviated pS1). This plasmid was cleaved at its unique
HindIII site, the ends "filled in" with the Klenow enzyme and then
religated in order to remove the HindIII site. The resulting plasmid
was designated pMTKβS1:2 and this was used in injection.

## Injection and sample preparation

Ovarian tissue was surgically removed from anaesthetized mature
female X.laevis (Xenopus Ltd., South Nutfield, Surrey), incubated in
$Ca^{2+}$-depleted medium containing 0.2% collagenase (Sigma) for 2hrs at
20° to 22°C, and then gently washed with modified Barth's medium
supplemented with 10μg/ml penicillin and 5μg/ml streptomycin.
Individual stage VI oocytes were selected for injection. In order to
obtain fertilized eggs, mature females were injected with 500IU of
gonadotrophin and 15 to 22 hours later eggs were squeezed out
through the cloaca. The eggs wer decapsulated in 2.0% cysteine
hydrochloride (pH 7.8), washed gently with MMR medium (32) supplemented with penicillin and streptomycin as above, and injected
immediately.

The DNA to be injected was purified by two bandings in CsCl
gradients and dissolved at the desired concentration in injection
buffer (0.1M NaCl, 0.01M Tris, pH 7.5). A volume of 15nl per oocyte
or egg was injected as described by Kressman and Birnstiel (33).
Oocytes were centrifuged prior to injection to bring the nucleus to
the surface where it could be easily visualized. In unfertilized
eggs, the DNA was injected into the cytoplasm because during
maturation of oocytes into eggs, the nuclear membrane disappears.
Injected oocytes or unfertilized eggs were incubated in modified
Barth's medium or MMR medium, respectively, at 18°C. Samples of
10 to 20 oocytes or eggs were taken after the indicated incubation
time and stored at -70°C. Samples were later homogenized in SET
(1% SDS, 5mM EDTA, 10mM Tris, pH 7.5) and treated with proteinase K
(100μg/ml, 37°C, 1hr). Nucleic acids were then isolated by phenol
extraction, chloroform extraction, and ethanol precipitation.

## Analysis of β1 globin gene transcription by primer extension

Transcripts of the X.laevis β1-globin gene were detected by
primer extension as previously described (10). RNA from three
injected oocytes or eggs was hybridized to a molar excess of a
single-stranded primer, a $^{32}$P-labelled 52-nucleotide BclI-Sau96 DNA
fragment derived from the first exon of the β1-globin gene (see
Fig.1). Using reverse transcriptase, the hybridized primers were
extended to the 5'-ends of the β1-globin gene transcripts. The
extension products were analyzed on 10% acrylamide-urea gels.

Correctly initiated X.laevis β1-globin gene transcripts give major
primer-extension products 127 and 129 nucleotides in length (10,
11,14).

Analysis of  1-globin gene transcription by nuclease S1 mapping

Nuclease S1 mapping was performed by the method of Berk and
Sharp (34) and Weaver and Weissmann (35) using single-stranded
probes which were end-labelled.

Analysis of replication

Following injection, oocytes or eggs were immediately transferred to medium (Barth's MMR). The oocytes or eggs were incubated
and samples collected and processed as described. Total DNA from the
equivalent of 0.5 oocytes or eggs was electrophoresed through a
0.8% agarose horizontal slab gel in 0.5x Tris-borate buffer
(0.045M Tris-borate, 0.045M boric acid, 0.001M EDTA) at 5.5V/cm for
4 hours. After electrophoresis, DNAs in the gel were depurinated,
denatured, transferred onto nitrocellulose membranes, and hybridized
to pAT153 DNA which was $^{32}$P-labelled by nick-translation. To obtain
quantitative results, areas of the filter hybridizing to the pAT153
DNA were cut out and radioactivity measured by liquid scintillation
counting.

REFERENCES

1.    J.B. Gurdon, "Control of Gene Expression in Animal Development,"
         Clarendon, Oxford (1974).
2.    C.C. Ford and H.R. Woodland, Dev. Biol. 48:189 (1975).
3.    J.B. Gurdon, M.L. Birnstiel and V.A. Speight, Biochim. Biophys.
         Acta 174:614 (1969).
4.    R.A. Laskey and J.B. Gurdon, Eur. J. Biochem. 37:467 (1973).
5.    R.M. Harland and R.A. Laskey, Cell 21:761 (1980).
6.    J.E. Mertz and J.B. Gurdon, Proc. Natl. Acad. Sci. U.S.A.
         74:1502 (1977).
7.    D. Rungger, P.D. Mathias and J.P. Huber, Transcription of
         complex structural genes in the Xenopus oocyte system,
         in: "International Cell Biology 1980-1981," H.G. Schweiger,
         ed., Springer Verlag, Berlin (1981).
8.    M.P. Wickens, S. Woo, B.W. O'Malley and J.B. Gurdon, Nature
         (London) 285:628 (1980).
9.    J.B. Gurdon and D.A. Melton, Ann. Dev. Genet. 16:189 (1981).
10.   M.M. Bendig and J.G. Williams, Proc. Natl. Acad. Sci. U.S.A.
         80:6197 (1983).
11.   M.M. Bendig and J.G. Williams, Mol. Cell Biol. 4:567 (1984).
12.   A.H. Wyllie, R.A. Laskey, J. Finch and J.B. Gurdon, Dev. Biol.
         64:178 (1978).
13.   R.A. Laskey, B.M. Honda, A.D. Mills, M.R. Morris, A.H. Wyllie,
         J.E. Hertz, E.M. DeRobertis and J.B. Gurdon, Cold Spring

Harbor Symp. Quant. Biol. 42:171 (1978).

14. R.K. Patient, R. Harris, M.E. Walmsley and J.G. Williams,
    J. Biol. Chem. 258:8521 (1983).
15. S.L. McKnight, E.R. Gavis and R. Kingsbury, Cell 25:385 (1981).
16. L.D. Etkin and R.E. Maxson Dev. Biol. 75:13 (1980).
17. S.L. McKnight and E.R. Gavis, Nucleic Acids Res. 24:5931 (1980).
18. J. Messing, New M13 vectors for cloning, in: Methods in
    Enzymology, Vol 101, R. Wu, L. Grossman and K. Moldave
    eds., Academic Press, New York (1983).
19. R.M. Kay, R. Harris, R.K. Patient and J.G. Williams, Nucleic
    Acids Res. 8:2691 (1980).
20. J.G. Williams, R.M. Kay and R.K. Patient, Nucleic Acids Res.
    8:4247 (1980).
21. M.M. Bendig, Nature (London) 292:65 (1981).
22. S. Rusconi and W. Schaffner, Proc. Natl. Acad. Sci. U.S.A.
    78:5051 (1981).
23. T. Igo-Kemenes, W. Horz and H.G. Zachau, Chromatin Ann. Rev.
    Biochem. 51:89 (1982).
24. G. Garguilo, W. Wasserman and A. Worcel, Cold Spring Harobor
    Symp. Quant. Biol. 47:549 (1983).
25. M. Ryoji and A. Worcel, Cell 37:21 (1984).
26. M.P. Wickens and J.B. Gurdon, J. Mol. Biol. 163:1 (1983).
27. J.P. Ford and M.-T. Hsu, J. Virol. 28:795 (1978).
28. J.R. Nevins, J.-M. Blanchard and J.E. Darnell, Jr, J. Mol.
    Biol. 144:377 (1980).
29. E. Hofer, R. Hofer-Warkinek and J.E. Darnell, Jr, Cell 29:887
    (1982).
30. R.K. Patient, J.A. Elkington, R.M. Kay and J.G. Williams, Cell
    21:565 (1980).
31. A.J. Twigg and D. Sherratt, Nature (London) 283:216 (1980).
32. S.J. Busby and R.H. Reeder, Dev. Biol. 91:458 (1982).
33. A. Kressmann and M.L. Birnstiel, Surrogate genetics in the frog
    oocyte, in: "Transfer of Cell Constituents into Eukaryotic
    Cells," J.E. Celis, A. Grassman and A. Loyter, eds.,
    Plenum Press, New York (1980).
34. A.J. Berk and P.A. Sharp, Cell 12:721 (1977).
35. R.F. Weaver and C. Weissman, Nucleic Acids Res. 7:1175 (1979).

# EXPRESSION OF CLONED MUSCLE-SPECIFIC GENES IN TRANSFECTED CELLS AND TRANSGENIC MICE

David Yaffe, Uri Nudel, Moshe Shani, Danielle Melloul,
Batya Aloni, Yitzhak Mayer and David Greenberg

Department of Cell Biology
The Weizmann Institute of Science
Rehovot 76100
Israel

## SUMMARY

The control of expression of muscle-specific genes introduced into myogenic cells and transgenic mice was studied. The expression of chimeric genes containing the 5' regions and flanking DNA of the genes coding for rat skeletal muscle actin and myosin light chain 2 was greatly increased during differentiation of stably transfected myogenic clones and in transiently transfected myogenic cells. Likewise, the expression of the chicken skeletal muscle actin gene was developmentally regulated in several stably transfected rat myogenic clones, indicating that the mechanisms controlling muscle-specific gene expression have been conserved for at least 300 million years. In contrast, the expression of a fused mouse/human $\beta$-globin gene, and of a chimeric gene containing the 5' region and flanking cDNA of the rat $\beta$-actin gene did not increase during differentiation of transfected myogenic clones. The expression of the rat MLC2 gene was tissue-specific and developmentally regulated in transgenic mice.

DNA sequence comparison reveals a high degree of sequence homology in the 5' flanking regions as well as in the 3' untranslated region between genes coding for homologous (isotypic) proteins in distantly related organisms. These sequences may be involved in the control of the tissue-specific expression of these genes.

## INTRODUCTION

During the differentiation of myogenic cells in culture, mononucleated myoblasts cease dividing, fuse and form multinucleated fibers. The transition from the proliferative state to cell fusion can be controlled by cell density and nutritional medium. Cell fusion is temporally correlated with a rapid accumulation of muscle-specific mRNAs and the synthesis of muscle-specific proteins. Using the myogenic cell line L8, it has been shown that during this transition the genes coding for myosin light chain 2 and skeletal muscle actin become preferentially sensitive to DNAase I, indicating a change in their transcriptional activity (Carmon et al., 1982). It was also found that the genes coding for myosin heavy chain, myosin light chain 2, skeletal muscle actin and cardiac actin are located on different chromosomes; thus the expression of these genes is not mediated by the activation of a single chromatin domain (Czosnek et al., 1982, 1983).

The possibility of cloning tissue-specific genes and of introducing them back into somatic cells or into the germ line now enables investigation into the control network of gene expression during terminal differentiation at the DNA and chromatin levels. In the present communication we demonstrate that the expression of cloned chimeric genes containing only the 5' flanking region of muscle-specific genes is developmentally regulated when introduced into myogenic cells. The results reveal that the 5' regions of two muscle specific genes contain sufficient information to confer stage- and tissue-specific expression of the genes in myogenic cells. We also show that the expression of a muscle-specific gene is tissue-specific and developmentally regulated following its introduction into the germ line.

EXPRESSION OF CHIMERIC GENES CONTAINING SKELETAL MUSCLE ACTIN OR MYOSIN LIGHT CHAIN 2 DNA SEQUENCES IN TRANSFECTED MYOGENIC CELLS.

We have reported previously on the isolation and the sequencing of the skeletal muscle actin gene and of the fast muscle myosin light chain 2 (MLC2) gene (Zakut et al., 1982; Nudel et al., 1984a). In order to study the control of expression of these genes following their introduction into myogenic cells and to be able to distinguish between the products of the introduced genes and the native genes, we have constructed and used for transfection a number of chimeric genes containing the 5' region of the muscle genes. Part of this work has been described elsewhere and will be reported here briefly (Melloul et al., 1984; Nudel et al., 1984b; Nudel et al., 1985a).

A chimeric gene containing about 2/3 of the skeletal muscle actin gene plus 730 bp of the 5' flanking region spliced to the 3' region of a human $\varepsilon$-globin gene (Fig. 1) was introduced into myogenic cells by cotransfection with a gene conferring neomycin resistance (plasmid pIPB1). Cells were grown in medium containing the neomycin derivative G418 and myogenic clones resistant to the drug were isolated and grown

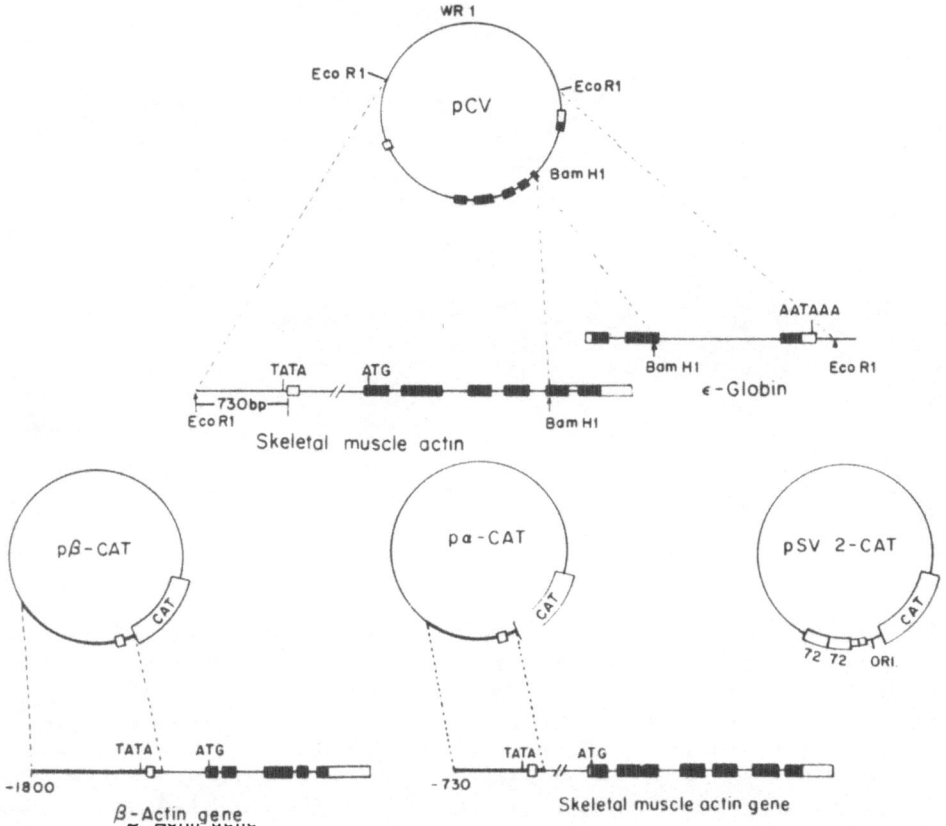

Fig. 1 The structure of the chimeric genes used for transfection.
The plasmid pCV contains a fused rat skeletal muscle actin/
human ε-globin gene (plus 730 bp 5' flanking sequences of the
actin gene and 172 bp 3' flanking sequences of the globin
gene). The plasmids pα-CAT, pβ-CAT and pSV2-CAT contain the
promoter regions of rat skeletal muscle actin gene, the rat
cytoplasmic β-actin gene, and the promoter-enhancer region
of SV40 DNA, respectively, spliced to the bacterial, (CAT)
gene. For more details see Melloul et al., (1984).

into mass cultures. Differentiation was induced by changing the
nutritional medium as described elsewhere (Melloul et al., 1984). In
the majority of the isolated clones the expression of the chimeric
gene increased many-fold during the process of cell differentiation
and formation of multinucleated fibers (Table 1). Furthermore, the
rapid accumulation of the chimeric gene transcripts was closely
correlated with the accumulation of the endogenous skeletal muscle
actin gene transcript, suggesting that the two genes respond to the
same transacting control signals (Melloul et al., 1984). Similar
results were obtained with a chimeric gene containing only the 730 bp

Table 1.  Expression of actin/globin gene in transfected cells

| Clone No. | Copy number of actin/globin gene | Expression* | | Induction fold |
|---|---|---|---|---|
| | | Mononucleated | Fibers | |
| 46 | 25-50 | 0.1 -0.3 | 3-10 | 50-80 |
| 36 | 10-20 | 0.05-0.2 | 2- 3 | 20-40 |
| 1 | N.D. | 0.05-0.1 | >1 | >20 |
| 51 | 2-3 | 0.02-0.05 | 0.1-0.2 | 5-20 |
| 8 | >500 | U.D. | 0.2-0.05 | >3 |
| 49 | 3- 5 | 0.1 -0.2 | 0.3-0.6 | 2- 6 |
| 47 | 3- 5 | U.D. | 0.05-0.1 | >3 |
| 33 | 1- 2 | U.D. | U.D. | |
| 20 | 1- 2 | U.D. | U.D. | |

* An estimation based on the intensity of bands formed on the
fluorograms of the endonuclease S1 analysis of the transcription
products, given in arbitrary units. 1 = the intensity of the
bands formed by the probe protected by the native muscle actin
mRNA in differentiated cultures of the same clone.  The numbers
indicate the range of values obtained in several experiments.
The range of fold of induction includes values obained also by
using the ε-globin derived DNA probe. (from Melloul et al., 1984)
U.D. undetectable
N.D. not determined

of 5' flanking DNA and the first untranslated exon of the actin gene
(plus 20 bp of the first intron) spliced to the bacterial structural
gene coding for chloramphenicol acetyl transferase (CAT), as described
in Fig. 1.  With this construct, up to 100-fold increase in CAT
activity during differentiation was observed (Fig. 2).  The temporal
relationship between cell fusion and increase in CAT activity was very
similar to that of the native muscle-specific creatine kinase (Fig.
3).

Another chimeric gene was constructed, containing 1.2 kb of the
5' flanking region of MLC2 gene spliced to the CAT gene as described
in Fig. 4.  The expression of this gene in myogenic cells was also
developmentally regulated (Fig. 2).

In contrast, high levels of constitutive CAT activity, with no
increase occurring with cell differentiation, were observed when cells
were transfected with a construct containing the 5' region of the non

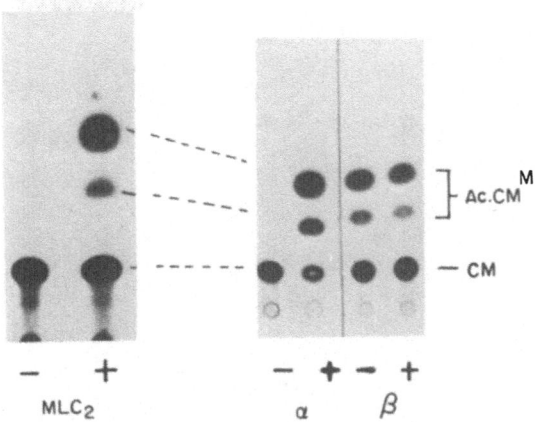

Fig. 2  Expression of pMLC-CAT (MLC), pα-CAT (α) and pβ-CAT (β) in
stably transfected L8 cells.  L8 cells were transfected with
the plasmids pMLC-CAT, pα-CAT or pβ-CAT as described in the
text and in Melloul et al., (1984).  After the selection with
G-418 clones of each experimental group were pooled (20-50
clones in each pool) and grown to confluency.  Cell extracts
were prepared from undifferentiated cultures (-) and
differentiated cultures containing multinucleated fibers (+).
CAT was assayed as described in Melloul et al., (1984).  The
$^{14}$C-chloramphenicol (CM) was separated from its acetylated
forms (AcCM) by thin layer chromatography and the thin layer
plate was autoradiographed.

muscle β-actin gene spliced to the CAT gene (Figs 1 and 2, Melloul et
al., 1984).

These results indicate that the 5' regions of the skeletal muscle
actin gene and the MLC2 gene used for the construction of the chimeric
gene contain DNA sequences which are sufficient to specify the differentiation associated expression of the two genes.  The results,
however, do not exclude the existence of additional DNA sequences at
other regions of the genes which may play a role in the
developmentally regulated expression of the native genes.  Indications
for the existence of such regulatory sequences in the β-globin gene
have been reported recently (Wright et al., 1985; Charnay et al.,
1985; see also Melloul et al., 1984, for further discussion).

The experiments described above were done with stably transfected
clones in which the transferred genes were integrated into the host
cell genome.  To exclude possible effects of host neighbouring DNA
sequences at the site of integration on the expression of the
transferred genes, we studied their expression in transient
transfection assays.  In these experiments the efficiency of

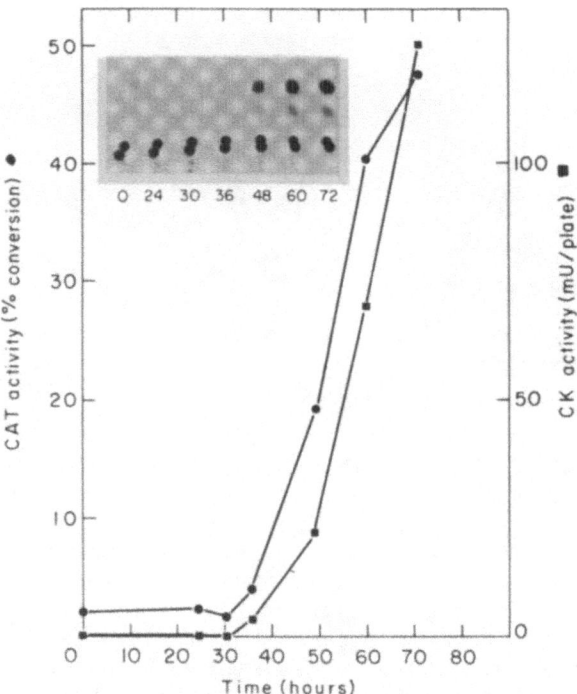

Fig. 3   Kinetics of accumulation of CAT (o) and CK (■) activity during
         differentiation of a myogenic clone stably transfected with
         the plasmid pα-CAT.   At zero time, cultures were stimulated to
         differentiate by changing the medium to a fusion-permissive
         medium.   Cell extracts were prepared at the indicated times,
         and CAT activity and creatine kinase activity were measured.
         The insert shows the autoradiogram of the thin layer chroma-
         tographic plate used in the CAT assay.   Cell fusion started
         about 30 h after the change of medium. (From Nudel et al.,
         1984b).

expression of several chimeric genes in nonmuscle cells and in
undifferentiated and differentiated L8 cells was assayed.   3T3 cells,
cultures of L8 mononucleated cells or differentiating L8 cultures were
transfected with the appropriate plasmid, harvested 24 h later and

assayed for CAT activity.  We found that pβ-CAT and pSV-CAT (CAT
structural gene controlled by an SV40 promoter and enhancer; Fig. 1)
are efficiently transcribed in 3T3 and in L8 cells.  In contrast, pα
-CAT is efficiently transcribed only in differentiated L8 cells.
These results demonstrate that the tissue- and stage-specific
expression of the transferred muscle genes does not depend on the
integration of the genes into the host chromosomes (Nudel et al.,
1985b).

    To study in more detail the structure of the control region, we
constructed a number of derivatives of the chimeric gene in which
deletions were introduced in the fragments derived from the 5'
flanking region of MLC2 and the actin genes. Preliminary results
indicate that the expression of chimeric genes containing only the
first 125 bp of the MLC2 5' flanking region is developmentally
regulated (Greenberg et al., unpublished).


THE EXPRESSION OF CHICKEN SKELETAL MUSCLE ACTIN GENE IN RAT MYOGENIC
CELLS IS DEVELOPMENTALLY REGULATED

    To determine whether the DNA sequences specifying the develop-
mentally regulated expression of the skeletal muscle actin gene are
evolutionarily conserved, we transfected cells of the line L8 with a
recombinant plasmid containing the chicken skeletal muscle actin gene
(in collaboration with C. Ordahl).  Myogenic clones containing this
gene were isolated and grown to mass cultures.  RNA was extracted from
undifferentiated cultures containing only proliferating mononucleated
cells and differentiated cultures containing multinucleated fibers.
The presence of chicken actin mRNA was assayed by the S1 endonuclease
mapping technique.  In the majority of the clones the amount of
chicken actin mRNA increased during differentiation (Nudel et al.,
1985a; Table 2).

    To test whether the increase in amounts of chicken actin mRNA in
differentiated myogenic cells was determined by conserved DNA
sequences specific for muscle gene expression, we investigated the
expression in myogenic cells of a cloned gene which is programmed to
be expressed during terminal differentiation of another tissue.  It
has been shown that the expression of a mouse/human β -globin chimeric
gene and of human β -globin gene introduced into mouse erythroleukemic
cells increased greatly after DMSO-induced differentiation (Chao et
al., 1983).  This plasmid was co-transfected with the plasmid pIBP1
(containing the neomycin resistance marker gene) into L8 cell cultures
and 11 neomycin resistant clones were isolated.  RNA was extracted
from undifferentiated and differentiated cultures.  The presence of β -
globin mRNA was assayed by S1 endonuclease mapping and by dot blot
hybridization.  In 8 out of 9 clones in which the gene was expressed
the amount of β-globin mRNA decreased during differentiation.  In one
clone a 2-fold increase in the amount of β -globin transcripts was
observed.

Table 2.  Expression of the chicken skeletal muscle actin
          gene in transfected rat myogenic cells.

| Clone No No. | Gene copy No. | Induction (fold) |
|---|---|---|
| 1a | 200-400 | 21.5 |
| 7a | 3-6 | 12.7 |
| 4c | 4-8 | 7.3 |
| 1d | 1-3 | 4.5 |
| 2a | 40-80 | 4.4 |
| 6b | 150-300 | 3.4 |
| 6a | 10-20 | 1.81 |
| 1b | 4-8 | 1.44 |
| 5b | 30-60 | 1.29 |
| 3a | 2-4 | U.D.* |
| 3b | 2-4 | U.D.* |

* U.D. = chicken actin mRNA was undetectable in undifferentiated
and differentiated cultures.
The transferred gene copy number was estimated from Southern blot
analysis of DNA extracted from each clone.  The amount of the
chicken actin gene transcript in undifferentiated and differentiated cultures of each of the clones was determined by endonuclease S1 analysis and by dot blot hybridization.  Induction
(fold) is the ratio between the amounts of chicken skeletal
muscle actin mRNA sequences in RNA prepared from differentiated
and undifferentiated cultures, (from Nudel et al., 1985a).

    These results indicate that the increase in expression of the
chicken skeletal muscle actin gene following differentiation of the
rat myogenic cells, is a specific response of a gene expressed during
myogenesis, and not a response to nonspecific changes associated with
terminal differentiation.  The regulated expression of the chicken
muscle gene in the rat myogenic cells demonstrated that the control
mechanisms have been conserved for at least 300 million years (the
divergence time between avians and mammals) (Nudel et al., 1985a).

    Comparison of the expression of the rat muscle actin/globin
chimeric gene with that of the chicken muscle actin gene reveals that
some clones containing the rat actin/globin chimeric gene showed a
greater differentiation associated increase in the amount of the
foreign gene transcripts than the increase in foreign gene transcripts
observed in differentiating cells containing the chicken muscle actin

gene (Tales 1 and 2).  The proportion of clones showing constitutive
expression of the transferred chicken actin gene was higher than in
the clones that contained the rat gene (data not shown).  This might
well be a statistical fluctuation.  However it is also possible that
although DNA sequences in the chick actin gene region involved in the
developmentally regulated expression interact with transacting factors
produced in the differentiating rat muscle cells, the interaction of
the presumptive chicken control DNA sequence with the rat muscle
cellular environment is not as efficient as that of the rat skeletal
muscle actin gene.


HIGHLY CONSERVED SEQUENCES IN THE 5' FLANKING REGION OF MUSCLE-
SPECIFIC GENES

    The rate of accumulation of spontaneous mutations in neutral DNA
sequences was estimated to be in the order of 0.5 - 1% per 1 million
years (MY).  A significant deviation from this rate indicates an
evolutionary constraint to conserve, or to change, the sequence.
Since the divergence time between chicken and rat is ca. 300 MY, the
expected homology between sequences which have no selective pressure
is about 25% (i.e., as the homology between unrelated DNA sequences)
The regulated expression of the chick skeletal muscle actin gene in a
significant number of transfected rat myogenic clones suggested the
conservation of DNA sequences involved in the regulation of expression
of the actin gene.  Sequence comparison indeed reveals a considerable
sequence homology between the two actin genes in the 5' flanking
regions.  Four blocks of highly conserved sequences are found in the
region extending from nucleotide -80 to nucleotide -230 (Nudel et al.,
1985a).

    Comparison of the nucleotide sequences of the 5' region of the
rat and human MLC2 gene showed that the region between the cap site
and ca. 200 bp upstream is highly conserved (>80% homology).  However,
no obvious sequence homology has been found in this region between the
rat skeletal muscle actin gene and the MLC2 gene except for a 100%
homology in a sequence of 12 nucleotides which included the TATAAA
box and 6 nucleotides upstream (Nudel et al., 1984a and unpublished).
The significance of the conservation of this sequence is being tested.


SEQUENCE CONSERVATION IN THE 3' UNTRANSLATED REGION

    Another interesting finding resulting from sequence comparison
was the existence of a very high degree of sequence homology in the 3'
untranslated regions (3'UTR) between mRNAs coding for isotypic actins
in distantly related vertebrates (e.g., rat and chicken β-actin (Yaffe
et al., 1985), human and rat cardiac actin (Mayer et al., 1984 and
Fig. 5), but not between the 3' UTRs of mRNAs coding for very similar
actins, which differ in their mode of expression (e.g. skeletal muscle

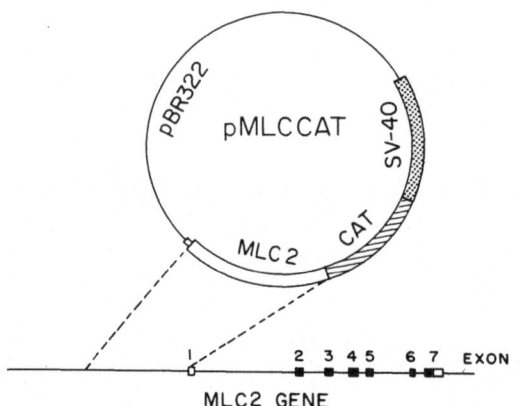

Fig. 4    The structure of plasmid pMLCCAT.  pMLCCAT consists of a 1210
          bp long DNA fragment of the 5' flanking sequences of rat MLC2
          gene (from the HindIII site at position -1206 to the Hinf1
          site at position +4 (Nudel et al., 1984a)) inserted into the
          BgIII site of the plasmid pCAT-3N (obtained from P. Gruss).
          The plasmid pCAT-3N is a CAT expression vector containing the
          coding region of the bacterial CAT gene, the SV40 T antigen
          intron and poly (A) addition signal, pBR322 sequences and
          polylinker (thin open bar).  In the scheme of the MLC2 gene
          exons containing untranslated and translated regions are
          presented by open and black bars, respectively.

and cardiac actins; Mayer et al., 1984).  Surveying and analysing the
published data on other genes revealed a similar pattern of homology
in a number of genes coding for non-muscle proteins (Fig. 6).

     Furthermore, it was noted that while there was a great varia-
bility in the size of the 3' UTRs, even in the same gene family, mRNAs
coding for isotypic proteins in distantly related organisms usually
have 3' UTRs of a similar size.  These observations suggest the
involvement of 3' UTR in transcriptional or post transcriptional
regulation of expression of these genes (Yaffe et al., 1985).
Experiments are now being conducted to examine the possible role of
the 3' UTR in the regulation of expression of muscle-specific genes.


THE EXPRESSION OF MUSCLE-SPECIFIC GENES IN TRANSGENIC MICE.

     Although the experiments described above showed developmentally

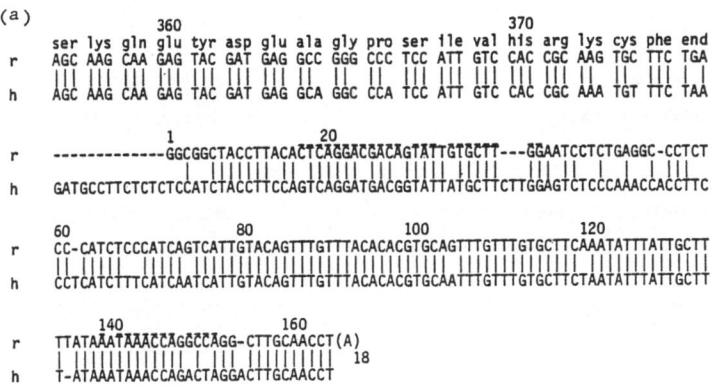

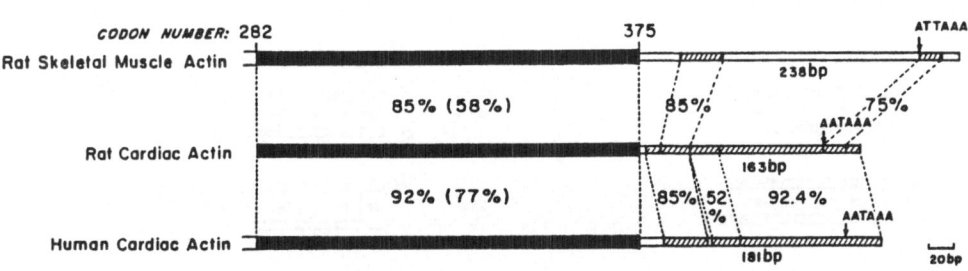

Fig. 5   (a) Sequence homology between the 3' UTRs of rat (r) and human
         (h) cardiac actin mRNA.   The numbering of the amino acid
         sequence (above) is according to Vanderkerckhove and Weber
         (1979).   Identical nucleotides are marked by vertical dashes.
         Sequences which share high homology also with sequences in the
         3' UTR of skeletal muscle actin mRNA are marked with
         horizontal dashed lines.

         (b) Schematic presentation of sequence homologies in the 3'
         regions between rat and human cardiac actin genes and rat
         skeltal muscle and cardiac actin genes.   Heavy solid bars,
         coding regions; thin bars, 3' untranslated regions.   Thin
         dashed lines connect regions that show sequence homology; the
         percentage of homology between these regions is indicated.
         The homology in the silent sites in the coding region is given
         in parentheses.   Empty bars, no significant homology was
         found. (From Mayer et al., 1984).

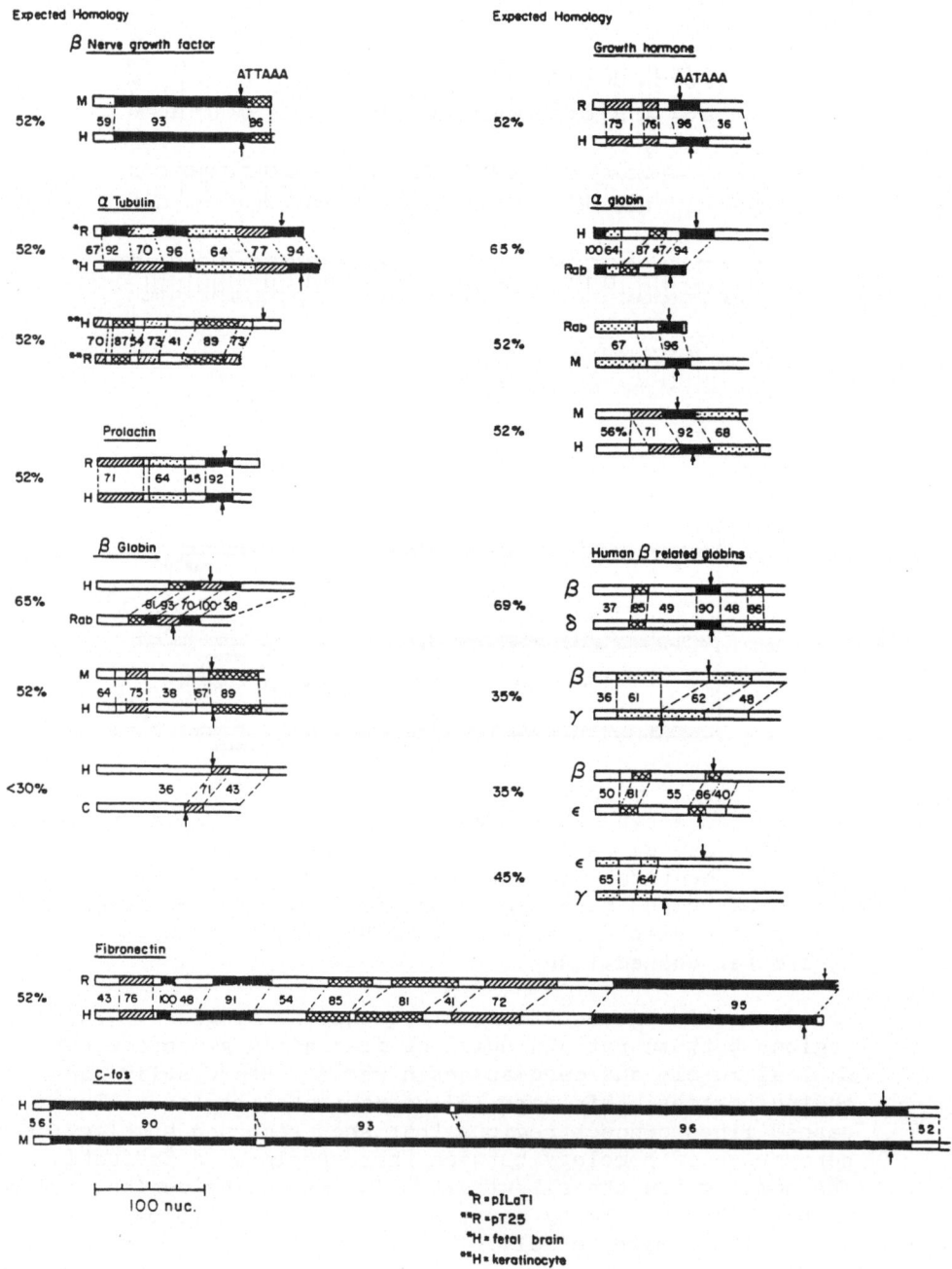

Expected Homology
β Nerve growth factor

Expected Homology
Growth hormone

Fig. 6  A schematic representation of sequence homologies in the 3'
◄──────  untranslated region between evolutionarily related genes.

    Thin dashed lines connect regions that show sequence homology
and the percentage of homology between the regions is
indicated (only when the homology is >30%).  The arrows
indicate the polyadenylation signals; the poly(A) addition
sites are 20-30 nucleotides downstream from the polyadenylation signal.  Bars describing data derived from cDNA clones
are closed in the 3' end while bars describing data from
genomic clones are open in the 3' end.  The numbers to the
left indicate the expected homology between neutral sequences
which had been diverged at the time of divergence between each
pair of genes.  The rate of divergence of neutral sequences is
about 1% per million years.  The calculation of expected
homology for neutral sequences includes a correction for
multiple changes.  The estimated divergence times between the
compared genes are as follows:  man/rodent 75 my;  man/rabbit
46 my;  mouse/rabbit 75 my;  mammals/birds 300 my.  The
divergence times between the various human β-type globins were
taken from Efstratiadis et al. (1980) and are as follows:
β/γ, ε, 200 my;  δ/ε, 100 my;  β/δ, 40 my.  The sources of the
data were indicated in Yaffe et al. (1985)

regulated expression determined by DNA sequences in the 5' region of
the two muscle specific genes, there are several reasons to suspect
that by introducing the cloned genes into somatic cells, we circumvent
important processes taking place early in development, which are
involved in the programing of expression of these genes.  Thus, for
example, in most cases, small amounts of the transcripts of the
introduced genes are detected before differentiation or in cells in
which the expression of the native gene is undetectable (Chao et al.,
1983; Melloul et al., 1984; Kurtz et al., 1981; Nudel et al., 1985a).
It is therefore important to compare the expression of genes
introduced into somatic cells with their expression following
introduction into the germ line, where the genes are exposed to all
developmental stages.  Moreover, this system allows the comparison of
the expression of the gene in different tissues following a single
integration event.

    To investigate the regulation of expression of cloned muscle-
specific genes following their introduction into the germ line, a
recombinant plasmid containing the rat skeletal muscle MLC2 gene
including 1.2 kb of its 5' flanking region and about 0.8 kb of its 3'
flanking DNA (Nudel et al., 1984a and Fig. 4) was injected into
fertilized mouse eggs, which were then implanted back into pseudo-
pregnant females and allowed to develop.  Four transgenic mice were
obtained (designated MLC/1, MLC/2, MLC/3 and MLC/4) containing about
20, 10 <1 and 16 copies of the rat gene, respectively.  When mice

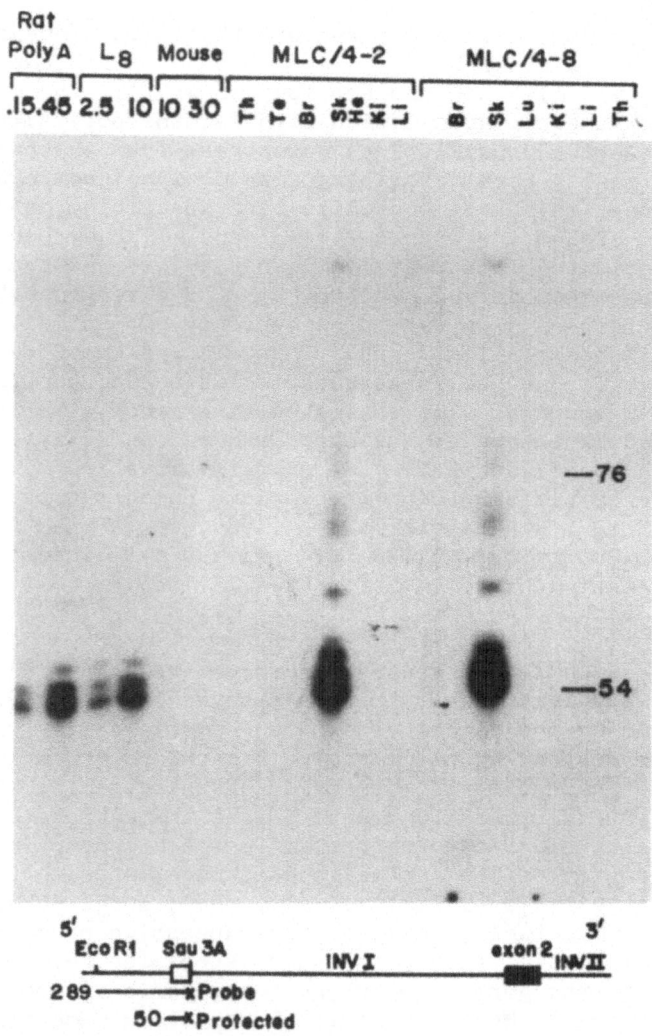

Fig. 7 Expression of the rat MLC2 gene in skeletal muscle and other
tissues of 2 of the offspring of transgenic mouse MLC/4.
Total RNA (20 μg) from the indicated tissues, and the
indicated amounts of total RNA from mouse skeletal muscle,
differentiated cultures of the rat myogenic cell line L8, or
poly (A) RNA of rat skeletal muscle were hybridized with 5'-
end labelled Sau3A-EcoR1 DNA fragments (see scheme, bottom
part). Thy, thymus; Te, testes; Br, brain; Sk, skeletal
muscle; He, cardiac muscle; Ki, kidney; Li, liver; Lu, lung

After treatment with S1 nuclease, the resistant hybrids were
sized on a 6% polyacrylamide/7 M urea gel. Bottom part: map
of the 5' region of the rat MLC2 gene and the probe used for
the hybridisation. Open box: The 5' untranslated exon.
Solid box: the first coding exon. The lengths of the probe
and the protected fragment are indicated. The labelled 3' end
of the probe is indicated by an asterisk. (From Shani and
Yaffe, 1985).

---

MLC/1, MLC/2 and MLC/4 were bred with normal mice, the gene was
transmitted to about 50% of their offspring, indicating the integration of the genes into a single chromosomal site. This conclusion
was also supported by Southern blot analysis of DNA taken from these
mice. The fourth mouse, MLC/3, which did not transmit the rat DNA to
any of its 60 first offspring, seems to be a mosaic mouse (Shani,
1985).

To investigate the mode of expression of the rat MLC2 gene in the
transgenic mice, RNA was extracted from muscle and from several other
tissues of offspring of transgenic mice MLC/1, MLC/2 and MLC/4. The
presence of rat MLC2 transcripts in the RNA preparation was determined
by S2 endonuclease mapping analysis, using as a probe a DNA fragment
derived from the 5' untranslated exon of the rat gene. No rat
transcripts could be detected in RNA prepared from skeletal muscle or
any of the other tissues of transgenic mouse MLC/1. However, in the
offspring of mice MLC/2 and MLC/4, rat transcripts were detected in
skeletal muscle but not in RNA prepared from thymus, testes, brain,
heart, lung, kidney and liver. The relative amounts of the rat MLC2
transcripts found in the skeletal muscle of the offspring of
transgenic mice MLC/2 and MLC/4 were about 0.02 and 2 to 4 times,
respectively, those found in rat skeletal muscle. Figure 7 shows the
S1 analysis of RNA prepared from several tissues of two offspring of
the transgenic mouse MLC/4. The S1 analysis also demonstrates the
correct initiation of transcription (Shani 1985).

We have previously shown that in proliferating rat myoblasts
there are undetectable levels of MLC2 mRNA, and that the main increase
in the amount of this mRNA occurs during the stage of cell fusion
(Yablonka and Yaffe, 1977; Shani et al., 1981). To test whether the
introduced gene is expressed specifically in differentiated cells,
primary skeletal muscle cultures were prepared from the homozygous
progeny of transgenic mouse MLC/2. RNA was isolated from proliferating mononucleated myoblasts and from differentiated cultures harvested
at early and advanced stages of formation of multinucleated fibers and
assayed for the presence of rat MLC2 transcripts using the S1
analysis. No rat MLC2 mRNA was detected in cultures consisting mostly
of mononucleated cells. However, increasing amounts of this mRNA were
found in differentiating cultures containing multinucleated fibers,
demonstrating that the expression of the introduced rat gene is stage-

specific. The expression of the MLC2 gene in the two transgenic mouse strains which expressed the gene seemed to be more stringently controlled than the expression of the other muscle gene constructs which were tested by transfecting myogenic cells. It is of importance to compare the expression of cloned genes which are developmentally regulated in transgenic mice with the expression of the same gene constructs in stably transfected myogenic cells.

Recently we have microinjected into fertilized mouse eggs the actin/globin chimeric gene. As described above, the expression of this gene was developmentally regulated when introduced into myogenic L8 cells (Melloul et al., 1984). Out of 36 mice born, 5 transgenic mice were identified. The number of copies of the inserted DNA was estimated at 15, 8, 8 and 4 copies per cell for mice CV/1, CV/2, CV/3 and CV/4 respectively. The fifth mouse (CV/5) carried an incomplete plasmid.

The presence of the chimeric gene transcripts in the offspring of transgenic mice CV/1-4 was determined by the S1 endonuclease mapping, using as a probe a 187 bp DdeI DNA fragment derived from the human $\varepsilon$-globin region of the construct. No detectable signal could be seen with skeletal muscle RNA of the offspring of all 4 transgenic mice. In three of the transgenic mice no transcripts could be detected in any other of the tissues examined. However, transcripts were detected in RNA from testes, thymus and lung of mouse CV/3. Such transcripts were most abundant in testes and at a lower level in thymus and lung. No transcripts were detected in the liver or kidney RNA. These transcripts protected the same size fragment of the probe as that protected by RNA from differentiated cultures of L8-46, containing the same gene construct, indicating that they possess the correct 3' end. No information is yet available on the initiation of transcription of the chimeric gene in these tissues.

If the differences between the expression of the MLC2 gene and that of the actin/globin chimeric gene are maintained in a larger number of transgenic mouse lineagews they would suggest a difference in the control of expression of the two cloned genes. They may also indicate a difference between the control of expression of genes introduced into somatic cells and genes introduced into the germ line, since the same construct was developmentally regulated in transfected myogenic cells. It should be mentioned that while the entire MLC2 structural gene including its 5' and 3' flanking sequences, was used for microinjection, in the actin/globin chimeric gene the 3' third of the actin gene was replaced with the equivalent region of the human $\varepsilon$-globin gene. As discussed earlier, this region of the gene may contain important DNA sequences involved in the control of expression of the gene (see also Yaffe et al., 1985; Shani and Yaffe, 1985; Charnay et al., 1984; Wright et al., 1984). Experiments are being conducted to investigate these possibilities.

CONCLUSIONS

The experiments reported here as well as similar experiments with other tissue-specific genes (e.g. β-globin and insulin; Chao et al., 1983; Wright et al., 1984; Walker et al., 1983) have shown that the expression of tissue-specific genes introduced directly into the appropriate somatic cells is developmentally regulated as measured by enhanced expression in the right cell type or at the right stage of development. This indicates that the DNA sequences of the structural gene and its close flanking sequences contain sufficient information for responding to the transacting cellular signals. In order for this information to be expressed the gene does not need to be exposed to the earlier stages of ontogenesis. The regulated expression of the α-CAT gene in transiently transfected cells show that the transferred gene does not have to be integrated into the host chromosomes in order to respond to the cellular regulatory signals operating at this level.

Transfected or microinjected DNA usually integrates at random, into a single or very few chromosomal sites; the sites of integration are different in each clone or animal (de Saint Vincent et al., 1981; Lacy et al., 1983). Yet, clonal analysis of transfected myogenic cells showed that in the majority of the clones the inserted muscle-specific gene is expressed and developmentally regulated. The high frequency of expression could be explained by the fact that by selection for neomycin resistance one may be selecting for clones in which the donor DNA happened to integrate into chromatin domains permissive for gene expression. However, this is not applicable to the microinjection experiments, because no selection was made and offspring of all transgenic mice containing the donor DNA in the germ line were examined for gene expression. Nevertheless, in the offspring of two out of the three transgenic mice carrying the rat MLC2 gene this gene was expressed specifically in muscle tissue and developmentally regulated during cell differentiation. This high frequency of regulated expression shows that the interaction between DNA sequences in the structural gene region and the changing cellular milieu plays an important role in the control of expression of the gene. On the other hand, the lack of expression of the MLC2 gene in one transgenic lineage; the >100-fold difference in the expression between the progeny of MLC/2 and MLC/4 transgenic mice and the expression of the actin/globin chimeric gene in the testis and lung of the offspring of one of the transgenic mice carrying this gene may reflect the effect of the site of integration or other important factors involved in the control of gene expression. Lacy et al. (1983) described a transgenic mouse strain in which a human β-globin was expressed specifically in inappropriate tissues.

More experiments are required to study the nature and significance of the differences in expression between the native and the inserted tissue-specific genes, as well as the possible differences between the expression of genes introduced into the germ line and

those introduced into somatic cells.  The observations that the
expression of the transfected genes is developmentally regulated
enable a search for the transacting cellular factors which interact
with DNA sequences contained in the gene constructs which are included
in the plasmids.  Experiments are currently being carried out which
aim at identifying the transacting regulatory factors and the genetic
system which controls their synthesis.

## ACKNOWLEDGEMENTS

The excellent technical assistance of Ms. Sara Neuman, Ms. Ora
(Saxel) Fuchs, Ms. Zehava Levy and Ms. Olla Yoffe and the editorial
assistance of Mrs M. Baer and Dr R. Aft are greatly appreciated.  We
thank Dr T. Maniatis for plasmid pMH , Dr P. Gruss for the plasmid
pCAT-3N, Dr C. Ordahl for the plasmid pG -actin-1, Drs C.M. Gorman and
P.E. Howard for plasmids pSVO-CAT and pSV2-CAT, Dr S. Silverstein for
plasmid pIPB1.  This investigation was supported by the Muscular
Dystrophy Association, Inc., USA, by the National Institutes of Health
(Grant No. GM-22767), and by the U.S.-Israel Binational Science
Foundation.  U. Nudel is the incumbent of the A. and E. Bloom Career
Development Chair for Cancer Research.

## REFERENCES

Carmon, Y., Czosnek, H., Nudel, U., Shani, M. and Yaffe, D., 1982,
    DNAase I sensitivity of genes expressed during myogenesis.
    Nucl. Acids Res., 10:3085
Chao, M.V., Mellon, P., Charnay, F., Maniatis, T. and Axel, R., 1983,
    The regulated expression of β-globin genes introduced into eryth-
    roleukemia cells, Cell, 32:483.
Charnay, P., Treisman, R., Mellon, P., Chao, M., Axel, R. and Maniatis
    T., 1984, Differences in human α- and β-globin gene expression in
    mouse erythroleukemia cells:  The role of intragenic sequences,
    Cell, 38:251.
Czosnek, H., Nudel, U., Shani, M., Barker, P.E., Pravtcheva, D.,
    Ruddle, F.H. and Yaffe, D., 1982, The genes coding for the muscle
    contractile proteins, myosin heavy chain, myosin light chain 2
    and skeletal muscle actin are located on three different mouse
    chromosomes, EMBO J., 1:1299.
Czosnek, H., Nudel, U., Mayer, Y., Barker, P.E., Pravtcheva, D.D.,
    Ruddle, F.H. and Yaffe, D., 1983, The genes coding for the
    cardiac muscle actin, the skeletal muscle actin and the cyto-
    plasmic β-actin are located on three different mouse chromosomes.
    EMBO J., 11:1977.
de Saint Vincent, B.R., Delbruck, S., Eckhart, W., Meinkoth, J.,
    Vitto, L. and Wahl, G., 1981, The cloning and reintroduction into
    animal cells of a functional CAD gene, a dominant amplifiable
    genetic marker, Cell, 27:267.

Efstatiadis, A., Pasakony, J.W., Maniatis, T., Lawn, R.M., O'Connell,
    C., Spritz, R.A., DeRiel, J.K., Forget, B.G., Weissman, S.M.,
    Slightom, J.L., Blechl, A.E., Smithies, O., Baralle, F.E.,
    Schoulders, C.C. and Proudoot, N.J., 1980, The structure and
    evolution of the human β-globin gene family, Cell, 21:653
Kurtz, D.T., 1981, Hormone inducibility of $\alpha_2\mu$-globulin genes in
    transfected mouse cells, Nature, 261:629.
Lacy, E., Roberts, S., Evans, E.P., Burtenshaw, M.D. and Costantini,
    F.D., 1983, A foreign β-globin gene in transgenic mice: integra-
    ticn at abnormal chromosomal positions and expression in in-
    appropriate tissues, Cell, 34:343.
Mayer, Y., Czosnek, H., Zeelon, P.E., Yaffe, D. and Nudel, U., 1984,
    Expression of the gene coding for the skeletal muscle and cardiac
    actin in the heart, Nucl. Acids Res., 12:1087.
Melloul, D., Aloni, B., Calvo, J., Yaffe, D. and Nudel, U., 1984,
    Developmentally regulated expression of chimeric genes containing
    muscle actin DNA sequences in transfected myogenic cells, EMBO J.
    3:983,
Nudel, U., Calvo, J.M., Shani, M. and Levy, Z., 1984a, The nucleotide
    sequence of rat myosin light chain 2 gene, Nucl. Acids Res., 12:
    7175.
Nudel, U., Melloul, D., Aloni, B., Greenberg, D. and Yaffe, D., 1984b,
    Developmentally regulated expression of chimeric muscle genes
    transferred into myogenic cells, In, Molecular Biology of
    Development, E. Davidson and R. Firtel, eds., p647, Alan R. Liss,
    Inc., New York.
Nudel, U., Greenberg, D., Ordahl, C.P., Saxel, O., Neuman, S. and
    Yaffe, D., 1985a, Developmentally regulated expression of a
    chicken muscle-specific gene in stably transfected rat myogenic
    cells, Proc. Natl. Acad. Sci. USA, 82:3106.
Nudel, U., Melloul, D., Aloni, B., Greenberg, D. and Yaffe, D., 1985b,
    The promoter regions of two muscle-specific genes containing DNA
    sequences which confer tissue- and stage-specific expression of
    chimeric genes in transfected myogenic cells, In, Molecular
    Biology of Muscle Development, UCLA Symp. on Molecular and
    Cellular Biology, New Series, Vol. 29, C. Emerson, D.A. Fischman,
    B. Nadal-Ginard and M.A.Q. Siddiqui, eds., Alan R. Liss, Inc.,
    New York.
Shani, M., 1985, Tissue-specific expression of rat myosin light chain
    2 gene in transgenic mice, Nature, 314:283.
Shani, M. and Yaffe, D, 1985, Expression of rat skeletal muscle genes
    in transgenic mice, In, Molecular Biology of Muscle Development,
    UCLA Symp., Molecular and Cellular Biology, New Series, Vol. 29,
    Alan R. Liss, Inc., New York.
Shani, M., Zevin-Sonkin, D., Saxel, O., Carmon, Y., Katcoff, D.,
    Nudel, U. and Yaffe, D., 1981, The correlation between the
    synthesis of skeletal muscle actin, myosin heavy chain, and
    myosin light chain and the accumulation of the corresponding mRNA
    sequences during myogenesis, Dev. Biol., 86:483.
Vanderkerckhove, J. and Weber, K., 1979, The complete amino acid

sequence of actins from bovine aorta, bovine heart, bovine fast
skeletal muscle and rabbit slow skeletal muscle.  A protein-
chemical analysis of muscle actin differentiation,
Differentiation, 14:124.

Walker, M.D., Edlund, T., Boulet, A.M. and Rutter, W.J., 1983, Cell-
specific expression controlled by the 5'-flanking region of
insulin and chymotrypsin genes, Nature, 306:557.

Wright, S., Rosenthal, A., Flavell, R. and Grosveld, F., 1984, DNA
sequences required for regulated experession of β-globin genes in
murine erythroleukemia cells, Cell, 38:265.

Yablonka, Z. and Yaffe, D., 1977, Synthesis of myosin light chains and
accumulation of translatable mRNA coding for light chain-like
polypeptides in differentiating muscle cultures, Differentiation,
8:133.

Yaffe, D., Nudel, U., Mayer, Y. and Neuman, S., 1985, Highly conserved
sequences in the 3'-untranslated region of mRNAs coding for
homologous proteins in distantly related species, Nucl. Acids
Res., 13:3723.

Yaffe, D. and Saxel, O., 1977, A myogenic cell line with altered serum
requirements for differentiation, Differentiation, 7:159.

Zakut, R., Shani, M., Givol, D., Neuman, S., Yaffe, D. and Nudel, U.,
1982, Nucleotide sequence of the rat skeletal muscle actin gene,
Nature, 298:857.

# EXPRESSION OF THE EXOGENOUS CHICKEN δ-CRYSTALLIN GENES

# INCORPORATED IN MOUSE TERATOCARCINOMA CELLS

T.S. Okada, Y. Takahashi and H. Kondoh

Institute for Biophysics, Faculty of Science
University of Kyoto, Kyoto 606, Japan

## INTRODUCTION

There is little doubt that the examination of expression of cloned foreign genes transferred into cells is one of the most powerful approaches to the elucidation of the mechanism of cell differentiation in terms of gene expression. Three different cell systems are provided for studies along this line. Studies on the expression of chick δ-crystallin genes (δ-genes), which are active very specifically in the lens tissue in situ, are one of the examples toward this goal (Kondoh et al., in this volume). Although such a system deals with the expression of a single specific gene in artificial conditions, there is little doubt that the results will provide basic knowledge for understanding coordinated gene expression in the normal process of cell differentiation. In the article by Kondoh et al., transitory expression has been thoroughly investigated after nuclear injection of the δ-crystallin genes. Naturally, it is also interesting to examine the expression of foreign genes which are stably integrated into host chromosomes.

Two other experimental systems seem to be of particular interest to this end. First, the use of transgenic mice which are derived from fertilized eggs that received foreign genes and stably incorporated them, is of unusual potentiality not only for genetic studies, but also for approaching the mechanism of gene expression in different tissues in developing embryos in situ (Palmiter and Brinster, 1985). Second, the use of teratocarcinoma (TCC) stem cells incorporating exogenous genes must also be promising for the same purpose (Pellicer et al., 1980; Wagner and Mintz, 1982; Bucchini et al.,1983). TCC stem cells are

undifferentiated but have a potential for giving
rise to a variety of cell types.  They can be easily propagated
in vitro as such and, the differentiation can be readily induced
in some other conditions.  Thus, by using transformed TCC stem
cells with exogenous genes, the expression of the genes can be
compared in undifferentiated and differentiated phases.  Such
transformed TCC stem cells are able to produce chimeras by
combining them with early mouse embryos and thus it is also
possible to study the gene expression in developing embryos in
situ.

Recently, we have established several cell lines of TCC stem
cells so transformed as to incorporate chicken genes in a stable
manner (Kondoh et al., 1984).  It was disclosed that the expression of the exogenous gene is highly "differentiation-dependent".
These cells are expected to be a useful vehicle for studying the
expression of genes in the developmental process.

EXPERIMENTAL SYSTEM

As the gene to be transferred, we choose the gene coding for
chick δ-crystallin (δ-gene).  This protein is highly "lens-
specific" in avians and reptilians (Piatigorsky, 1984).  In
mammals, δ-gene is totally absent.  However, our previous
results demonstrate that the expression is predominant in lens
cell after micro-injection of the gene into mouse cell nuclei in
xenoplastic manner (Kondoh et al., 1983).  In this system the

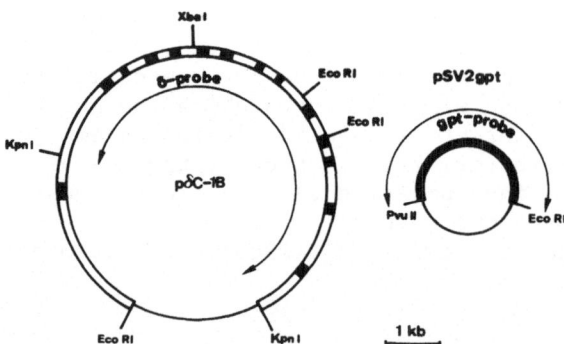

Fig. 1. Structure of the recombinant plasmids, pδC-1B and
        pSV2gpt.  Solid bars represent exon DNA sequences of
        chicken δ-crystallin gene and the bacterial gpt gene
        joined to SV40 segments.  Open bars represent flanking
        and intron sequences.  The thin lines represent vector
        sequences.

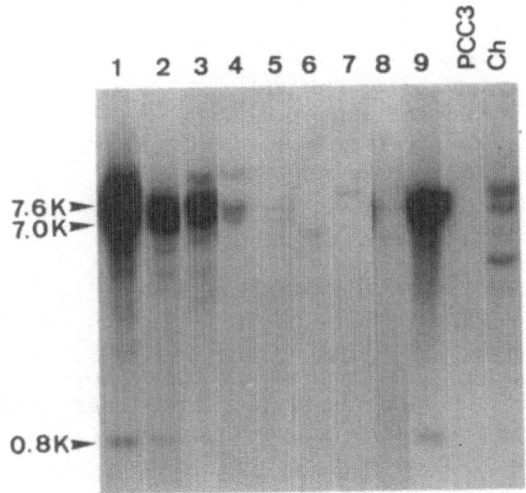

Fig. 2.    Southern blot analysis of the transformant DNAs.    10 µg
           of the EcoRI digest of the DNA of each line was electro-
           phoresed.    The numbers 1 to 9 indicate transformed lines,
           Yδ-1 to Yδ-9, respectively.    DNA of a non-transformed TCC
           line, (PCC3), and of the chickens (Ch) were also electro-
           phoresed.    DNA was transferred to a nitrocellulose sheet
           and hybridized with the $^{32}$P-labelled δ-probe.    The po-
           sitions of the 7.6-, 7.0- and 0.8kb EcoRI fragments of
           pδC-1B are shown.

expression, though occurring in high frequency, is considered to
be transitory (Kondoh et al., 1983) and there is no evidence for
the stable incorporation of the injected gene   (Hayashi et al.,
1985).

     For the transfer of δ-gene into TCC stem cells, the calcium
phosphate technique was adopted.    PCC3 mouse TCC stem cells were
cotransfected with a plasmid carrying the δ-gene and with the
plasmid pSV2gpt containing the selectable bacterial xanthine-
guanine phosphoribosyl-transferase (XGPRT) gene (Figure 1).
After a brief treatment with the selection-medium, 9 clonal lines
which appeared to incorporate δ-gene stably were isolated from
initially cotransfected $5 \times 10^{6}$ cells.

THE PRESENCE OF THE EXOGENOUS DNAs

    The total cellular DNA was extracted from each of these 9
lines (Yδ-1 to Yδ-9) and was subjected to Southern blot analysis
(Figure 2). The DNAs were digested with EcoRI and hybridized with
δ- and gpt-probes (Figure 1). The results demonstrated that the
exogenous genes were actually present in all these 9 cell lines and
they are recombined with mouse DNA and are, perhaps, integrated
into a chromosome of the host cells.

    The multiplicity of the exogenous DNA copies is highly variable
among different clonal lines, ranging from 1 to 500 copies of δ-
genes per diploid mouse genome (Table 1). Lines with a large
copy number of δ-gene contain proportionally more gpt sequence
also. The multiplicity and the different patterns of integration
of δ-gene in each clonal line is very stably maintained after
recloning followed by passages over 100 cell generations.

    When $1 \times 10^7$ transformed cells were injected into the syn-
genic mice, 129/Sv, they formed large solid tumors with a variety
of differentiated tissues including cartilage, nervous tissues,
glandular epithelial structures, muscles and other tissues. The total
cellular DNA extracted out of these tumors showed the same hybridization pattern characteristic for each clone as observed in
assays  of DNA of transformed stem cells.


EXPRESSION OF δ-GENE IN TRANSFORMED TCC CELLS

    The expression of δ-gene in transformed TCC cells was assayed
immunologically by using mono-specific antibody against δ-
crystallin. Undifferentiated stem cells which propagated in
vitro up to a subconfluent density did not contain δ-crystallin
as assayed by both immunohistological staining with PAP and
immuno-blot analysis of an electrophoreogram of the extracts.

    When cultures reached confluence, the differentiation of
fibroblasts, neuron-like cells, epithelial cells and other unidentifiable cells occurred together with a number of stem cells
The presence of positive cells was detected by immunohistological
staining. Some clusters of small round cells which were morphologically distinct from TCC stem cells and resemble immature
neuroblasts were stained in confluent cultures of the Yδ-3 line
(Figure 3a). However, such positive cells appeared only in this
particular line. In cultures of all other lines, all cells were
negative, though clusters of such round cells often appeared.

    The appearance of positive cells was extensively examined by
immunohistological method in histological sections of solid

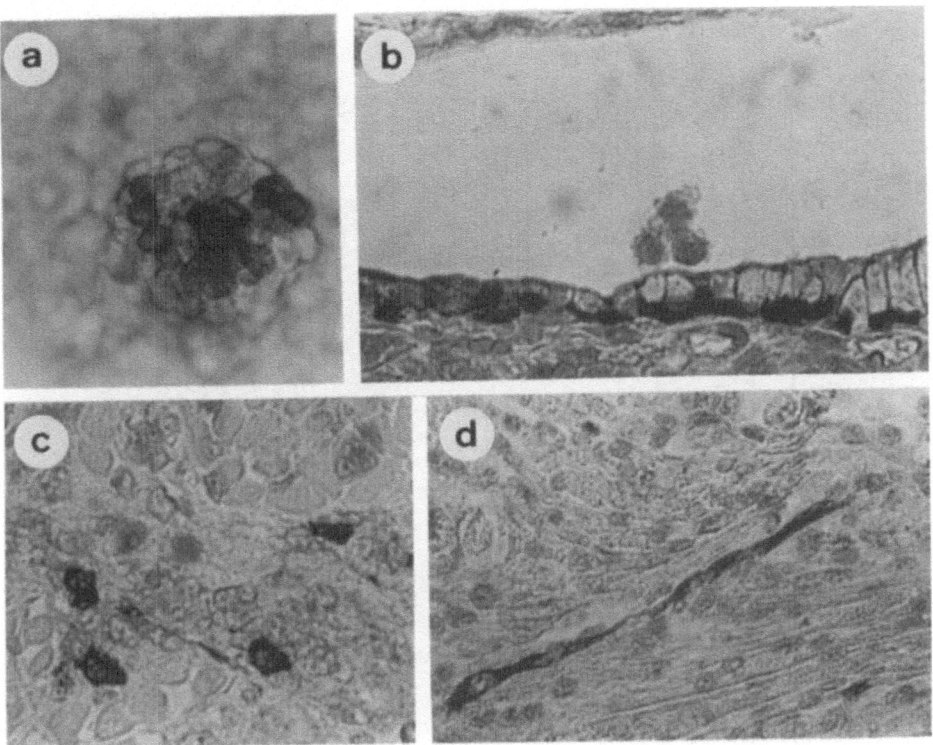

Fig. 3.    Immunohistological detection of δ-crystallin in differ-
           entiated tissues of the transformed cell lines.    The
           specimens were stained using anti-δ and PAP. (a) Cell
           clusters found  in  a confluent Yδ-3 culture with δ-
           crystallin synthesizing cells.   (b) In a solid tumor of
           line Yδ-2, columnar epithelial cells facing the lumen
           are stained with anti-δ.   (c) δ-Crystallin synthesizing
           cells found in sections of solid tumors of Yδ-3.   (d) An
           area wherein many skeletal muscle fibers are produced in
           the tumor of Yδ-9.   One of the fibers with multiple
           nuclei is stained.

tumors formed after injection of transformed TCC stem cells into
mice.   Although cells of all lines equally produced solid tumors
with a variety of differentiated tissues as in the cases of
injection of non-transformed parental cells, cells stained with
antibody against δ-crystallin were found in three lines, Yδ-2,
Yδ-3 and Yδ-9 (Figure 3b, c and d).

Table 1. Characterization of the transformed TCC lines.

| Cell line | δ-crystallin gene copies per diploid mouse genome[a] | EcoRI fragment of pδC-1B | | | pSV2gpt | δ-crystallin gene expression in culture[c] | δ-crystallin gene expression in solid tumor[d] |
|---|---|---|---|---|---|---|---|
| | | 7.6 kb | 7.0 kb[b] | 0.8 kb[b] | 5.1 kb | | |
| Yδ-1 | 500 (B) | + | + | + | + | − | 0/3 |
| Yδ-2 | 130 (B) | + | + | + | + | − | **5/5** |
| Yδ-3 | 60 (B) | + | + | + | + | + | **9/9** |
| Yδ-4 | 4 (B) | + | + | + | + | − | 0/3 |
| Yδ-5 | 2 (B) | + | − | + | + | − | 0/2 |
| Yδ-6 | 1 (B) | − | − | − | + | − | 0/2 |
| Yδ-7 | 1 (B) | − | − | − | + | − | 0/2 |
| Yδ-8 | 1 (B) | + | − | − | − | − | 0/2 |
| Yδ-9 | 240 (A) | + | + | + | + | − | **4/5** |

a. As determined by Southern blot analysis of EcoRI digest of DNAs after serial dilution with digested PCC3 DNA. (A) and (B) indicate pδC-1A and pδC-1B, respectively, for the gene-carrying plasmid.
b. The 7.0 kb fragment of pδC-1B is replaced by a 7.3 kb fragment in pδC-1A.
c. +, positive; −, negative.
d. The number of tumors containing expressing cells/total number of tumors examined.

It is noteworthy that positive cells were found in different tissues in each line.  In tumors derived from Yδ-2, cells with δ-crystallin were found in the columnar epithelium.  In tumors from Yδ-3, some large, spindle-shaped cells were stained, whereas a small population of multinucleated skeletal muscle cells were stained in tumors from Yδ-9.

The extracts of Yδ-3 tumors, in which positive cells were most frequently observed, were subjected to the immuno-blotting analysis using antibody against δ-crystallin.  This analysis demonstrated that authentic δ-crystallin polypeptides with the m.w. of 50,000 are actually present in such tumors derived from the transformed line (Figure 4). No such polypeptides was found in tumors from the non-transformed PCC3 TCC stem cells.

These results showed that cells of some transformed lines can express the activity of the exogenous genes.  But, the activity seems to be totally repressed as long as the transformed cells propagate as undifferentiated stem cells.  Therefore, we can say that the expression is "differentiation-dependent". There are no correlation between the capability of expression and the copy number of exogenous genes incorporated.

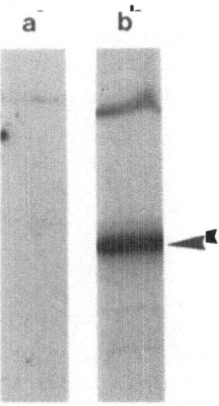

Fig. 4.    Detection of δ-crystallin in an immuno-blot of tumor extract.  δ-Crystallin in soluble extract from the solid tumors were immunoprecipitated, electrophoresed and processed for immuno-blotting. Immunoprecipitates from (a), a PCC3 tumor lysate and (b), lysate of the tumors of Yδ-3. δ-Crystallin band (arrow) is indicated.

SOME FUTURE PROSPECTS

There are several immediate questions to be raised from the
cellular properties of the transformed stem cells so far investigated.  The first question is to ask what is the mechanism for
repressing the activity of $\delta$-genes in undifferentiated TCC stem
cells.  Second, we have to seek any biological implication of the
expression of $\delta$-genes in several non-lens tissues differentiated
from TCC stem cells.  As reviewed in other articles of the
present volume(by Clayton and by Kodama), a low level accumulation
of $\delta$-crystallin has been shown in various non-lenticular tissues
of chicken embryos.  The possibility that these $\delta$-crystallin
positive cells are provided with the capability of transdifferentiation into lens is also discussed by Clayton (see also Okada, 1983).
However, it is still doubtful if the expression of $\delta$-genes in such
highly artifical conditions as in the present case may reflect the
situations in normally  developing embryonic cells.

Perhaps, the most unambiguous results in relation to cell
differentiation is that the expression of $\delta$-genes occurred only
in particular cell types in the manner unique to each line.  Such
specificity in the expression of exogenous genes in "inappropriate tissues" can be partly ascribed to the position effect of
the integrated chromosome.  In fact, recent observation on in
situ hybridization techniques can localize the $\delta$-genes in different chromosomes in the three lines which express the genes in
different cell types.  Further studies are necessary before con-
cluding that the specificity in cell types in the expression is
due to the position effect.  In order to approach the elucidation
 of the mechanism of coordinated gene activity by use of such
artificially transformed cells, it is necessary to see the
expression of $\delta$-genes in lens cells differentiated from TCC cells.
We are expecting the production of chimeric mice, in which the
$\delta$-gene-containing TCC cells may contribute to the lens differentiation.

REFERENCES

Bucchini, D., Lasserre, C., Kunst, F., Lovell-Badge, R., Pictet,
        R., and Jami, J., 1983, Stable transformation of mouse
        teratocarcinoma stem cells with the dominant selective
        marker Eco.gpt and retention of their developmental
        potentialities, EMBO J., 2:229.
Hayashi, S., Kondoh, H., Yasuda, K., Soma, G., Ikawa,Y., and
        Okada, T.S., 1975, Tissue-specific regulation of a chicken
        $\delta$-crystallin gene in mouse cells: involvement of the 5'
        end region, EMBO J., 4:2201.
Kondoh, H., Yasuda, K., and Okada, T.S., 1983, Tissue-specific

expression of a cloned chick δ-crystallin gene in mouse
cells, Nature, 301:440.

Kondoh, H., Takahashi, Y., and Okada, T.S., 1984, Differentiation-
dependent expression of the chicken δ-crystallin gene
introduced into mouse teratocarcinoma stem cells, EMBO J.,
3:2009.

Okada, T.S., 1983, Recent progress in studies of the transdifferentiation of eye tissues in vitro, Cell Differ., 13:177.

Palmiter, R.D., and Brinster, R.L., 1985,  Transgenic mice, Cell,
41:343.

Pellicer, A.E., Wagner,F., El Kareh, A., Dewey, M.J., Reuser,
A.J., Silverstein, S., Axel, R., and Mintz, B., 1980,
Proc. Natl. Acad. Sci. U.S.A., 77:2098.

Piatigorsky, J., 1984, δ-Crystallin and their nucleic acids, Mol.
Cell. Biochem., 59:33.

Wagner, E.F., and Mintz, B., 1982, Transfer of non-selectable
genes into mouse teratocarcinoma cells and transcription
of the transferred human β-globin gene, Mol. Cell. Biol.,
2:190.

# DEVELOPMENTAL EVENTS AT THE CELLULAR LEVEL

## INTRODUCTION

Experimental embryology has long accustomed us to think both of
the competence of the responding system and the nature of the signal
which induces it to respond. It is evident that the selection of a
system which may be readily manipulated and in which important
products are readily characterisable is a prerequisite for the
application of the techniques which will enable us to study the
molecular basis for competence, the nature of the signals and the
characteristics of the response.

Some of our understanding of cellular decisions have come from the
study of the differentiation of the cell types from a stem cell
population, as for example haemopoeitic cells (e.g. Lord, 1982). In
other cases the cellular decisions appear to be taken amongst members
of a large cell population which is itself steadily changing with
time, such as the differentiation of neurones (for example Black et
al., 1984), or the development of epidermal derivatives.

Several lines of evidence suggest that a third type of cell
decision, transdifferentiation, appears to be a multistep phenomenon
(Clayton 1979a,b, Okada et al., 1983, Eguchi and Itoh, 1982).

An example of each of the three types of system is dealt with in
this section. Further discussion of the switching of cellular
phenotypes both during normal differentiation and transdifferentiation
will be found in the report of the final discussion.

## REFERENCES

Black, I.B., Adler, J.E., Dreyfus, C.F., Jonakait, G.M., Katz, D.M.,
    La Gamma, E.F., and Markey, K.M., 1984, Neurotransmitter
    plasticity at the molecular level, Science, 225:1266.
Clayton, R.M., 1979a, Regulatory factors for lens fibre formation in
    cell culture. I. Possible requirements for pre-existing cell
    culture, Ophthal. Res., 11: 324

Clayton, R.M., 1979b, Regulatory factors for lens fibre formation in
    cell culture. II.  The role of growth conditions and factors
    affecting cell cycle duration, Ophthal. Res., 11:329
Eguchi, G. and Itoh, Y., 1982, Regeneration of the lens as a
    phenomenon of cellular transdifferentiation.  Regulability of the
    differentiated state of the vertebrate pigment epithelial cells.
    Trans. Ophthal. Soc. U.K., 102:374
Lord, B.I., 1982, The murine haemopoeitic stem cell: patterns of
    proliferation and differentiation, in, Stability and Switching in
    Cell Differentiation, R.M. Clayton and D.E.S. Truman, eds.,
    p275, Plenum Press, New York, London.
Okada, T.S., Nomura, K. and Yasuda, Y., 1983, Committment to trans-
    differentiation into lens occurs in neural retina cells after
    brief spreading culture of dissociated cells, Cell Differ., 122:85

# EXTRA-LENTICULAR CRYSTALLINS

R.M. Clayton

Department of Genetics
University of Edinburgh
West Mains Road
Edinburgh EH9 3JN

## INTRODUCTION

The detection of lens crystallin proteins in non-lens tissues, and the events during transdifferentiation of non-lens cells to lens cells raise questions concerning the role of the crystallins, and the regulation of their expression. Since some of the data from this laboratory is presented elsewhere in this volume (Bower et al., Errington et al., and Patek and Clayton) it may be permissible to speculate on some of these general questions in the light of this data, and of other reports in the literature.

Transdifferentiation from a single melanin-containing pigmented retina cell, to produce crystallin-containing lens cells amongst its progeny, was first shown by Eguchi and Okada (1973). This experiment made it clear that transdifferentiation involves a genuine switch from one differentiated cell type to another, normally characteristic of tissues of quite different developmental origin. Since that time a large number of possible pathways to lens cells have been demonstrated. In the chick embryo, examples include iris, neural retina, pigmented retina, early brain, epiphysis, adenohypophysis and early limb bud (Clayton, 1982a; Eguchi and Itoh, 1982; Okada, 1983; Kodama and Eguchi, 1982; Watanabe et al., 1985). Other exchanges of fate are also possible between this group of tissues, both in vivo and in vitro (Clayton, 1982a,b). Examination of the data on transdifferentiation from neural retina to lens shows that transdifferentiation is a multistep process (Clayton, 1982a,b; Okada et al., 1983). Cell dissociation is required to initiate the transdifferentiation process, but new cell-cell contacts are required for the later stages and increasing the degree of cell contact accelerates crystallin synthesis

(Moscona and Degenstein, 1981) and lentoid formation (Clayton et al., 1977). An increase in transcription of crystallin RNA occurs during transdifferentiation of neural retina or pigment epithelium to lens (reviewed Clayton, 1978, 1982a). Processing capacity increases more slowly so that nuclear transcripts accumulate until towards the end of the pre-lentoid period, (Bower et al., 1983a).

Transdifferentiation-type changes in cell differentiation are not confined to the pigment cell neuronal epithelium lens cell triad of tissues. Muscle cells can transdifferentiate to chondrocytes when grown in contact with bone matrix (Nogami and Urist, 1974), and this is also a multistep phenomenon (Nathanson and Hay, 1980). Transdifferentiation from epithelial cells to mesenchyme (Greenburg and Hay, 1982, 1984) and between different types of amphibian chromatophores (Ide, 1978) may also be obtained. It also seems likely that some at least of the range of ectopic hormone tumours represent transdifferentiation events. These tumours produce large amounts of hormones in tissues in inappropriate locations, and of different developmental origins from the organs normally producing these hormones. The tissue of origin of the tumour generally already normally expresses low levels of the product which, when superabundant, defines the tumour (Baylin and Mendelsohn, 1980; Ratcliffe, 1982; Wyllie et al., 1982). Chick tissues which can transdifferentiate to lens cells all express δ-crystallin RNA at appreciable levels. Tissues which do not have transdifferentiation capacity express δ-crystallin RNA at neglible or trace levels (Clayton et al., 1979; Bower et al., 1983b; Agata et al., 1983). Low levels of crystallin antigenicity may also be detected in some of these tissues (Clayton et al., 1968; 1979). Thus both in ectopic hormone tumours and transdifferentiation to lens there is an apparent relationship between the prior expression at moderate levels of a gene product (whether polypeptide or RNA) and the capacity for conversion to a tissue synthesising that product at superabundant levels.

## The Locations and Possible Roles of Extra-Lenticular Crystallins

We argued that comparisons of the rate of increase of crystallin RNAs during transdifferentiation to lens from neural retina of different ages and from pigment epithelium were best explained if the tissues in question were heterogeneous with respect to crystallin RNA expression, both in terms of the numbers of cells per tissue and the levels of expression per cell (Thomson et al., 1981). In situ hybridisation with a cDNA probe to translatable sequences of δ-crystallin has confirmed this prediction, (Jeanny et al., 1984, 1985, in press).

Certain questions follow from these observations. Except for lens, where all cells were labelled, all embryonic tissues examined had some cells transcribing δ-crystallin RNA, surrounded by cells of similar morphology, which were negative. The moderate levels of

transcription found in tissues such as neural retina therefore
represents a subpopulation of cells with quite high levels of δ-
crystallin RNA (Jeanny et al., 1984, 1985). Tissues which can
transdifferentiate to lens have a higher proportion of cells
expressing δ-crystallin RNA, forming larger cell groups than tissues
which do not transdifferentiate (Bower et al., this volume). The
grouping of positive cells implies either a clonal origin, or the
existence of localised factors, affecting cells in that area.

A discussion of the evidence for a relationship between the
levels of extralenticular crystallin RNA expression in vivo and
transdifferentiation capacity has been presented elsewhere (Clayton
1982a,b; Clayton et al., 1979). This however leaves aside the
question of the factors controlling such extra-lenticular expression
in the first place. The expression of crystallins in the retina
appears to be specifically localised in putative glial cells (Bower et
al., 1983a and this volume): we do not yet know whether positive
cells in general are distinguished from negative cells by their future
fate.

Apart from the puzzling example of the cells in the limb bud,
(Kodama and Eguchi, 1982), which might originate in the neural crest,
tissues with transdifferentiation potential which express δ-crystallin
RNA are topologically homologous outpushings of the neural tube and
topologically homologous invaginations of head ectoderm (Clayton
1978).

A working hypothesis may be suggested for critical investigation:
that the expression of non-lenticular crystallins at significant
levels is not random and is conserved as strongly as the cellular
capacity for transdifferentiation potential.

Some feature of the regulation of expression of genes other than
crystallins in these tissues may tend to make contiguous crystallin
DNA sequences more susceptible to the occasional access of
transcription enzymes (Yamada, 1982). Alternatively, the evolution of
the crystallins themselves may be relevant.
Proteins of the myosin and the globin families which, at high
concentrations, characterise the highly specialised muscle and red
cells respectively, evolved from molecular species of similar
properties which were already available, and which function in various
other cells at much lower levels.

A comparison between all known vertebrate αA and αB crystallin C-
terminal halves with four small heat shock proteins (hsp) of
Drosophila shows that 77% of the positions are the same in at least
some of the crystallins and one or more of the hsp, while 19% are
identical in all α-crystallins and all hsp. The βγ-crystallin
superfamily has homologies with the C myc oncogene and the S spore
coat proteins of Myxococcus Xanthus (these homologies are reviewed by

de Jong, this volume). The antigenic similarity between feather keratin and δ-crystallin also implies strong similarity between some part of these molecules (Kodama and Eguchi, this volume). Parallels between properties of hsp and crystallins have been discussed elsewhere (Wistow 1985; Clayton 1985). It is possible that extra-lenticular crystallins might be functional because of properties of relative water exclusion, binding to the plasma membrane and to cytoarchitectural elements, and the capacity for forming ordered arrays.

δ-crystallin protein is synthesised in the early avian embryo in structures derived from neural tube and head ectoderm (Barabanov,1982; Watanabe, et al., 1985) and a number of authors have found α-crystallin protein in the retina and iris of several vertebrate species (reviewed Clayton. et al., 1968; Clayton 1978).

If any of the ectopic crystallins have a function in the tissues in which they appear, there may be some genetic consequences. The expression of a molecular species in several tissues is one of the several mechanisms of pleiotropy. Mutants with stationary cataract or with a failure of lens fibre formation not secondary to failures of induction may include crystallin mutants. Other genetic cataracts with this type of cataract morphology in rodents have pleiotropic effects including ophthalmic effects, sterility, reduced viability or body weight, vestibular defects, and deficient pigmentation. (reviewed Clayton, 1985). One such mutant, Wh in the Syrian hamster, exhibits a cilium defect in the early development of ocular and neuroectodermal structures, including lens, retina, pituitary, pineal, labyrinth and neural tube (Asher and James, 1982). Other mutants with broadly similar or partially overlapping syndromes are known, and some of these might be expected to involve various other molecular species which are also expressed in this group of tissues.

## Implications of Differentiation and Transdifferentiation for the Regulation of Crystallin Expression

Several levels of regulation are required to provide even a parsimonious explanation of the observed changes in the presence, distribution and quantitative levels of the various crystallins during development and transdifferentiation.

Although the sequence of changes overall in crystallin compo-sition during lens development appears to be conserved under various conditions and in different lens genotypes (Patek and Clayton, 1985 and in preparation,) independent regulation of the crystallins is demonstrated by the range of effects on their synthesis in lens epithelial cells under different growth conditions (reviewed Clayton, 1979), by the decline of δ-crystallin transcription and synthesis and the differential augmentation of the transcription and synthesis of the various β- crystallins over the same developmental period (Clayton, 1979; Piatigorsky 1981) and by the different sequences of transcriptional events for $\alpha$A-, $\beta$25kd- and $\delta$-crystallin RNAs when transdifferentiating tissues are compared with normal lens development (Errington et al., this volume, and unpublished). $\delta$-crystallin is the first to be transcribed in the developing lens, but the last to be transcribed in transdifferentiating pigment epithelium: $\alpha$A crystallin is the first to be transcribed in the transdifferentiating neural retina.

Although the sequence of crystallin synthesis during lens fibre formation appears to depend on the tissue of origin, there also appears to be an overriding effect on crystallin synthesis of conditions affecting the rate of mitosis: factors which increase this also increase the relative contribution of $\delta$-crystallin in the cell, those which depress the rate of mitosis favour $\beta$-crystallin synthesis (reviewed Clayton, 1979, 1982a). Agencies such as retinoic acid, which affect $\delta$-crystallin preferentially and prevent its loss during long term culture (Patek and Clayton, this volume) may operate, at least in part, through the effect on cell division but retinoids also affect the cell membrane and cytoarchitecture, and such structures bind crystallins (see Benedetti et al., 1984; Alcalá et al., 1982): further, anomalies of the cell membrane may be associated with changes in crystallin ontogeny (McDevitt and Clayton, 1979)

Other conditions affecting crystallin expression include the wide range of agencies which affect transdifferentiation, including hormones (Connelly, 1980) cell-cell contacts, (Clayton et al., 1977; Moscona and Degenstein, 1981; Okada et al, 1983) or contact with lens epithelium (Lopashov 1983), or neuronal tissues (Reyer 1977) and agencies affecting specific syntheses (Eguchi et al., 1982).

The injection of chick $\delta$-crystallin DNA into mouse cells (Kondoh et al., 1983) showed high expression in lens cells, low in epithelia, but no expression in fibroblasts, (although tissue specific expression may be abrogated by location when incorporated into a chromosome: Kondoh et al., 1984). Thus the expression of $\delta$-crystallin RNA is tissue specific but is neither species nor crystallin class specific. The expression of $\alpha$-crystallin is also tissue specific but not species specific (Kondoh et al., this volume). However the presence of some $\alpha$-crystallin in retina and iris has been reported by many investigators (reviewed Clayton et al., 1968, Clayton 1978) but although traces of $\alpha$ crystallin RNA are detectable in embryo neural retina (Errington et al., this volume), the cellular location has not yet been examined. Kondoh et al., (this volume) have shown that tissue-specific transcription requires the presence of a 30kb sequence in the 5' untranslated region of the $\delta$-crystallin gene, but low level expression is associated with a different but contiguous 20kb sequence. The absence of crystallin and species specific effects implies that similar sequences may be found in the 5' regulatory regions of both chick $\delta$-and mouse $\gamma$-crystallins. It would seem necessary, however, to postulate the existence of other regulatory

sequences which distinguish the crystallins from each other in the
lens itself.

Yet another regulatory region of crystallin genes is implied by
the temporal succession of transcription,during lens development, of
members of a gene family:  for example the γ-crystallins (Schoenmakers et al., 1984; Lok et al., 1984) or β- crystallins (Ostrer et
al., 1981; Piatigorsky et al., 1984).  Quantitative regulation might
be explained by changes in the level or status of cytoplasmic signals
affecting transcription, processing, or both, but the relevant DNA
sequences which permit differential crystallin regulation must be
separate from those described by Kondoh et al.this volume.  Few of the c
conditions and agencies mentioned above are likely to operate directly
on the genes - some at least may act on crystallin gene expression via
a chain of intra-cellular events, which converge on the same eventual
mechanism.

Processing is largely incomplete in ectopic sites (Agata et al.,
1983; Bower et al., 1983a), but is evidently greater in the transcribing cells of adenohypophysis, for example, than in some other
ectopic sites (Jeanny et al., 1984, 1985; Bower et al., this volume).
Since 8 day embryo neural retina has latent processing capacity (Bower
et al., this volume), it would appear that cellular conditions act as
a regulator for the activation of processing and must do so
independently of the regulation of transcription. δ -crystallin
processing lags behind transcription in the early embryo lens (Bower
et al., 1981) and during neural retina transdifferentiation (Bower et
al., 1983b).  Changes in translational efficiency and mRNA stability
have also been reported (see Piatigorsky 1981; Clayton, 1982a).


## REFERENCES

Agata, K., Yasuda, K. and Okada, T.S., 1983, Gene coding for a lens
        specific protein, δ-crystallin, is transcribed in non lens
        tissues of chicken embryos, Dev. Biol., 100:222
Alcala, J., Maisel, H., Katar, M. and Ellis, M., 1982, δ-crystallin
        in a chick lens fibre cell membrane extrinsic protein, Exp. Eye
        Res., 35:379
Asher, J.H. and James, S.I., 1982, The primary ultrastructural defect
        caused by anophthalmic White (Wh) in the Syrian hamster, Proc.
        Natl. Acad. Sci. USA, 79:437
Barabanov, V.M., 1982, Extra lenticular localisation of δ-crystallins
        in Japanese quail embryos. Doklad. Akad. Nauk. SSSR., 262:1491
Baylin, S.B. and Mendelsohn, G., 1980, Ectopic (innapropriate) hormone
        production by tumours: mechanisms involved and the biological and
        clinical implications, Endocrin. Rev., 1:45
Benedetti, E.L., Dunia, I., Ramaekers, F.C.C. and Kibbelaar, M.A.,
        1981, Lenticular plasma membranes and cytoskeleton, in: Molecular
        and Cellular Biology of the Eye Lens, H. Bloemendal, ed., p137,
        J. Wiley & Sons, New York.

Bower, D.J., Errington, L.H., Wainwright, N.R., Sime, C., Morris, S.
    and Clayton, R.M., 1981, Cytoplasmic RNA sequences complementary
    to cloned chick δ-crystallin cDNA show size heterogeneity,
    Biochem. J., 201:339
Bower, D.J., Errington, L.H., Pollock, B.J., Morris, S. and Clayton,
    R.M., 1983a, The pattern of expression of chick δ-crystallin
    genes in lens differentiation and transdifferentiating cultured
    tissues, EMBO J., 2:333
Bower, D.J., Errington, L.H., Cooper, D.N., Morris, S. and Clayton,
    R.M., 1983b, Chicken lens δ-crystallin gene expression and
    methylation in several non lens tissues, Nucl. Acid Res., 11:2513
Bower, D.J., Jeanny, J-C., Errington, L.H. and Clayton, R.M.,
    Quantitation and localisation of chick δ-crystallin gene
    transcription in developing non-lens tissue, this volume.
Clayton, R.M., 1978, Divergence and Convergence in lens cell differ-
    entiation: regulation of the formation and specific content of
    lens fiber cells in stem cells and tissue homeostasis, B.I. Lord
    C.S. Potten and R.J. Cole, eds., p115, Cambridge University Press
    Cambridge.
Clayton, R.M., 1979, Genetic regulation in the vertebrate lens cell,
    in: Mechanisms of Cell Change, J.D. Ebert and T.S. Okada, eds.,
    p129, John Wiley & Sons, New York.
Clayton, R.M., 1982a, Cellular and molecular aspects of differentia-
    tion and transdifferentiation of ocular tissues in vitro, in:
    Differentiation in Vitro, M.M. Yeoman and D.E.S. Truman, eds.,
    p83, Cambridge University Press, London, New York.
Clayton, R.M., 1982b, The molecular basis for competence, determina-
    tion and transdifferentiation: a hypothesis, in: Stability and
    Switching in Cellular Differentiation, R.M. Clayton and D.E.S.
    Truman, eds., Adv. Exp. Med. Biol., 158:23, Plenum Press, New
    York.
Clayton, R.M., 1985, Developmental Genetics of the Lens, in: The
    Ocular Lens Structure, Function and Pathology, H. Maisel, ed.,
    p61, Marcel Dekker, New York and Basel.
Clayton, R.M., Campbell, J.C. and Truman, D.E.S., 1968, A re-examina-
    tion of the organ specificity of lens antigens, Exp. Eye Res.,
    7:11
Clayton, R.M., de Pomerai, D.I. and Pritchard, D.J., 1977,
    Experimental manipulation of alternative pathways of differentia-
    tion in cultures of embryonic chick neural retina, Dev. Growth
    Differ., 19:319
Clayton, R.M., Thomson, I. and de Pomerai, D.I., 1979, Relationship
    between crystallin mRNA expression in retina cells and their
    capacity to re-differentiate into lens cell, Nature, 282:628
Connely, T.G., 1980, The influence of hormones and other substances on
    lens regeneration in vitro, Differentiation., 85:91
Eguchi, G. and Okada, T.S., 1973, Differentiation of lens tissue from
    the progeny of chick retinal pigment cells cultured in vitro.
    A demonstration of a switch of cell type in clonal cell culture,

Proc. Natl. Acad. Sci. USA, 70:1495

Eguchi, G. and Itoh, Y., 1982, Regeneration of the lens as a phenomenon of cellular transdifferentiation. Regulability of the differentiated state of the vertebrate pigment epithelial cell. Trans. Opthal. Soc. U.K., 102:374

Eguchi, G., Masuda, A., Karasawa, Y., Kodama, R. and Itoh, Y., 1982, Microenvironments controlling the transdifferentiation of vertebrate pigmented epithelial cells in in vitro culture, in: Stability and Switching in Cellular Differentiation, R.M. Clayton and D.E.S. Truman, eds., Adv. Exp. Med. Biol., 158:209, Plenum Press, New York,

Errington, L.H., Bower, D.J. and Clayton, R.M., Identification and characterization of a chick αA2 crystallin genome clone and preliminary identification of a chick  crystallin cDNA clone, this volume.

Greenburg, G. and Hay, E.D., 1982, Epithelium suspended in collagen can lose polarity and express characteristics of migrating mesenchymal cells, J. Cell Biol., 98:333

Greenburg, G. and Hay, E.D., 1984, The formation of mesenchyme-like cells from thyroid follicular epithelium cultured in collagen gels, J. Cell Biochem. Suppl., 8B.

Hayes, B.P. and Fisher, R.F., 1981, Epithelial invasion and secretion of banded collagen in the regenerating lens capsule of the rat, Curr. Eye Res., 1:85

Ide, H., 1978, Transformation of amphibian xanthophores into melanophores in clonal culture, J. Exp. Zool., 203:287

Jeanny, J-C., Bower, D.J., Errington, L.H., Morris, S. and Clayton, R.M., 1984, δ-crystallin mRNA presence in non lens tissues, Biol. Cell., 51:309

Jeanny, J-C., Bower, D.J., Errington, L.H., Morris, S. and Clayton, R.M., 1985, Cellular heterogeneity in the expression of the δ-crystallin gene in non lens tissues, Dev. Biol., 112:94

de Jong, W.W., Crystallin: the families of eye lens proteins, this volume.

Kodama, R. and Eguchi, G., 1982, Dissociated limb bud cells of chick embryos can express lens specificity when reaggregated and cultured in vitro, Dev. Biol., 91:221

Kodama, R. and Eguchi, G., Immunological analysis of δ-crystallin expressed in various tissues of the chick in vivo and in vitro, this volume.

Kondoh, H., Yasuda, K. and Okada, T.S., 1983, Tissue-specific expression of a cloned chick δ-crystallin gene in mouse cells, Nature, 301:440

Kondoh, H., Takahashi, Y. and Okada, T.S., 1984, Differentiation-dependent expression of the chicken δ-crystallin gene introduced into mouse teratocarcinoma stem cells, EMBO J., 3:2009

Kondoh, H., Hayashi, S., Okazaki, K., Yasuda, K. and Okada, T.S., Tissue-specific expression of cloned chicken crystallin genes in mammalian cells, this volume.

Lok, S., Tsui, L-C., Shinohara, T., Piatigorsky, J., Gold, R. and

Breitman, M., 1984, Analysis of the mouse γ-crystallin gene
family: assignment of multiple cDNAs to discrete genomic
sequences and characterisation of a representative gene, Nucl.
Acid Res., 12:4517

Lopashov, G.V., 1983, Transdifferentiation of pigmented epithelium
induced by the influence of lens epithelium in frogs,
Differentiation, 24:27

McDevitt, D.S. and Clayton, R.M., 1979, Ontogeny and localisation of
the crystallins during lens development in normal and Hy-1 (hyper
plastic lens epithelium) chick embryos, J. Embryol. Exp. Morph.,
50:31

Moscona, A.A. and Degenstein, L., 1981, Lentoids in aggregates of
embryonic neural retina cells, Cell Differ., 10:39

Nathanson, M.A. and Hay, E.D., 1980, Analysis of cartilage differentiation from skeletal muscle grown on bone matrix, Dev. Biol.,
78:301

Nogami, H. and Urist, M.R., 1974, Substrata prepared from bone matrix
for chondrogenesis in tissue culture, J. Cell. Biol., 62:510

Okada, T.S., 1983, Recent progress in studies of the transdifferentiation of eye tissue in vitro, Cell Differ., 13:177

Okada, T.S., Nomura, K. and Yasuda, Y., 1983, Committment to transdifferentiation into lens occurs in neural retina cells after
brief spreading culture of dissociated cells, Cell Differ., 122:
85

Ostrer, H., Beebe, D.C. and Piatigorsky, J., 1981,  crystallin mRNAs
differential distribution in the developing chicken lens, Dev.
Biol., 86:403

Patek, C.E. and Clayton, R.M., 1985, A comparison of the changing
patterns of crystallin expression in vivo, in long term primary
cultures, in vitro, and in response to a carcinogen, Exp. Eye Res
40:357

Patek, C.E. and Clayton, R.M., Retinoic acid is lentoidigenic but
differentially affects δ-crystallin expression by chick lens
cells in vitro, this volume.

Piatigorsky, J., 1981, Lens differentiation in vertebrates. A review
of cellular and molecular features, Differentiation, 19:134

Ratcliffe, J.G., 1982, Ectopic hormones, in: Stability and Switching
in Cellular Differentiation, R.M. Clayton and D.E.S. Truman, eds.
Adv. Exp. Med. Biol., 158:155, Plenum Press, New York.

Reyer, R.w., 1977, The amphibian eye: Development and Regeneration,
Handbook of Sensory Physiology VII 5:311

Schoenmakers, J.G.G., den Dunnen, J.T., Moorman, R.J.M., Jongbloed,
R., van Leen, R.W. and Lubsen, N.H., 1984, The crystallin gene
families, J. Nugent, and J. Whelan, eds., CIBA Found. Symp. 20:
208, Pitmans, London.

Thomson, I., Yasuda, K., de Pomerai, D.I., Clayton, R.M. and Okada,
T.S., 1981, The accumulation of lens-specific protein and mRNA
in cultures of eye cups from 3  day embryos, Exp. Cell Res.,
135:445

Watanabe, K., Aoyama, H., Tamamaki, N., Yasujima, M., Nojyo, Y.,

Ueda, Y. and Okada, T.S., 1985, Oculopotency of embryonic quail
    pineals as revealed by cell culture studies, Cell Differ., 16:251
Wistow, G., 1985, Domain structure and evolution in $\alpha$ crystallins and
    small heat shock proteins, FEBS Lett., 181:1
Wyllie, A.H., Clayton, R.M. and Truman, D.E.S., 1982, Introductory
    review:  tumours transposition and transdifferentiation, in:
    Stability and Switching in Cellular Differentiation, R.M. Clayton
    and D.E.S. Truman, eds., Adv. Exp. Med. Biol., 158:143, Plenum
    Press, New York.
Yamada, T., 1982, Transdifferentiation of lens cells and its
    regulation, in: Cell Biology of the Eye, D.S. McDevitt, ed., p193
    Academic Press, Orlando, Florida, USA

# GLIAL CELL LINEAGES AND DIFFERENTIATION IN THE RAT OPTIC NERVE

Martin C. Raff

Medical Research Council Neuroimmunology Project
Zoology Department
University College London
London WC1E 6BT

My colleagues and I are interested in the problem of cell diversification in the mammalian central nervous system (CNS): how does the relatively simple neuroepithelium of the embryonic neural tube give rise to the large numbers of different types of neurons and glial cells of the adult CNS? To overcome the technical problems associated with cell identification, inaccessibility to experimental manipulation and the intimidating cellular complexity of the CNS, we have employed three strategies: (i) we have used antibodies to identify and manipulate specific types of neural cells and their precursors; (ii) we have studied cell diversification in culture so that we can manipulate the cells and their environment, and (iii) we have studied one of the simplest parts of the CNS, the rat optic nerve, which contains astrocytes and oligodendrocytes but no intrinsic neurons, so that glial cell development can be studied without the complication of neuronal development. Rather than review the experiments we have done, many of which have been published, I will briefly summarize some of the conclusions we have drawn from our studies so far.

The rat optic nerve contains three types of macroglial cells that develop in a precise sequence: type-1 astrocytes first appear at embryonic day 16 (E16), oligodendrocytes at the time of birth (E21) and type-2 astrocytes at around postnatal day 8-10 (P8-10). These three cell types develop in culture from two different precursor cells: type-1 astrocytes develop from a type-1 astrocyte precursor cell, while both oligodendrocytes and type-2 astrocytes develop from a common, bipotential progenitor cell, which differentiates into an oligodendrocyte if cultured in serum-free medium, but into a type-2 astrocyte if cultured in 10% fetal calf serum (FCS). Presumably,

early in development, the neuro-epithelial cells of the optic stalk,
which give rise to the macroglial cells of the optic nerve, must
choose between developing into type-1 astrocyte precursor cells or
0-2A progenitor cells, but so far this decision point has been
inaccessible to study. For this reason we have concentrated our
efforts on the 0-2A progenitor cells in an attempt to understand what
controls their differentiation into oligodendrocytes and type-2
astrocytes.

In the embryonic optic nerve, 0-2A progenitor cells apparently
proliferate until the end of gestation, when some of them stop
dividing and differentiate into oligodendrocytes. Post-mitotic
oligodendrocytes continue to be produced from dividing 0-2A progenitor
cells during the first two weeks after birth. Although the evidence
is still indirect, it seems that 0-2A progenitor cells differentiate
into type-2 astrocytes beginning at P8-P10 and that the production of
these astrocytes then continues for at least another two weeks.

The 0-2A progenitor cells behave very differently in vitro: in
cultures of perinatal optic nerve, the majority of these cells
prematurely stop dividing and differentiate within a day or two into
oligodendrocytes in serum-free medium, or into type-2 astrocytes in
10% FCS.      They do so even when cultured on their own in single cell
microcultures, indicating that they do not need to interact with other
cells in order to differentiate and that FCS acts directly on 0-2A
progenitor cells to induce their differentiation into type-2
astrocytes. The 0-2A progenitor cells can differentiate along either
pathway in culture without dividing  or synthesizing DNA.   Their
choice of differentiation pathway is reversible, but only for a day or
two:  for example, many cells that develop into type-2 astrocytes in
10% FCS change their developmental course and develop into oligodendrocytes if switched to serum-free medium after two days, but not
if they are switched after 3 days. Moreover, cells can switch from
the astrocyte to the oligodendrocyte pathway without dividing,
suggesting that DNA synthesis is not requried for the switch.

If 0-2A progenitor cells rapidly stop dividing and differentiate
in culture, what keeps them from doing so in the nerve? The answer
seems to be the type-1 astrocytes. Noble and Murray have shown that
type-1 astrocytes in culture release a growth factor that stimulates
0-2A progenitor cells to divide in serum-free medium.     Furthermore,
type-1 astrocytes prevent the premature differentiation of 0-2A
progenitor cells into oligodendrocytes: if E17 optic nerve cells are
cultured in serum-free medium, oligodendrocytes develop within two
days, which is two days before they develop in vivo; however, if they
are cultured on type-1 astrocytes or in medium conditioned by type-1
astrocytes, oligodendrocytes first appear after four days, equivalent
to the time they first appear in the nerve. On the other hand,
type-1 astrocytes do not prevent the premature differentiation of 0-2A
progenitor cells into type-2 astrocytes in the presence of 10% FCS.

The simplest interpretation of these findings is that:  (i) type-1 astrocytes secrete a growth factor that stimulates 0-2A progenitor cells to divide and thereby expands their numbers;  (ii) if the progenitor cells are deprived of growth factor, they stop dividing and, as a result, differentiate into oligodendrocytes, unless FCS is present to induce them to become type-2 astrocytes;  (iii) even in the presence of growth factor, some 0-2A progenitor cells stop dividing and differentiate into oligodendrocytes beginning around birth, probably because the progenitor cells become unresponsive to the growth factor;  (iv) while 0-2A progenitor cells seem to differentiate into oligodendrocytes constitutively when they stop dividing;  an additional signal (which can be provided by FCS in culture) is required for them to differentiate into type-2 astrocytes;  this signal apparently does not appear in vivo until P8-10.

Many questions concerning macroglial cell diversification in the rat optic nerve remain to be answered.  For example, what is the nature of the growth factor(s) released by type-1 astrocytes, or the endogenous signal that induces type-2 astrocyte differentiation in vivo; or the intrinsic clock that is responsible for oligodendrocyte differentiation beginning at E21?  We are hopeful that the relative simplicity of the optic nerve will make it possible to obtain answers to these questions and that, when they are available, they will be useful for understanding cell diversification in the more complex regions of the CNS, and perhaps in other tissues as well.


ACKNOWLEDGEMENTS

I thank my colleagues who participated in the experiments whose results I have briefly summarized here.


REFERENCES

1.   M.C. Raff, E.R. Abney, J. Cohen, R. Lindsay and M. Noble, Two types of astrocytes in cultures of developing rat white walker. Differences in morphology surface gangliosides and growth characteristics.  J. Neurosci., 3:1289 (1983).

2.   R.H. Miller, S. David, R. Patel, E.R. Abney, and M.C. Raff, A quantitative immunohistochemical study of microglial cell development in the rat optic nerve: in vivo evidence for two distinct astrocyte lineages. Dev. Biol., 111:35 (1985).

3.   M.C. Raff, E.R. Abney and R.H. Miller, Two glial cell lineages diverge prenatally in rat optic nerve. Dev. Biol., 106:53 (1984).

4.   M.C. Raff, R.H. Miller and M. Noble, A glial progenitor cell that develops in vitro into an astrocyte or an oligodendrocyte depending on culture medium, Nature, 303:390 (1983)

5.   R.P. Skoff, D.L. Price and A. Stocks, Electron microscope auto-
        radiographic studies of gliogenesis in rat optic nerve. II.
        Time of origin.  J. Comp. Neurol., 169:313. (1976).
6.   S. Temple and M.C. Raff, Differentiation of a bipotential
        glial progenitor cell in single cell microculture,
        Nature, 313:223 (1985).
7.   M.C. Raff, E.P. Williams and R.H. Miller, The in vitro differ-
        entiation of a bipotential glial progenitor cell,
        EMBO J., 3:1857 (1984).
8.   M. Noble and K. Murray, Purified astrocytes promote the in
        vitro division of a bipotential glial progenitor cell,
        EMBO J., 3:2243 (1984).
9.   J. Fok-Seang, E.R. Abney and M.C. Raff, in preparation.

# REGULATION OF KERATINIZATION DURING THE DEVELOPMENT OF THE AVIAN FEATHER AND SCUTATE SCALE

Roger H. Sawyer and Anne Reeves Haake

Department of Biology
University of South Carolina
Columbia, South Carolina    29208

## INTRODUCTION

Unlike other vertebrates birds and reptiles produce beta keratins, in addition to the alpha keratins which appear in the epidermis of all vertebrates.  The alpha and beta keratins can be distinguished by their X-ray diffraction patterns, for which they are named (Bell and Thathachari, 1963; Baden and Maderson, 1970), ultrastructural characteristics (Parakkal and Matoltsky, 1968; Sawyer et al., 1974a; b), molecular weights (Walker and Bridgen, 1976), immunological identities (O'Guin et al., 1982), and nucleotide sequences (Molloy et al., 1982).  The alpha keratin polypeptides of mammals are products of a multigene family (Moll et al., 1982), which are expressed in a tissue-specific manner (Sun et al., 1983).  O'Guin and Sawyer (1982) and O'Guin (1984) have shown that the alpha keratins of birds are also expressed in a tissue-specific manner, and are recognized, on Western Blots, by at least one of the monoclonal antibodies made against human alpha keratins (Sun et al., 1983).

The beta keratins, originally called feather keratins because they were first isolated from feathers, are the major epidermal proteins of beaks, claws, feathers, and most types of scales in birds (Sawyer et al., 1985).  Alpha keratins are present in developing feathers (Dhouailly et al., 1978; Haake et al., 1984), and it is now apparent that alpha keratins are also present in developing and adult scutate scales (O'Guin and Sawyer, 1982; O'Guin et al., 1982; O'Guin, 1984; Sawyer et al., 1985).  More specifically, in relation to the present discussion, the beta keratins comprise the hard plate-like outer epidermal surface (Beta Stratum) of the overlapping scutate scales (O'Guin et al., 1982) and are the major components of

the rachis, calamus, barbs and medulla of feathers (Rudall, 1947;
Kemp and Rogers, 1972; Kodama and Eguchi, 1983; Haake et al., 1984).
The beta keratins of feathers and scales comprise multigene families, related to those of the beak and claw, which probably arose
from a common ancestral gene by tandem duplication (Walker and
Bridgen, 1976; Lockett et al., 1979; Molloy et al., 1982).  Different beta keratin genes are expressed in different tissues and at
different times during development (Molloy et al., 1982; O'Guin and
Sawyer, 1982; Haake et al., 1984; Sawyer et al., 1985).

   The integument of the chick embryo has been used extensively in
studies of the role of epidermal-dermal interactions in regulating
morphogenesis, histogenesis and cytodifferentiation (Sengel, 1958;
1976; Rawles, 1963; Kato, 1969; Kemp and Rogers, 1972; Linsenmayer,
1972; Novel, 1973; Brotman, 1977a,b; Dhouailly et al., 1978; Sawyer,
1979; 1983; McAleese and Sawyer, 1982; O'Guin and Sawyer, 1982;
Sawyer and Fallon, 1983; Dhouailly and Sawyer, 1984; Haake et al.,
1984; König and Sawyer, 1985; Sawyer et al., 1985).  Although very
little is known about the actual mechanism by which these tissue
interactions occur, they result in the formation of epidermal
appendages which display regional specificity in terms of pattern
formation, biochemical differentiation (the expression of alpha and
beta keratins) and function.  In the case of down feathers and
scutate scales, pattern formation and morphogenesis of the basic
structures precede histogenesis, which in turn precedes production
of the tissue-specific keratins.  Kemp and Rogers (1972) raised the
question as to whether the interactions which controlled tissue
morphology also regulated keratinization.  Based on their results
that the keratins of feathers differed from those of scutate scales
and that differences in the production of keratins also existed
between the adult and embryonic tissues of these structures, they
suggested that the keratinization of each appendage was dependent on
morphogenesis of the particular appendage.  A biochemical analysis
of the keratins found in heterotopic recombinations between the
epidermal and dermal components of presumptive feather and scale
tissues led Dhouailly et al. (1978) to reach similar conclusions.
Furthermore, studies of the scutate scales have shown that disruption of the normal sequence of morphogenesis (either by experimental
means or through genetic mutation) alters tissue-specific keratinization (Abbott and Asmundson, 1957; Sawyer and Abbott, 1972; Sawyer
et al., 1974b; Sawyer, 1975; 1979; McAleese and Sawyer, 1981; 1982;
Fisher et al., 1984; O'Guin, 1984).

   Are the differences seen in the expression of keratin genes for
feathers and scutate scales reflected in differences in their mode
of development?  Our intent in this article is to review the recent
work which relates to this question and to draw some conclusions.
To do this, we will first describe the tissue-specific keratinization of feathers and scutate scales.  Then we will compare the
early morphological development of feathers and scutate scales,

including the results of cell proliferation studies. And finally, we will examine experiments in which the terminal differentiation of feathers and scutate scales has been altered by modifying morphogenesis and/or histogenesis of these appendages. It is our hope that this article will add further support to the contention that morphogenesis and histogenesis play a role in regulating the tissue-specific expression of feather and scutate scale keratins.

## TISSUE-SPECIFIC KERATINIZATION OF FEATHERS AND SCUTATE SCALES

Bell and Thathachari (1963) showed that feathers completed much of their development before mature feather beta keratins could be detected with X-ray diffraction techniques. Keratinization first took place in the sheath of the feather near its distal end, progressed to the barbule cells and then to the barb cells. Later, Matulionis (1970) confirmed the apico-basal gradient of feather differentiation of Bell and Thathachari (1963) with a thorough electron microscopic study of developing feathers. Matulionis (1970) also identified several different cell types that underwent keratinization in the developing feather germ. Kemp and Rogers (1972) determined that the keratins of feathers were different from those of scutate scale, by comparing reduced and S-carboxymethylated keratin polypeptides (Schroeder and Kay, 1955) by polyacrylamide gel electrophoresis. With their 10% gel system, at pH 9.5, they found that the bands of intermediate mobility, designated Beta 1-5, contained the major proteins of feathers and scales. Peptide mapping, immunodiffusion, amino acid analysis and in vitro filamentation studies demonstrated that the Beta group was a family of proteins related to beta (feather) keratin. With slight modification of the procedures of Kemp and Rogers (1972), Dhouailly et al. (1978) showed that feathers and scutate scales from embryos of 17- to 21-days of incubation also differed significantly in their electrophoretic banding patterns. In that study, the major feather keratins of intermediate mobility were designated Bf, while the major scale keratins of intermediate mobility were designated Bs. With this information, Dhouailly et al. (1978) then demonstrated that the epidermis from presumptive feather-forming regions was capable of making the scutate scale-specific keratins when heterotopically recombined with scutate scale dermis. Likewise, the epidermis from presumptive scutate scale forming regions made the feather-specific keratins when heterotopically recombined with dermis from a presumptive feather-forming region.

The alpha keratins of slow mobility in feather and scale tissues were designated Af and As, respectively (Dhouailly et al., 1978). The Af keratins were considered to be in the feather sheath, while the As keratins were believed to be in the hinge region of the overlapping scales. In order to be better able to evaluate both alpha and beta keratins in the same preparation, O'Guin and Sawyer (1982) modified, slightly, the procedures of Dhouailly et al.

(1978). Basically, the S-carboxymethyl (SCM) derivatives of the
epidermal proteins were separated by sodium dodecyl sulfate-
polyacrylamide gel (10%) electrophoresis (SDS-PAGE) with a 4.4%
acrylamide stacking gel, both at pH 8.3.   Comparison of the alpha
and beta keratins found in the scutate scales, scutellate scales,
reticulate scales, spurs and feathers of normal and scaleless
chickens resulted in the conclusion that alpha keratins were major
components of scales, showing tissue-specificity for the individual
scale types (O'Guin and Sawyer, 1982; McAleese and Sawyer, 1981;
1982; Smoak and Sawyer, 1982).   In fact, O'Guin et al. (1982) used
indirect immunofluorescence with antiserum to avian alpha and beta
keratins to demonstrate that alpha keratins are present in the outer
plate-like surface of scutate scales, as well as the hinge region
and inner scale surface.   O'Guin (1984) has also demonstrated that
alpha keratins are still major components of the outer surface of
scutate scales from 2 week old hatched birds.   Recently, Haake et
al. (1984) used SDS-PAGE analysis (O'Guin and Sawyer, 1982) and
indirect immunofluorescence (O'Guin et al., 1982) to characterize
keratinization in developing down feathers.   In this case, the
feather beta keratins were designated Bf 1-5 following the nomencla-
ture of Dhouailly et al. (1978), O'Guin and Sawyer (1982), and
Sawyer et al. (1985).   The electrophoretic analysis confirmed the
studies of Bell and Thathachari (1963) by showing that polypeptides
BF 1-5 became the major components of feathers at stage 39 (13 days
of incubation), and it confirmed the observation of Dhouailly et al.
(1978) that some alpha keratins are present in developing feathers.
In addition, antiserum to beta keratins allowed Haake et al. (1984)
to demonstrate, cytohistochemically, the apical-basal (see Bell and
Thathachari, 1963) and peripheral-central (see Matulionis, 1970)
gradients of beta keratinization, while antiserum to alpha keratins
allowed their cytohistochemical localization to the feather sheath.
Thus, feathers and scutate scales show differences not only in the
types of alpha and beta keratins they make but also in the distribution of these keratins and their time of appearance.

## MORPHOGENESIS AND CELL PROLIFERATION IN FEATHERS AND SCUTATE SCALES

Early studies suggested that the initial stages of feather and
scutate scale morphogenesis were virtually identical (Rawles, 1963;
Thomson, 1964); with these appendages described as arising from
epidermal thickenings which formed above aggregations of dermal
cells.   More extensive histological studies have demonstrated
differences in the morphogenesis of feathers and scutate scales.
Feathers arise as round epidermal placodes just before the formation
of dermal condensations (Sengel and Rusaouen, 1968).   The condensations are 235 micrometers in diameter and contain 5.52 nuclei/1000
micrometers cubed, as compared to 2.60 nuclei/1000 micrometers cubed
in the surrounding dermis (Wessells, 1965).   The cells of the
feather dermal condensation undergo a non-labeling phase of about 20
to 30 hours as determined by autoradiography with tritiated

thymidine (Wessells, 1965). Wessells (1965) also suggested that the cells of the overlying epidermal placodes did not incorporate tritiated thymidine during this period.

In contrast, scutate scales arise as oblong epidermal placodes which measure 150 to 170 micrometers by 250-300 micrometers (Sawyer 1970; 1972a; b). Dwyer (1971) showed that the overall density of the scale dermis, just before placode formation, was 3.31 nuclei/1000 micrometers cubed, while the preplacode dermis of feather regions was found to contain 2.60 nuclei/1000 micrometers cubed (Wessells, 1965). The actual scale placode dermis only attains a density of 3.24 nuclei/1000 micrometers cubed, never reaching the level found in feather dermal condensations. Also of significance, a non-labeling phase was not found in the dermis of scutate scales (Sawyer, 1970; 1972b). After the definitive scale ridge had formed, at 12 days of incubation, a small dermal condensation was seen in the distal most tip of the scale (Dwyer, 1971).

Even though the scutate scale dermis does not show any non-labeling phase during morphogenesis, the epidermal placodes of scales undergo a definite non-labeling period (Sawyer, 1970; 1972b). Tanaka and Kato (1983a), have now provided an extensive qualitative and quantitative characterization of the epidermal cells which give rise to the scutate scale. They described the characterization of the epidermal placode and interplacode regions, two distinct cell populations, whose coordinated activities give rise to the scutate scale epidermis. They have also carried out a detailed analysis of the role of cell proliferation and migration in the morphogenesis and differentiation of the scutate scale epidermis (Tanaka and Kato, 1983b). Several significant observations were made in their studies. First, cell division occurred only in the interplacode regions from day 9.25 to day 11. After mitosis, interplacode cells moved into the more distal placode region. During this time the mitotic figures of the single layer of basal cells are oriented with their long axis parallel to the proximodistal axis of the scales. The first sign of histodifferentiation occurred on day 11 with the initial appearance of suprabasal cells, which were the result of renewed proliferation of the basal cells from day 11 to day 11.75 (Tanaka and Kato, 1983b). This population of suprabasal cells then increased through cell proliferation of its own cells. It is tempting to speculate that this population of cells, located beneath the peridermal cells and increasing itself through cell proliferation, gives rise to the well-developed subperiderm of scutate scales. The cell layers beneath the subperiderm, which most likely originate from further proliferation of the basal cells, differ considerably from the subperidermal cells and those of the Beta Stratum (Sawyer et al., 1974a; 1985).

Unfortunately, such detailed cell proliferation and cell lineage studies are not available for developing feathers.

Matulionis (1970), however, examined the developing feather germ
with the electron microscope, and concluded that the columnar basal
cells of the 8 day feather germ, divided mitotically from 9-10 days
of incubation and formed 2-3 cell layers.  These cell layers then
gave rise to the peridermal and epidermal cells of the feather germ.
Thus, again significant differences exist in the early morphogenesis
and cell proliferation of feathers and scutate scales.

## EXPERIMENTAL APPROACHES TO FEATHER AND SCUTATE SCALE DEVELOPMENT

In the final sections of this article, we will discuss the
results of three experimental approaches which have provided further
information on the relationships between morphogenesis and the
biochemical differentiation of skin appendages in birds.

### Epidermal-Dermal Recombination Experiments

The existence of epidermal-dermal interactions during both
feather and scale morphogenesis has been shown by several tissue
recombination studies.  One of the most informative studies concerned with differences in the inductive nature of feathers and
scutate scales is that of Rawles (1963).  She showed that the
inductive capacity of the dermis and the competence of the epidermis
vary with both developmental stage and tissue location.  In recipro-
cal epidermal-dermal recombination experiments between prospective
feather and scale regions, feather dermis was a strong feather
inducer throughout stages 27-34 (5-8.5 days of incubation), while
scale dermis appeared to be bipotential in its inductive ability;
first supporting feather development from stages 35-38 (9-12 days of
incubation) and then inducing scales from stages 39-41 (13-15 days
of incubation) (Rawles, 1963).

Fisher and Sawyer (1979) then repeated Rawles (1963) work using
the chorionic epithelium (CE) as the responding tissue.  As demonstrated by Kato and Hayashi (1963), the CE, which has not undergone
the inductive influences of epidermis, readily forms normal feathers
or beak when recombined with presumptive dermis from the feather and
beak forming regions, respectively.  Furthermore, Kato (1969) showed
that the CE forms normal scutate scale epidermis when recombined
with stage 41 (15 days) scutate scale dermis.  Like Kato (1969),
Fisher and Sawyer (1979) found that the CE formed normal scutate
scale epidermis in combination with stage 39-41 scutate scale
dermis, but formed only feather-like structures with dermis younger
than stage 38.

The results of Fisher and Sawyer (1979) suggested again that
the scutate scale dermis was bipotential during development, first
inducing feathers then scales.  However, Rawles (1963) had also
suggested an alternative hypothesis; that the responding tissue
might have a feather bias.  This point of view was further supported
by Dhouailly's (1978) observation that the chorion (ectodermal and

mesodermal components together) can form normal feathers when exposed to embryonic mouse dermis. Recently, Dhouailly and Sengel (1983) showed that scutate scale dermis, younger than stage 38, does in fact have the ability to induce complete scutate scale morphogenesis in apteric epidermis, which normally does not form any appendages. Earlier, Linsenmayer (1972) had demonstrated that presumptive reticulate scale epidermis could also make scutate scales in combination with stage 36-37 scutate scale dermis. Thus the formation of a feather or a scale depends not only on the inductive nature of the dermis but also on the ability of the epithelium to respond. While the CE fails to.undergo scale morphogenesis when recombined with scutate scale dermis younger than stage 38, it apparently can form feathers de novo. It is possible that the CE has a bias for making feathers, yet it is also possible that the inductive phenomena of presumptive feather and scutate scale dermises are different.

Further information regarding the role of scutate scale morphogenesis in regulating biochemical differentiation is gained from tissue recombination studies using an unique line of chickens known as scaleless, sc/sc, (Abbott and Asmundson, 1957). Scaleless embryos are defective in the morphogenesis of several of the integumental derivatives, including feathers and scutate scales. Tissue recombinations indicated that the defect in the mutant skin initially resides in the ectodermal component of feathers and scales (Sengel and Abbott, 1963).

Later, Sawyer and Abbott (1972) demonstrated that the epidermal placodes did not form in scaleless embryos. Subsequently, the beta stratum failed to form (Sawyer et al., 1974b) and the characteristic alpha and beta keratins were not expressed (O'Guin & Sawyer, 1982). Dhouailly and Sawyer (1984) have now shown that the scaleless, dermis becomes defective at a stage (9.5 days) which coincides with the appearance of epidermal placodes in the normal embryo. They concluded that failure of the scaleless dermis to be associated with the placode resulted in the inability of the dermis to participate in later events of scale development. McAleese and Sawyer, (1981; 1982) showed that scaleless epidermis, in fact, can undergo normal scutate scale differentiation if recombined with a normal dermis which had completed early scale morphogenesis (stage 38 or later). In this case the normal histodifferentiation and tissue-specific keratin expression was achieved in the scaleless epidermis by by-passing the defective morphogenesis in scaleless.

Transfilter Experiments

A second approach to analysis of the relationship between morphogenesis and cytodifferentiation has involved the placement of a Nuclepore Filter between epidermis and dermis of presumptive feather and scutate scale tissues. This procedure has been

particularly useful for the study of feather development. While
scale tissues can easily be separated into epidermis and dermis, at
late stages of development, this is not true of feathers. Therefore, it is difficult to assess the developmental competence of
feather components at later stages of development. The transfilter
technique provides a means by which one can disrupt normal tissue
interactions and observe the effect on both morphogenesis of feathers and the subsequent expression of feather beta keratins. The
availability of thin (25 micrometers) Nuclepore filters with a wide
range of pore sizes, allows different approaches to be taken. For
example, a Nuclepore filter with a pore size of 12 micrometers
readily allows dermal cells to traverse the filter and reorganize
into a new dermis beneath the epidermis; while smaller pore sizes
(i.e., 0.4 micrometers) will only allow contact between the cell
processes of the dermis and epidermis. Using the first approach
with presumptive feather tissues, König and Sawyer (1985) obtained
normal feathers distributed in a normal feather pattern. The
presumptive feather dermis (Stages 27-29, Hamburger and Hamilton,
1951) simply migrates through the filter and forms a new dermis,
which then induces feather morphogenesis. The same experiment with
embryonic scutate scale tissues (Stages 38-40, H & H) gives different results. Although the dermal cells easily migrate through the
filter and form a new dermis beneath the epidermis, the scutate
scale ridges do not form and a Beta Stratum does not form (O'Guin,
1984). Using the second approach, König and Sawyer (1985) found
that feather-like filaments could form in the presumptive feather
epidermis, even when recombined with its dermis across an interpos-
ing filter of 0.4 micrometers which does not allow the passage of
dermal cells. While resembling feathers, these feather-like filaments did not undergo barb ridge morphogenesis or differentiation of
barb ridge cells. The cells of the feather-like filaments as well
as the cells of the surrounding epidermis were positive for alpha
keratin, by indirect immunofluorescence. In a few recombinants,
beta keratin could be detected in some cells of the feather-like
filaments and the subperidermal cells of the adjacent epidermis, by
indirect immunofluorescence. Since the antiserum against beta
keratin recognizes the beta keratins of the subperiderm, scutate
scale beta stratum (O'Guin et al., 1982; Sawyer et al., 1985),
feather barb ridge, feather sheath (Haake et al., 1984) and claw
(unpublished observation); and since electrophoresis could not be
carried out on individual feather-like filaments, König and Sawyer
(1985) could not identify the beta keratin as feather-specific. At
present, König and Sawyer (1985) favor the hypothesis that the beta
keratins found in the feather-like filaments are present in sheath-
like cells or unidentifiable cells which formed from aborptive barb
ridges, and are not the beta keratins which characterize the barb
ridge cells of normal feathers.

Hopefully, further analysis of this relationship will be
possible with the development of monoclonal antibodies against the

feather and scale beta keratin polypeptides and by 2-dimensional gel
electrophoretic analysis.  Our goal is to be able to distinguish
individual beta keratin polypeptides and to localize these to
particular cells or cell layers in feathers and scales.  An in-depth
developmental analysis of beta keratin expression may then allow us
to elucidate the requirements, in terms of morphogenesis and histogenesis, for a feather or scutate scale epidermal cell to express
its appropriate keratin genes.

## Hydrocortisone Treatment

Experimental treatments of presumptive feather or scutate scale
tissue with corticosteroids have demonstrated the role of tissue
interactions in feather and scale development and the importance of
morphogenesis for the tissue-specific expression of keratins.
Moscona and Karnovsky (1960) first showed that cortisone, applied to
the chorioallantoic membrane of the chick embryo, inhibits the
formation of both feathers and scutate scales.  Furthermore, this
effect was dependent on the developmental stage of the embryo.
Stuart et al. (1972), carried out a more detailed analysis of the
effects of hydrocortisone on feather development, in which they
showed that inhibition of feather formation was associated with
disruption of early morphogenetic events.  Thus, no epidermal
placodes or dermal condensations formed, and the typical organization of extracellular fibrous components was not present.  Recipro-
cal epidermal-dermal recombination experiments, involving both
hydrocortisone-treated and non-treated skin components, indicated
that hydrocortisone primarily affected the morphogenetic capacity of
the epidermis, since treated epidermis could not participate in
normal feather development even when recombined with an untreated
dermis.  The fact that an untreated epidermis, recombined with a
treated dermis resulted in the formation of feathers and restored a
dermal organization similar to that of normal skin, was considered
evidence of epidermal-dermal interaction.  Demarchez et al. (1984)
have recently carried out a study of the effect of hydrocortisone on
dorsal skin.  They have examined the ultrastructure of the treated
skin, as well as the distribution of the extracellular matrix
materials, such as fibronectin, laminin, and Types I and III
collagen.  These authors concluded that hydrocortisone treatment
resulted in an early maturation of both the epidermis and dermis,
perhaps affecting the morphogenetic competence of the epidermis and
disrupting normal tissue interactions.  While this study did not
include a biochemical analysis of keratin expression in the treated
skin, the effect of hydrocortisone on scale development and keratinization was carried out by Fisher et al. (1984).  Like previous
studies, the effect of hydrocortisone on the epidermal derivatives
was found to be both stage and dose dependent.  In addition, the
effect on different types of scales and feathers was not the same.
While scutellate and interstitial scales were completely inhibited,
scutate and reticulate scale development was only partially blocked.

Immunohistochemical and biochemical analysis of the hydrocortisone-
treated scutellate scale region showed that the Beta Stratum was
absent and the beta keratins, BS 1 to 3, were greatly reduced.
While it is not known whether hydrocortisone has any direct effect
on beta keratin expression (Obinata et al., 1982), these results
suggested that it can act indirectly by inhibiting morphogenesis of
the scale. Furthermore, these results supported the hypothesis that
there may be differences in the tissue interactions governing the
morphogenesis of structurally distinct scale types, and that each
scale type has its own distinctive temporal, morphological and
biochemical pattern of development.

CONCLUSIONS

Since the early observation that the inductive interactions of
feathers differ from those of scales (Sengel, 1958; Rawles, 1963)
and the observation of Kemp and Rogers (1972) that the keratins of
feathers differ from those of scutate scales, evidence continues to
accumulate that these appendages differ significantly in several
aspects of their morphogenesis, histogenesis and biochemical differentiation. With the ever increasing evidence that morphological and
histological events in skin development are causally related to
keratinization, it is not surprising that two skin appendages which
elaborate different keratins, do, in fact, differ in aspects of
their morphogenesis and histogenesis.

In the future, with the rapidly developing technology of
genetic engineering, it is not inconceivable that we will have
cloned gene fragments specific for all the keratins of the chicken
integument (Wilton, 1984). The techniques of in situ hybridization
will then allow us to make meaningful correlations between morphogenetic or histogenic events and the appearance of specific mRNAs in
individual cells.

REFERENCES

Abbott, U.K., and Asmundson, V.S., 1957, Scaleless, an inherited
    ectodermal defect in the domestic fowl, J. Hered., 18:63.
Baden, H.P., and Maderson, P.F.A., 1970, Morphological and bio-
    physical identification of fibrous proteins in the amniote
    epidermis, J. Exp. Zool., 174:225.
Bell, E., and Thathachari, Y.T., 1963, Development of feather
    keratin during embryogenesis of the chick, J. Cell. Biol.,
    16:215.
Brotman, H.F., 1977, Epidermal-dermal tissue interactions between
    mutant foot skin and normal backskin: A comparison of the
    inductive capacities of scaleless low line and normal anterior
    foot dermis. J. Exp. Zool., 200:125.
Brotman, H.F., 1977, Epidermal-dermal tissue interactions between
    mutant and normal embryonic back skin: site of mutant gene

activity determining abnormal feathering in the epidermis, J. Exp. Zool., 200:243.

Démarchez, M., Mauger, A., Herbage, D., and Sengel, P., 1984, Effect of hydrocortisone on skin development in the chick embryo: ultrastructural, immunohistological and biochemical analysis, Dev. Biol., 106:15.

Dhouailly, D., Rogers, G.E., and Sengel, P., 1978, The specification of feather and scale protein synthesis in epidermal-dermal recombinations, Dev. Biol., 65:58.

Dhouailly, D., and Sengel, P., 1983, Feather forming properties of the foot integument in avian embryos, in: "Epithelial-mesenchymal interactions in development", R.H. Sawyer and J.F. Fallon, eds., Praeger Press, NY.

Dhouailly, D., and Sawyer, R.H., 1984, Avian scale development: XI. Initial appearance of the dermal defect in scaleless skin, Dev. Biol., 105:343.

Dwyer, N.K., 1971, Chick scale morphogenesis: Early events in the formation of overall shank and individual scale shape, Master's Thesis, Univ. of Massachusetts, Amherst, Mass.

Fisher, C., and Sawyer, R.H., 1979, Response of the avian chorionic epithelium to presumptive scale-forming dermis, J. Exp., Zool., 207:505.

Fisher, C.J., O'Guin, W.M., and Sawyer, R.H., 1984, Altered keratin biosynthesis follows inhibition of scale morphogenesis by hydrocortisone, Dev. Biol., 106:45.

Haake, A.R., König, G., and Sawyer, R.H., 1984, Avian feather development: Relationships between morphogenesis and keratinization, Dev. Biol., 106:406.

Kato, Y., and Hayashi, Y., 1963, The inductive transformation of the chorionic epithelium into skin derivatives, Exp. Cell Res., 31:599.

Kato, Y., 1969, Epithelial metaplasia induced on embryonic membranes. I. Induction of epidermis from chick chorionic epithelium, J. Exp. Zool., 170:229.

Kemp, D.J., and Rogers, G.E., 1972, Differentiation of avian keratinocytes: Characterization and relationship of the keratin proteins of adult and embryonic feathers and scales. Biochemistry, 11:969.

Kodama, R., and Eguchi, G., 1983, Characterization of an antiserum against feather keratins of the chick: Its cross-reaction with lens protein, (delta)-crystallin, Dev., Growth and Differ., 25(3):261.

König, G., and Sawyer, R.H., 1985, Analysis of feather morphogenesis and cytodifferentiation, Dev. Biol., in press.

Linsenmayer, T.F., 1972, Control of integumentary patterns of the chick, Dev. Biol., 27:244.

Lockett, T.J., Kemp, D.J., and Rogers, G.E., 1979, Organization of the unique and repetitive sequences in feather keratin messenger ribonucleic acid, Biochemistry, 18:5654.

Matulionis, D.H., 1970, Morphology of the developing down feather of chick embryos, Z. Anat. Entw.-Gesch, 132:107.

McAleese, S.R. and Sawyer, R.H., 1981, Correcting the phenotype of the epidermis from chick embryos homozygous for the gene scaleless (sc/sc). Science 214:1033.

McAleese, S.R., and Sawyer, R.H., 1982, Avian scale development, IX. Scale formation by scaleless (sc/sc) epidermis under the influence of normal scale dermis, Dev. Biol., 89:493.

Moll, R., Franke, W.W., Schiller, D.L., Geiger, B., and Krepler, R., 1982, The catalog of human cytokeratins: Patterns of expression in normal epithelia, tumors and cultured cells, Cell, 31:11.

Molloy, P.L., Powell, B.C., Gregg, K., Barone, E.D., and Rogers, G.E., 1982, Organization of feather keratin genes in the chick genome. Nucleic Acids Res., 10:6007.

Moscona, M.H. and Karnofsky, D.A., 1960, Cortisone-induced modifications in the development of the chick embryo, Endocrinology, 66:533.

Novel, G., 1973, Feather pattern stability and reorganization in cultured skin, J. Embryol. Exp. Morphol., 30:605.

Obinata, A., Kawanda, M., and Endo, H., 1982, Heterogeneity of low molecular weight epidermal structural proteins of chick embryonic tarsometatarsal skin. Effect of hydrocortisone on its accumulation with reference to differentiation of epidermal cells, Biochim. Biophys. Acta, 708:33.

O'Guin, W.M., and Sawyer, R.H., 1982, Avian scale development. VIII. Relationships between morphogenetic and biosynthetic differentiation, Dev. Biol., 89:485.

O'Guin, W.M., Knapp, L., and Sawyer, R.H., 1982, Biochemical and immunohistochemical localization of alpha and beta keratins in avian scutate scale, J. Exp. Zool., 220:371.

O'Guin, W.M., 1984, Relationships between morphogenetic and biosynthetic differentiation in the development of the avian integument, Ph.D. Dissertation, University of South Carolina.

Parakkal, P.F., and Matoltsy, A.G., 1968, An electron microscopic study of developing chick skin, J. Ultrastruct. Res., 23:403.

Rawles, M.E., 1963, Tissue interactions in scale and feather development as studied in dermal-epidermal recombinations, J. Embryol. Exp. Morphol., 2:765.

Rudall, K.M., 1947, X-ray studies of the distribution of protein chain types in the vertebrate epidermis, Biochim Biophy. Acta, 1:549.

Sawyer, R.H., 1970, An analysis of avian scale morphogenesis, Ph.D. Dissertation, University of Massachusetts.

Sawyer, R.H., 1972a, Avian scale development. I. Histogenesis and morphogenesis of the epidermis and dermis during formation of the scale ridge, J. Exp. Zool., 181:365.

Sawyer, R.H., 1972b, Avian scale development. II. A study of cell proliferation, J. Exp. Zool., 181:385.

Sawyer, R.H., and Abbott, U.K., 1972, Defective histogenesis and morphogenesis in the anterior shank skin of the scaleless mutant, J. Exp. Zool., 181:99.

Sawyer, R.H., Abbott, U.K., and Fry, G.N., 1974a, Avian scale development. III. Ultrastructure of the keratinizing cells of the outer and inner epidermal surfaces of the scale ridge, J. Exp. Zool., 190:57.

Sawyer, R.H., Abbott, U.K., and Fry, G.N., 1974b, Avian scale development. IV. Ultrastructure of the anterior shank skin of the scaleless mutant, J. Exp. Zool., 190:71.

Sawyer, R.H., 1975, Avian scale development. V. Ultrastructure of the chorionic epithelium induced by anterior shank dermis from the scaleless mutant, J. Exp. Zool., 191:133.

Sawyer, R.H., 1979, Avian scale development: Effect of the scaleless gene on morphogenesis and histogenesis, Dev. Biol. Biol., 68:1.

Sawyer, R.H., and Fallon, J.G.F., eds., Epithelial-mesenchymal interactions in development, Praeger, New York.

Sawyer, R.H., 1983, The role of epithelial-mesenchymal interactions in regulating gene expression during avian scale morphogenesis, in: "Epithelail-Mesenchymal Interactions in Development", R.H. Sawyer and J.F. Fallon, eds., Praeger Press, NY.

Sawyer, R.H., Knapp, L.W., and O'Guin, W.M., 1985, Avian Skin, in: "Biology of the Integument, Vol. II Vertebrates", Bereiter-Hahn, J., Maltolsy, A.G, and Richards, K.S. ed., Springer-Verlag, Berlin, in press.

Schroeder, W.A., and Kay, L.M., 1955, The amino acid composition of certain morphologically distinct parts of white turkey feathers, and of goose fetaher barbs and goose down, J. Amer. Chem. Soc., 7:3901.

Sengel, P., 1958, Recherches experimentales sur la differenciation des germes plumaires et du pigment de la peau de l'embryon de poues en culture in vitro, Ann. Sci. Zool., 20:421.

Sengel, P., and Abbott, U.K., 1963, In vitro studies with the scaleless mutant: Interaction during feather and scale differentiation, J. Hered. 54:254.

Sengel, P., and Rusaouen, M., 1968, Aspects histologiques de la differenciation precoce des ebauches plumaires chez le Poulet. C r Acad. Sci., D266:795.

Sengel, P., 1976, Morphogenesis of skin, in: "Developmental and cell biology series", Abercrombie, M., Newth, D.R., and Torrey, S.G., eds., University Press, Cambridge.

Smoak, K.D. and Sawyer, R.H., 1983, Avian spur development: abnormal morphogenesis and keratinization in the scaleless (sc/sc), Mutant BioScience, 33(8):514.

Stuart, E.S., Garber, B., and Moscona, A.A., 1972, An analysis of feather germ formation in the embryo and in vitro, in normal development and in skin treated with hydrocortisone, J. Exp. Zool., 179:197.

Sun, T-T., Eichner, R., Nelson, W.G., Tseng, S.C.G., Weiss, R.A., Jarvinen, M., and Woodcock-Mitchell, J., 1983, Keratin classes: Molecular markers for different types of epithelial differentiation, J. Invest. Dermatol., 81(1):109.

Tanaka, S., and Kato, Y, 1983, Epigenesis in developing avian scales. I. Qualitative and quantitative characterization of finite cell populations, J. Exp. Zool., 225:257.

Tanaka, S., and Kato, Y., 1983, Epigenesis in developing avian
    scales. II. Cell proliferation in relation to morphogenesis
    and differentiation in the epidermis, J. Exp. Zool., 225:271.

Walker, I.D., and Bridgen, J., 1976, The keratin chains of avian
    scale keratin genes, Eur. J. Biochem., 67:283.

Wessells, N.K., 1965, Morphology and proliferation during early
    feather development, Dev. Biol., 12:131.

Wilton, S.D., 1984, Molecular studies of keratin genes expressed in
    avian epidermal tissue, Ph.D. Dissertation, University of
    Adelaide, South Australia.

# COMMUNICATIONS BETWEEN CELLS AND THE CONSTRUCTION OF TISSUES

## INTRODUCTION

There is a tendency to circularity in the events of regulation of gene expression which has to be accomodated within the linear organisation of a conference and its published proceedings. The signals between cells can be seen either as a beginning of a sequence of events in differentiation triggering and regulating gene expression, or they can be seen as the end product of one stage of the continuing process of tissue differentiation, in which a specific tissue or group of cells synthesises a signal molecule, which is taken up by other cells or tissues.

Communications between cells in development are clearly hetero-geneous in nature, and range from the production of diffusible substances, which may elicit response from certain cell types only, to the formation of intimate cell-cell contacts. The earliest investiga-tions into this group of phenomena was the study of the primary organiser, followed by the study of systems with secondary and tertiary inductions (Reviewed, Browder 1980).

Although work on the physiology of ductless glands has developed extensively in this century, it could be claimed that the role of the testis in development was empirically well understood in ancient times by all cultures which required the production of eunuchs and castrati, and was also important in animal husbandry. The chemical characterisation of the hormones and the identification of their targets has permitted a comparatively detailed understanding of the mechanism of their action, the nature of their receptors and, particularly in the case of the steroid hormones, has enabled this understanding to be brought to the level of DNA and the control of transcription (Harrison, 1983; Anderson, 1984).

The diffusibility of growth factors has similarly led to their isolation and to the characterisation of many of them (Gospodarowicz, 1976; Courtois et al., 1982; Hunter and Cooper, 1985). Part, at least, of the distinction between growth factors and hormones stems from the history of the technology of the detection and there is no clear dividing line between them. Chemically growth factors are peptide in nature, as are many, but not all, hormones.

Oncogene products include substances that have growth factor effects and other substances which appear to be growth factor receptors (Bishop, 1983; Heldin and Westermark, 1984).

Cell-cell signals which depend upon intimate cell contact clearly do not depend upon diffusible substances and are much more difficult to investigate. The discovery that the growth of cells in vitro could be markedly affected both by conditioned medium and by growth in dishes which had previously supported the growth of another cell population, opened up the possibility of extracting the substances responsible. Subsequent research has shown that the extracellular material includes many high molecular weight polymers of low solubility which may severally act upon cellular differentiation by triggering it, directing it, or stabilizing it in a particular pathway and, directly or indirectly affecting gene expression (for example, Spiegelman and Ginty, 1983). The extracellular matrix may also have the function of orienting cells in particular spatial relationships to one another, and thus initiating tissue architecture. (Nathansen and Hay, 1980; Greenberg et al., 1981; Linkhart et al., 1981; Loring et al., 1982; Wicha et al., 1982; Turner et al., 1983).

The association of cells into structures which are incipient tissues has three consequences: members of the cell population come to occupy locations in the mass which have different physiological characteristics; the signals to which they can respond become different from those to which they could respond as individual cells, (for example Moscona and Degenstein, 1982), and they become increasingly unable to enter upon alternative pathways of differentiation or to transdifferentiate.

Selective cell-cell adhesion appears to be an important morpho- genetic factor throughout development (reviewed Edelman, 1985) and affects cell relationships and orientation even as early as the blastula (Shirayoshi et al., 1983). The significance of cell-cell contacts in maintaining the stability of a differentiated cell is implied by the requirement for their disruption before transdifferen- tiation can occur (Moscona & Degenstein, 1982; Clayton, 1982; Eguchi et al., 1982; Okada, 1983).


REFERENCES

Anderson, J.N., 1984, The effect of steroid hormones on gene trans- cription, in 'Biological Regulation and Development', R.F. Goldberger, and K.R. Yamamoto, eds., Vol 3B, p169 Plenum Press New York, London
Bishop, J.M., 1983, Cellular oncogenes and retroviruses, Ann. Rev. Biochem., 52:301.

Browder, L.W., 1980, Developmental Biology, Chapt. 13, Saunders,
    Philadelphia.
Clayton, R.M., 1982, Cellular and molecular aspects of differentia-
    tion and transdifferentiation of ocular tissues in vitro, in,
    Differentiation in Vitro, M.M. Yeoman and D.E.S. Truman, eds.,
    p83, Cambridge University Press, London, New York.
Courtois, Y., Arruti, C., Barritault, D., Courty, J., Tassin, J.,
    Olivie, M., Plouet, J., Laurent, M. and Perry, M., 1982, The
    role of a growth factor derived from the retina (EDGF) in
    controlling the differentiated stages of several ocular and non
    ocular tissues, in Stability and Switching in Cellular Different-
    iation, R.M. Clayton and D.E.S. Truman, eds., p289, Plenum
    Press, New York, London.
Edelman, G.M., 1985, Cell adhesion and the molecular processes of
    morphogenesis, Ann. Rev. Biochem., 54:135
Eguchi, G., Masuda, A., Karasawa, Y., Kodama, R. and Itoh, Y., 1982,
    Microenvironments controlling the transdifferentiation of
    vertebrate pigmented epithelial cells in in vitro culture, in
    Stability and Switching in Cellular Differentiation, R.M. Clayton,
    and D.E.S. Truman, eds., p209, Plenum Press, New York, London
Gospodarowicz, D. and Moran, J.S., 1976, Growth factors in mammalian
    cell culture, Ann. Rev. Biochem. 45:531
Greenberg, J.H., Seppa, S., Seppa, H. and Hewitt, A.T., 1981, Role of
    collagen and fibronectin in neural crest cell adhesion and
    migration, Dev. Biol., 87:259.
Harrison, R.W., III, 1983, Cellular factors which modulate hormone
    responses: glucocorticoid action in perspective, in Int. Rev.
    Cytol, Suppl. 15, Aspects of Cell Regulation, G.H. Bourne, J.F.
    Danielli and K.W. Jeon, eds., p1, Academic Press, New York,
    London.
Heldin, C-H. and Westermark, B., 1984, Growth factors:  mechanism of
    action and relation to oncogenes, Cell 37:9.
Hunter, T. and Cooper, J.A., 1985, Growth factors and receptors, Ann.
    Rev. Biochem., 54:897.
Loring, J., Glimetius, B. and Weston, J.A., 1982, Extracellular matrix
    material influences quail neural crest cell differentiation in
    vitro, Dev. Biol., 90:165.
Linkhart, T.A., Clegg, C.H., and Hauschka, S.D., 1981, Myogenic
    differentiation in permanent clonal mouse myoblast cell lines:
    Regulation by macromolecular growth factors in the culture medium,
    Dev. Biol., 86:19.
Moscona, A.A. and Degenstein, L., 1982, Formation of lentoids from
    neural retina cells:  glial origin of the transformed cells, in,
    Stability and Switching in Cell Differentiation, R.M. Clayton and
    D.E.S. Truman, eds., p187, Plenum Press, New York, London.
Nathanson, M.A. and Hay, E.D., 1980, Analysis of cartilage differ-
    entiation from skeletal muscle grown on bone matrix, Dev. Biol.,
    78:301.
Okada, T.S., 1983, Recent progress in studies of the transdifferentia-
    tion of eye tissue in vitro, Cell Differ., 13:177.

Shirayoshi, Y., Okada, T.S. and Takeichi, M., 1983, The calcium-
    dependent cell-cell adhesion system regulates inner cell mass
    formation and cell surface polarisation in early mouse development
    Cell, 35:631.
Spiegelman, B.M. and Ginty, C.A., 1983, Fibronectin modulation of cell
    shape and lipogenic gene expression in 3T3 adipocytes, Cell, 35:
    657.
Turner, D.C., Lawton, J., Dollenmeier, P., Ehrishmann, R., Chiquet, M.
    1983, Guidance of myogenic cell migration by oriented deposits of
    fibronectin, Dev. Biol., 95:497
Wicha, M., Lowrie, G., Kohn, E., Bagavandoss, P. and Mahn, T., 1982,
    Extra cellular matrix promotes mammary epithelial growth and
    differentiation in vitro, Proc. Natl. Acad. Sci. 79:3213.

# RESPONSES OF METASTATIC RHABDOMYOSARCOMA CELLS AND NORMAL MYOBLASTS TO GROWTH FACTORS DERIVED FROM NORMAL TISSUES

M. Becker, M-F. Poupon and Y. Courtois*

I.R.S.C. du CNRS, ER 278 - 94802 Villejuif Cedex
France;

* INSERM U.118, Unite de Recherches Gerontologique
29 rue Wilhem, 75016 Paris, France

ABSTRACT

During metastasis tumor cells may be affected by a variety of
environmental factors including intercellular substances and growth
factors of host origin. We have studied this relationship on several
cloned cell lines derived from a rat rhabdomyosarcoma selected on the
basis of their metastatic potential. We show that the parental cell
line (9-4/0) was stimulated to proliferate in vitro by Epidermal
Growth Factor (EGF), pituitary Fibroblast Growth Factor (pFGF) and Eye
Derived Growth Factor (EDGF) in the presence of 10% fetal calf serum
(FCS). Six sublines which differed in their doubling time and
metastatic potential were studied. These growth factors stimulate all
these cells to some extent but some cell lines were more responsive to
EGF than to EDGF or to FGF, while other cell lines were more
responsive to EDGF and very little to EGF. One cloned cell line (14)
was chosen to study the different parameters playing a role in growth
factor stimulation. This growth factor-increased proliferation was
independent on the FCS concentration and on the initial cell density.

The effect of growth factors on proliferation was also studied
on cells grown on collagen type IV, fibronectin, laminin and
extracellular matrix (ECM). The results showed that the growth
factors enhanced the different proliferative response of the cells
to different substrata except for ECM.

The non-tumorigenic, myoblastic cell line L6 was stimulated by
FGF and EDGF, and not by EGF. The growth of L6 cells differed on
plastic and ECM, was stimulated by EDGF and FGF on plastic, but was

not stimulated by these growth factors on ECM.

Fibronectin expression was decreased in the presence of the growth factor(s). We conclude from these experiments that exocrine growth factors (EGF, FGF, EDGF) associated or not to culture substrata modulate the in vitro behaviour of tumor cells, add a new parameter to their diversity and we hypothesize that they could regulate their metastatic behaviour.


INTRODUCTION

Growth factors have been implicated in the cancer process by many investigators. Among the various aspects, one is the decreased serum dependence of tumor cells (Cherington et al., 1979; Moses and Robinson, 1982) leading to the discovery of transforming growth factors (TGF) produced by tumor cells in culture (Chua et al., 1983; De Larco and Todaro, 1978; Kaplan et al., 1982; Roberts et al., 1983). These TGF(s) were able to transform the phenotype of normal cells and influence that of transformed cells. Furthermore, growth factors extracted from normal tissues can influence the growth and phenotype of normal and transformed cells (Balk et al., 1982; Jetten et Goldfarb, 1983; Keski-Oja et al., 1980; Lim et al., 1981).

Many spontaneous, chemically or virally transformed cells have been shown to synthesize autocrine growth factors in vitro. Several of them have been purified to homogeneity (Marquardt et al., 1983). A link between these growth factors and growth factors extracted from normal tissue (Barritault et al., 1982; Cohen, 1983; Gospodarowicz et al., 1978; Ross et al., 1974) has been suspected. They induce a mechanism of membrane protein tyrosine kinase activation (Chambard et al., 1983), similar to the one described for the induction of cell proliferation in SSV transformed cells (Elk et al., 1982). This was further emphasized by the discoveries of sequence homologies between PDGF and the sis-onc gene (Robbins et al., 1983) and the homology between the receptor site of EGF and the erb-onc gene (Davonward et al., 1984).

In addition to the messages received through diffusible growth factors, cancer cells interact with the extracellular matrix (ECM) (review in Gospodarowicz, 1983). Cell division and differentiation are influenced by cellular shape and reactivity to ECM (Campisi and Medrano, 1983; Gospodarowicz et al., 1978; Vlodavsky et al., 1980). For instance, transformed cells cultured on the appropriate matrix can lose their in vitro phenotypic characteristics. Growth factors are also involved in the control of ECM expression by normal and tumor cells (Gospodarowicz, 1983; Kern et al., 1983; Moczar et al., 1983; Tassin et al., 1983). Reciprocally ECM can modify the shape and behaviour of cells and thereby determine their response to growth factors. Thus, while autocrine or exocrine growth factors may play a key role in tumor cell growth, their role in the maintenance of tumor heterogeneity and in the process of metastasis has thus far not been investigated. Primary tumor and metastatic cells are morphologically and functionally heterogeneous, in terms of growth pattern, invasive properties, cell surface glycoproteins, glycolipids, enzymes and antigenic determinants (Hart and Fidler, 1981; Nicolson, 1982; Nicolson, 1984). Previous studies have also shown a heterogeneity in cell response to environmental signals such as growth factors and hormones (Kaplan and Ozanne, 1983; Lifsmitz et al., 1983; Sirbasku, 1978; Shupnik and Tasnjian, 1982).

These processes are dependent on the intrinsic properties of tumor cells (Hart and Fidler, 1981; Nicolson, 1982; Nicolson, 1984) but may also be influenced by the extracellular environment (Ossowski and Reich, 1983). However, in the process of metastatic dissemination, it is possible to identify the steps in which growth factors could be involved by a pleiotropic action, in comparison to their action on normal cells.

Growth factors 1) activate the proliferation of cells and; 2) provoke detachment of cells from other cells and from the basement membrane through an effect on its components (Jetten and Goldfarb, 1983); 3) accelerate the chemotaxis and migration of cells (Glaser et al., 1980; Gospodarowicz, 1979; Grotendorst, 1984; Seppa et al., 1983; Westermark et al., 1983); 4) activate degradative enzymes, for instance the plasminogen activator (Gross et al., 1983) to disrupt blood vessel walls (Nicolson, 1982); 5) commit division in cells that have entered the blood circulation by circulating growth factors (Chambard et al., 1983). Indeed, "committment" factors such as PDGF are present in platelets and EGF in the serum; 6) contribute to tumor cell recognition of the different ECM components or eventually change the ECM properties to facilitate cell attachment (Gospodarowicz, 1983; Vlodavski and Gospodarowicz, 1981; Vlodavski et al., 1980). All these events have been implicated also in tumor formation and metastasis.

To investigate the different influences of growth factors on tumor cells, we have chosen to compare the response of a rhabdomyo-sarcoma primary tumor cell line and several derived sublines to three different tissue growth factors (EGF, FGF and EDGF). The rat nickel-induced rhabdomyosarcoma was recently developed in the laboratory of one of us (Sweeney et al., 1982). The primary cell line as well as its sublines have various metastatic and pulmonary colonizing potentials, various growth and differentiation properties in vitro as well as various fibronectin expression. L6 is considered to be a normal cell line of rat Wistar myoblasts. The three growth factors were selected because of their ability to stimulate normal and tumoral cell proliferation in culture (Barritault et al., 1981; Courtois et al., 1981).

In addition, both EDGF (Barritault et al., 1982) and GFG

(Gospodarowicz, 1977) can stimulate the proliferation of skeletal myoblasts, the putative normal counterpart of rhabdomyosarcoma cells. However, normal myoblasts are not stimulated by EGF (Lim et al., 1984) despite the presence of EGF receptor kinase in developing skeletal muscle of 13 day mouse embryo (Hortsch et al., 1983) or in mouse myoblasts in vitro (Lim and Hauschka, 1984).

We have employed this model to answer the following questions: 1) Do L6 cells and different sublines derived by cloning from a myoblastic tumor, express various responses to these three growth factors in terms of accelerated proliferation in culture?   2) Are these responses controlled by ECM and its components?   3) Are these responses accompanied by changes in the expression of fibronectin? 4) Could the observed results be related to the various metastatic potential of the sublines?

MATERIAL AND METHODS

A primary rhabdomyosarcoma (RMS) induced by nickel in a WAG male rat has been developed in our laboratory.  A series of cloned cell lines have been derived from an original 9-4/0 parental cell line. The behaviour of these cell lines has been studied in terms of the presence of fibronectin, growth parameters, tumorigenicity and metastatic potential by subcutaneous and intravenous routes (Pot-Deprun et al., 1983; Sweeney et al., 1982).  The data have been actualized and are presented in Table 1.  All these cloned cell lines will be further referred to as sublines (6, 8, 13, 14, 21, 22).  The parental cell line 9-4/0 has been cloned at the 10th and the 35th passages.  In these conditions, cloned cell lines maintained a stable phenotype as well in vivo, as in vitro.  L6 was kindly provided to us by Dr Leibovitch (IGR, Villejuif).  EGF was provided by Cliniscience, Paris, France.  pFGF by Kor, Biochemicals, England, EDGF was prepared by us.  The activity of EDGF was described as the amount of proteinic growth factor able to induce half of the maximum serum dependent stimulation of arrested bovine epithelial lens cells (Barritault et al., 1982).  The preparation used in these assays had an activity of 700 U/ml and 10  g/ml.  The rabbit anti-human fibronectin serum was obtained from Collaborative Research (USA), goat anti-rabbit serum from Institut Pasteur, Paris (France), human fibronectin from Kor. Laminin was prepared as described by Timpl (Timpl et al., 1979).  ECM, deposited in vitro by endothelial corneal cells was prepared according to a modification of Gospodarowicz (Gospodarowicz et al., 1978; Tassin et al., 1983).

The 35mm Falcon Petri dishes covered with type IV collagen from human liver were provided from CERAD, Lyon (France).

Cells were cultured in D-MEM (Dulbecco modified Eagle medium, Grand Island Biological Co., Grand Island, N.Y.) supplemented with

Table 1.  In Vitro Cell Characteristics and Lung Metastatic
Potential of a Rat Rhabdomyosarcoma Parental Cell Line
and its Cloned Cell Lines.

| Cell lines | | Doubling time (hours) | Individual count of lung tumoral nodules* | |
| --- | --- | --- | --- | --- |
| | | | After s.c. Tumor growth | After i.v. tumor cell injection |
| Parental line | 0 | 23 | 0,5,6,7,8,26,29, 40,40,56 | 110,110,120,135 150,175 |
| Sublines | 6 | 15 | 7,10,19,31,36, 45,51,66,107,155 | 23,44,49,51,51, 59,62,69,92,103 |
| | 14 | 21 | 1,1,4,4,10,29,90 | 43,46,68,78,78, 83,83,95,98,99 |
| | 13 | 18 | 0,0,8,13,16,17 | 98,99,101,110, 192,215 |
| | 21 | 27 | 0,0,0,1,2,2,2,59 25 | 0,0,0,0,0,0,2, 3,4,8 |
| | 22 | 30 | 0,0,0,0,0,0,0,1, 2 | 5,8,8,12,13,16, 19,23,24 |
| | 8 | 21 | 2,2,5,6,6,6,7,8,8 9 | 0,0,0,0,0,0,1, 1,3,6 |

* Groups of 10 rats received either subcutaneously (in the flank)
or intravenously (tail vein) $10^5$ cells for each cell line resus-
pended in 0.1ml of the culture medium.   Lung nodules were counted
at the lung surface on autopsy.

heat-inactivated FCS (Fetal calf serum, Gibco) and 1% of strepto-mycin
-penicillin solution (5 x $10^3$ units/ml), (Gibco Europe, Glasgow,
Scotland).  Cultures were grown at 37°C in humid atmosphere of 95%
air/5% $CO_2$.

A standard proliferation test was performed by seeding 25 x $10^3$
or 50 x $10^3$ cells in 60 mm Falcon petri dishes with 5ml D-MEM,
supplemented with 10% of FCS.  Four identical dishes were prepared for
every growth factor studied.  Growth factors were added every two
days, at a concentration of 20 ng/ml of medium for EGF, 40 ng/ml of
medium for FGF and 25 U/ml of medium for EDGF unless otherwise stated.
After 5 days, the cells were trypsinised and counted with a Coulter-

counter (Coultronic, France).  The culture conditions varied by the
inoculum size, the serum concentrations and the various substrata used
as supports as described in the results section for each experiment.
Falcon Petri dishes were coated with laminin, fibronectin, ECM as
previously described (Tassin et al., 1983).  For immunofluorescent
studies, cells were seeded on glass coverslips.  After fixation with
2% solution of formaldehyde, they were incubated with antifibronectin
serum (1:100) for 1 hour at 37°C, washed and incubated with an
antibody anti-rabbit immunoglobulin coupled with fluorescein (1:100)
for 1 hour at 37°C.  The statistical analysis of the data was done
using the Student's t test.


RESULTS

Effect of FGF, EDGF and EGF on the RMS Parental Cell Line 9-4/0
Compared to the L6 Myoblast.

    The RMS parental cells were stimulated to divide by the three
growth factors but to a different extent, as shown in Table 2.  FGF
had a slight but significant effect (p<.0008), EDGF a greater effect
and EGF the best effect.  The same pattern of stimulation was obtained
in the presence of 6% FCS (results not shown).  L6 was stimulated by
EDGF (p< $10^{-4}$) to the greatest extent, less by FGF (p< $10^{-5}$) and was
not stimulated by EGF.


Table 2.   Effect of Three Growth Factors on the
           Proliferation of the Parental Rhabdomyosarcoma
           Cell Line, Compared to the Stimulation of a
           Normal Myoblastic Cell Line.

| | No. of Cells x $10^{-3}$ ± s.e. | | | |
| Cell lines | Control | FGF | EDGF | EGF |
| --- | --- | --- | --- | --- |
| 9-4/0 | 1390 ± 59 | 1597 ± 50 | 1961 ± 48 | 2413 ± 60 |
| L6 | 911 ± 17 | 1432 ± 16 | 1534 ± 22 | 835 ± 19 |

$50$ x $10^{-3}$ cells were seeded in 60mm diameter Falcon Petri
dishes in a 10% FCS supplemented medium.

Table 3:   The Effect of Three Growth Factors on Various
           Rhabdomyosarcoma Sublines.
           Statistical Significance.

| | Control | Number of cells x $10^{-3} \pm$ s.e. | | |
| | | FGF | EDGF | EGF |
|---|---|---|---|---|
| Line 0 | 1390 | 1596** | 1961** | 2413** |
| | 59 | 50 | 48 | 60 |
| Subline 13 | 2791 | 3115* | 3576** | 3197** |
| | 41 | 180 | 38 | 46 |
| Subline 6 | 1856 | 2446* | 2452* | 2572* |
| | 196 | 145 | 22 | 102 |
| Subline 14 | 896 | 1411** | 1807** | 1942** |
| | 34 | 38 | 28 | 31 |
| Subline 8 | 2080 | 3062** | 4202** | 3563** |
| | 176 | 92 | 43 | 142 |
| Subline 21 | 1202 | 1993** | 2022** | 1590* |
| | 158 | 137 | 125 | 205 |
| Subline 22 | 1042 | 1528** | 1692** | 1087ns |
| | 42 | 37 | 62 | 75 |

1.) $50 \times 10^3$ were seeded in 60mm Petri dishes in a 10%
    FCS supplemented D-MEM in the presence of either of
    three growth factors. (FGF-40ng/ml; EDGF-25U/ml; EGF
    -20ng ml.  Cells were counted after 5 days culture
    (see: Materials and Methods).
2.) ns: no significance; * $p < 0.01$ $p < 0.05$; ** $p < 0.001$.
    For each line the statistical values compared the
    effect of the growth factors with the control.

Comparative Pattern of Stimulation of 6 RMS Sublines by EGF, FGF and
EDGF (Table 3).

    Since the original 9-4/0 cell line had given rise to the various
sublines with different growth and metastatic potential, it was of
interest to compare their response to the stimulation by the different
growth factors.  The results are represented on Table 3.  The fastest
growing lines (6, 8, 13) were stimulated to proliferate as well as the
slowest ones (14, 21, 22) but it can be seen that in our experimental

conditions, the effect of growth factors on proliferation was not a function of their doubling time.  Each individual subline had its own pattern of response to each growth factor studied.  In general, the response to the FGF treatment was weaker than to the EGF and EDGF.

To more precisely compare these data, we have performed a Student's t test statistical analysis comparing each treated cell culture to the control cells culture.

These results, compiled from three independent experiments for each subline, were highly reproducible giving the same pattern for both initial concentration of cells (25 x $10^3$ or 10 x $10^3$ cells per 60mm Petri dish) and for 6 or 10% serum concentration (data not shown).  It is noteworthy that the extent of stimulation varied considerably between the different sublines with no stimulation for one growth factor and 200% of increase for another one.

These results demonstrate that there was a different response of various sublines to three growth factors purified from normal tissues.

Since various conditions can modulate the response of cells to growth factors, we investigated the proliferation of the parental cells and of the various sublines by varying growth factor concentration, cell density, serum concentration and culture supports. The influence of all these parameters will be described below, using subline 14 as an example.

Effect of Growth Factors Concentration

We have treated subline 14 cells with two different growth factor concentrations.  The results (Table 4) demonstrated that subline 14 was stimulated by EGF and EDGF in a dose dependent manner. The results were highly reproducible as were the experiments carried out with other sublines.  The assays using increasing growth factors concentrations up to 500 ng.ml$^{-1}$ for EGF and 200 U.ml$^{-1}$ for EDGF revealed the same pattern of response and no toxic effects due to overdose.

Effect of Various FCS Concentration on Growth Factors Stimulation of Subline 14

The previous experiments were performed in the presence of 10% FCS.  As the serum contains various growth factors which may interfere with exogenous growth factors, we investigated the stimulation of subline 14, at different FCS concentrations, Table 5).

The results show that subline 14 growth was dependent upon FCS concentration.  In all serum concentrations studied, cells were stimulated by EGF, EDGF and to a lesser extent by FGF.  Student's t test analysis confirmed these results.  It thus seems that the

Table 4. Dose-dependent Growth Factor Induced Effect on the Proliferation of the RMS Subline 14 Cells.

| | Control | EDGF | | EGF | |
|---|---|---|---|---|---|
| | | 50u/ml | 20u/ml | 20ng/ml | 8ng/ml |
| No. of cells x $10^{-3}$ $\pm$ s.e. | 523 $\pm$ 29 | 807 $\pm$ 5 | 644 $\pm$ 4 | 980 $\pm$ 19 | 655 $\pm$ 23 |

25 x $10^{-3}$ cells were seeded in 60mm diameter Falcon dishes in a 10% FCS supplemented medium.

Table 5. FCS Concentration Dependence of Growth Factors Effect on theProliferation of RMS Subline 14 Cells.

| FCS Concentration % | No. of cells x $10^{-3}$ $\pm$ s.e. | | | |
|---|---|---|---|---|
| | Control | FGF | EDGF | EGF |
| 2 | 59 $\pm$ 2 | N.D. | 117 $\pm$ 1 | 91 $\pm$ 4 |
| 4 | 88 $\pm$ 2 | 124 $\pm$ 3 | 288 $\pm$ 3 | 181 $\pm$ 2 |
| 6 | 800 $\pm$ 52 | 1068 $\pm$ 28 | 1180 $\pm$ 20 | 1482 $\pm$ 19 |
| 10 | 896 $\pm$ 34 | 1411 $\pm$ 38 | 1807 $\pm$ 28 | 1942 $\pm$ 31 |

50 x $10^3$ cells were seeded in 60mm Petri dishes (FGF 40ng, EGF 20ng, EDGF 25U) per ml of medium.

promoting effect of the growth factors present in FCS had no effect on the hierarchy of stimulation induced by these three exogenous growth factors.

## Effect of the Initial Cell Inoculum Size on the Stimulation of Subline 14 Growth by EGF, FGF and EDGF

Tumor cells can frequently grow in low serum concentration or even in the total absence of serum if seeded at a concentration sufficient to autocondition their medium. The subline 14 stimulation was tested at three different initial cell densities as shown in Fig. 1. It was stimulated for all cell concentrations studied with the same stimulation pattern: EGF, EDGF, FGF. Thus we can conclude that if the cells produced a growth factor in these experimental conditions, it does not seem to interfere with their response towards these three growth factors.

It was previously shown (Courtois et al., 1981) that growth factors can modulate cell morphology and fibronectin expression, two parameters which are involved in tumor cells anchorage and growth.

## Effect of the Various Growth Factors on Cell Morphology and Fibronectin Expression in Rhabdomyosarcoma Cell Lines.

As an example, the RMS subline 13 cells were treated with the two growth factors at the optimal concentration in the presence of serum.

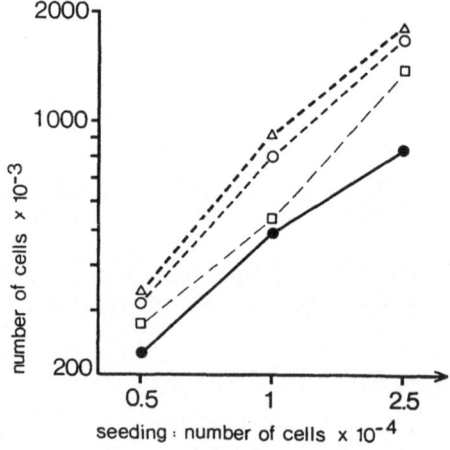

Fig. 1.    Stimulation of subline 14 cells by EGF 20ng ( Δ ),
           EDGF 25U (O) and FGF (40ng) ( □ ) compared to FCS
           (●) at different initial seeding concentration,
           as indicated in Materials and Methods.

**F4_9/13**

C                    EGF                    EDGF

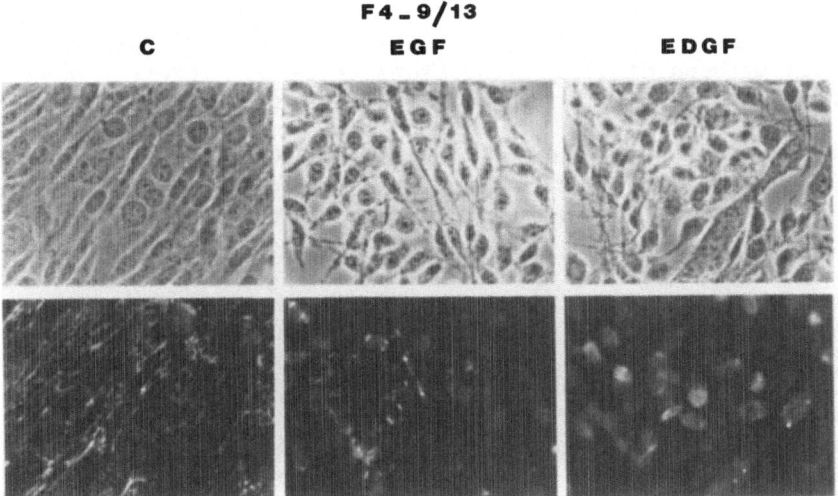

Fig. 2   Immunofluorescent localisation of fibronectin of rhabdo-
         myosarcoma subline 13 treated by EGF (20 ng/ml) and EDGF
         (25 U/ml).   Top phase contrast, bottom immunofluorescence

After fixation, their fibronectin expression was revealed by
immunofluorescent techniques (Fig. 2).

The subline 13 (Fig. 2) adopted a different configuration when
treated by the growth factors.  Cells formed long and thin processes.
The fibronectin pattern modification was much more apparent than in
the previous cells, with a strong decrease of fibronectin deposits in
comparison to the controls.  Thus fibronectin expression of
rhabdomyosarcoma cells was modulated in vitro by exogenous growth
factors.  Previous results (Courtois et al., 1981) on the effects of
EDGF on fibronectin expression in BEL cells have demonstrated that
fibronectin synthesis is directly suppressed by the growth factor.
Whether this is the same for rhabdomyosarcoma cells remains to be
established by quantitative analysis.

Effect of Various Substrata on the Stimulation of L6, Sublines 14 and
8 by EGF and EDGF

If the extracellular material deposition can be directly
influenced by growth factors, it was of interest to study if the
substratum on which the cells were deposited in vitro can also play

a role in their response to the action of growth factors (Kern et al., 1983; Moczar et al., 1983: Tassin et al., 1983). This was investigated by seeding various sublines cells on different substrata, made from isolated ECM or from several of its components.

Proliferation of two sublines was measured on plastic, ECM, collagen type IV, laminin, fibronectin and the growth capacity was compared after 5 days culture in the absence or presence of growth factors (Table 6).

Both sublines behaved similarly. Compared to plastic, they grew better on collagen type IV, ECM, fibronectin and laminin in this order. We can rule out the possibility that these data reflect a differential initial adhesion of these cells to these different substrata because we have shown that dissociated rhobdomyosarcoma cells adhere more rapidly on laminin than on fibronectin or collagen type IV (unpublished results). The main observation is that when these cells were simultaneously stimulated by EGF or EDGF, their growth was enhanced on all these substrata but ECM, on which they grow much more slowly. ECM did not promote the growth of L6 cells (Table

Table 6.   Effect of Growth Factors on the Proliferation of Two Cloned Cell Lines Maintained on Various Substrata.

Final number of cells x $10^{-3}$ ± s.e.

| Substratum | SUBLINE 14 | | SUBLINE 8 | |
| | Control Medium | EGF Completed Medium | Control Medium | EDGF Completed Medium |
| --- | --- | --- | --- | --- |
| Falcon Petri dish | 40 ± 2 | 77 ± 2 | 60 ± 1 | 81 ± 1 |
| ECM | 85 ± 4 | 47 ± 3 | 167 ± 4 | 83 ± 3 |
| Collagen IV | 99 ± 2 | 123 ± 3 | 172 ± 1 | 215 ± 2 |
| Laminin | 52 ± 2 | 85 ± 1 | 78 ± 2 | 117 ± 1 |
| Fibronectin | 80 ± 1 | 117 ± 2 | 142 ± 2 | 178 ± 2 |

$6 \times 10^3$ cells were seeded in 35mm Petri dishes.
Coating of plastic dishes were performed by one hour incubation with 1ml of 100ug/ml of purified collagen IV, laminin of fibronectin followed by washing.   ECM was deposited by cultivated endothial corneal cells, subsequently treated by Triton x 100 and washings as indicated in material and methods.

Table 7.  Proliferation of L6 Cells on Plastic and on ECM and
          Stimulated by EGF, EDGF and FGF.

| Substratum | Final number of cells x $10^{-3}$ ± s.e. | | | |
| --- | --- | --- | --- | --- |
|  | Control Medium | FGF Completed Medium | EDGF Completed Medium | EGF Completed Medium |
| Falcon Petri dish | 911 ± 17 | 1432 ± 16 | 1534 ± 22 | 835 ± 19 |
| ECM | 417 ± 14 | 313 ± 15 | 395 ± 22 | 300 ± 19 |

$50 \times 10^3$ were seeded on 6cm Petri dishes.  All the conditions
were similar to Table IV.

7).  In addition, none of the growth factors were able to stimulate
further cell growth in these conditions.  These data show that the
nature of the support can modify the stimulation of the cells by
growth factors, introducing a new parameter to the variation in tumor
cell behaviour.


DISCUSSION

     The experiments reported in this work have shown first that a
highly metastatic rat rhabdomyosarcoma cell line and several sublines
while being highly serum dependent are all sensitive to the action of
various growth factors isolated from normal tissue.  The transformed
phenotype of cells studied does not make them independent for their
growth from FCS or exogenous growth factors.  In this respect, some
RMS sublines react like their normal counterpart rat myoblast which
are stimulated by FGF (Gospodarowicz et al., 1977) and EDGF
(Barritault et al., 1981) but not by EGF (Linkhart et al., 1981).
However other sublines (subline 21, 8, 14, 13, 6, including parental
cell line 0) differed from L6 myoblasts since they respond to EGF to
some extent.  It was recently shown (Lim et al., 1984) that a variant
cell line derived from a non-EGF responsive murine myoblast cell line
MM 14, concomittantly lost its differentiation capacity and recovered
a response to EGF.  In our experiments, rhabdomyosarcoma sublines were
able to form myotubes, independently of their growth factor response.
Thus there was no relation between response to growth factor and the
state of spontaneous morphological differentiation in our model.

     The growth factor independence, although shared by most _in vitro_ transformed cells is not a general rule.  For instance, chemically transformed 3T3 hamster cells still require serum growth factor to undergo DNA synthesis.  Various reports in the literature show that tumor cells could be stimulated by either of the growth factors used in our study, i.e. rat PC-12 pheochromocytoma (Chandler and Herschman, 1983) and human colon carcinoma (Zenisek and Fernandez-pol, 1982) cell line by EGF, amelanotic human melanoma cell line (Richmond et al., 1982) by FGF; CCL 39 - a potentially tumorigenic hamster lung fibroblast cell line is stimulated by EGF, FGF and EDGF (Chambard et al., 1983).  The experiments performed on the 6 sublines and on the parental cell line show that they respond differently to the three different growth factors.  This pattern of response is characteristic of each of the cell lines and is relatively independent of the amount of FCS added in the culture medium or of the initial seeding density This means that the growth factors may act synergistically with the growth promoting activity present in FCS but also that they do not compete with a putative autocrine growth factor.  However, the presence of an autocrine growth factor or TGF synthesized by the rhabdomyosarcoma cells themselves is suspected from the preliminary experiments performed on subline 6.  It was recently shown that a human rhabdomyosarcoma produces a TGF (Todaro et al., 1982).  It is noteworthy that the extent of stimulation for each individual clone was independent of the initial doubling time determined in the presence of 10% FCS.

Differences in growth factor response was observed between different lines of the same histologic type of tumor i.e:  human mammary tumor reacting with EGF (Imai et al., 1982) and human osteosarcoma with EGF (Shupnik and Tasnjian, 1982) but the hetero geneous clonal response both of normal and transformed cells has not been exhaustively studied.  Normal cells such as aortic endothelial cells in culture were shown to display a clonal variability in their EGF response (Longenecker et al., 1983).  Human epidermoid carcinoma A-431 cloned cells were tested for EGF stimulation and three types of response were found:  stimulation, growth unchanged and inhibition.  The EGF induced morphological changes of colony appearance was the same for all three types of response (Lifsmitz et al., 1983). Kaplan (Kaplan and Ozane, 1983) found a clonal difference in the serum, EGF or TGF reactivity of rat fibroblast line F2400.  The clones were either highly or weakly stimulated by all the three factors studied in colony forming assay in soft agar.  In our study, we observed the differential response of every clone to each of three factors studied but the two approaches differed in the cell source, the factors studied and the assays applied.

To be clear, we should raise an important problem,concerning the interpretation of growth factors proliferative effect on tumour cells. In our experiments the amplitude of growth factor action varied from one line to another and from one factor to another one.  This effect was observed after a relatively long time culture and suggested the average shorter cell doubling time.  Unfortunately we cannot know whether this effect was due to the stimulation of small cell fraction drowned in non-stimulated cell mass or to the stimulation of whole cell population.  If the second hypothesis is true then such a stimulation could have a heavy consequence on the behaviour of cells in vivo.

Some authors (Hill et al., 1984; Price et al., 1984) have shown that the cells having a true metastatic potential are very few even in a highly metastatic whole population and we cannot exclude that this cell population is specially sensitive to the GF induced stimulation of proliferative response.  Nobody is able to select those cells efficiently and we have worked (as the others) on whole cell population and with indirect method of analysis.

However, an interesting, albeit limited, observation results when comparing the metastatic properties of rhabdomyosarcoma cells and their ability to be stimulated by one of the three growth factors. Out of 7 cell lines studied, the ones which have the higher capacity to form pulmonary colonies (0, 14, 13, 6) are those which are the more sensitive to EGF  The other sublines (8, 21, 22) have the lower pulmonary colonizing potential and are optimally stimulated by EDGF. This correlation needs to be extended to other sublines and primary tumour cell lines but it seems to suggest a new mechanism of regulation which would add a new parameter to explain the variability of the metastatic process for this tumour.

The experiments performed to assess the effect of the various growth factors on the expression of fibronectin by rhabdomyosarcoma cells indicate that when the cells are stimulated, the fibronectin is diminished on their surface.  Since fibronectin is involved in cell adhesion, it is tempting to propose that growth factor action on the one of the components of the extracellular matrix synthesized by the cells may play a role in the detachment of cell from the primary site. To complete this study on the role of the extracellular matrix (ECM), we have performed stimulation experiments on ECM and several of its various components: laminin, collagen IV and fibronectin.  The results demonstrate a parallel cooperation between these supports and different growth factors on two different clones.  The biological substrata increased the rate of division of the two clones.  There was a slight but statistically significant difference in their efficacy to induce proliferation, which was not related to the adhesive capacity of the cells.  In unpublished experiments performed on short term adhesiveness of RMS cells on these substrata we have shown that these supports allowed a rapid attachment of the cells with an optimal affinity to laminin.

Growth factors (EGF and EDGF) did not support the cell growth on ECM, while they support it on purified ECM components.  We have

described a similar phenomenon on bovine lens epithelial (BEL) cells
treated with EDGF and grown on ECM (Kern et al., 1983; Moczar et al.,
1983; Tassin et al., 1983). In this case, we have attributed the
failure of cooperative effect of EDGF and ECM on BEL cells to an
induction of differentiation. In our model, further studies are
needed to elucidate this observation.

In these experiments, exogenous growth factors have been added to
rhabdomyosarcoma cells. However, as for many other tumour cells (Chua
et al., 1983; De Larco and Todaro, 1978; Kaplan et al., 1982; Roberts
et al., 1983; Todaro et al., 1982), there is also a possibility that
at least some of these cells synthesize an autocrine growth factor.
To test this possibility, we have performed a preliminary experiment
with a conditioned medium prepared from the serum free supernatant of
subline 6 characterized by the shortest doubling time (15h). This
conditioned medium when added to the standard medium (1:3) on subline
22 increased the number of cells by 170% in 5 days. These results,
while still preliminary, indicate that this conditioned medium
contains a growth promoting activity which could be an endogenous
growth factor the nature of which is currently under investigation.

We thus proposed that rhabdomyosarcoma cells are susceptible to
environmental factors with respect to their growth. The experiments
performed in this study allow us to imagine that the variability of
metastatic potential should probably take into account two more
parameters. One is the different susceptibility of cell
subpopulations to the stimulation of their growth by various growth
factors which they may meet in situ, either in the primary tumour or
during their trip to other sites in the body. The differential
response of the cells to the growth factors could permit the selection
of these cells in order to metastasize. The second parameter is the
mutual interaction between the cells and the extracellular matrix that
they can meet and/or they can synthesize.

ACKNOWLEDGEMENTS

We are grateful to D. Barritault and J. Courty for preparing and
testing EDGF throughout this work, and J. Tassin for preparing ECM.

Note.
An abstract form of this work has been presented at the Thirty
Seventh Annual M.P. Anderson Symposium on Fundamental Cancer Research
(Houston, Texas, USA) March 6-9th, 1984.
Recently, R. Allen, M. Dodson and L.S. Luitten (Exp. Cell Res.
152: 154, 1984,) demonstrated that FGF stimulates rat skeletal muscle
satellite proliferation.

REFERENCES

Balk, S.D., Shiu, R.P., La Fleur, M.M., and Young, L.L., 1982,
    Epidermal growth factor and insulin cause normal chicken heart
    mesenchymal cells to proliferate like their sarcoma virus-
    infected counterparts. Proc. Natl. Acad. Sci. USA, 79:1154.
Barritault, D., Arruti, C. and Courtois, Y, 1981, Is there an
    ubiquitous growth factor in the eye? Differentiation 18:29.
Barritault, D., Plouet, J., Courty, J. and Courtois, Y., 1982,
    Purification, characterisation and biological properties of the
    eye-derived growth factor from retina.   Analogies with brain
    derived growth factor. J. Neuroscience Res., 8:477.
Campisi, J. and Medrano, E.E., 1983, Cell cycle perturbation in normal
    and transformed fibroblasts caused by detachment from the
    substratum, J. Cell Physiol., 114:53.
Chambard, J.C., Franchi, A., Le Cam, A and Pouyssegur, J., 1983,
    Growth factor-stimulated protein phosphorylation in Go/G1-
    arrested fibroblasts. J. Biol. Chem., 258: 1706.
Chandler, C.E. and Herschman, H.R., 1983, Binding, sequestration and
    processing of epidermal growth factor and nerve growth factor by
    PC12 cells. J. Cell Physiol., 114:321.
Cherington, P.V., Smith, B.L. and Pardee, A.B., 1979,  Loss of
    epidermal growth factor requirement and malignant transformation,
    Proc. Natl. Acad. Sci. USA, 76:3937.
Chua, C.C., Geiman, D. and Ladda, R.L., 1983, Transforming growth
    factors released from Kirsten sarcoma virus transformed cells do
    not compete for epidermal growth factor membrane receptors.
    J. Cell Physiol., 117:116.
Cohen, S., 1983, The epidermal growth factor. Cancer, 51:1781.
Courtois, Y., Arruti, C., Barritault, D., Tassin, J., Olivie, M. and
    Hughes, R.C., 1981, Modulation of the shape of epithelial lens
    cells in vitro directed by a retinal extract factor.  A model of
    interconversion and the role of actin filaments and fibronectin.
    Differentiation 18:11.
Davonward, J., Yarden, Y., Mayes, E., Scrace, G., Totty, N.,
    Stockwell, P., Ullricht, S., Schlessinger, J. and Waterfield,
    M.D., 1984, Close similarity of epidermal growth factor receptor
    and v-erb B oncogene protein sequences, Nature, 307:521.
De Larco, J.E. and Todaro, G.J., 1978, Growth factors from murine
    sarcoma virus transformed cells, Proc. Natl. Acad. Sci. USA, 272:
    4001.
Elk, B., Westermark, B., Wasteson, A. and Heldin, C.H., 1982,
    Stimulation of tyrosine-specific phosphorylation by platelet-
    derived growth factor, Nature 419-420.
Glaser, B.M., d'Amore, P., Seppa, H., Seppa, S. and Shiffmann, E.,
    1980, Adult tissues contain chemoattractants for vascular
    endothelial cells, Nature, 288:483.
Gospodarowicz, D., 1983, The control of mammalian cell proliferation
    by growth factors, basement lamina, and lipoproteins, J. Invest.
    Dermatol., 81:40s.

Gospodarowicz, D., Bialecki, H. and Greenberg, G., 1978, Purification of fibroblast growth activity from bovine brain, J.Biol. Chem., 253:3636.

Gospodarowicz, D., Bialecki, H. and Thakral, T.K., 1979, The angiogenic activity of the fibroblast and epidermal growth factor, Exp. Eye Res., 28:501.

Gospodarowicz, D., Greenburg, G. and Birdwell, C.R., 1978, Determination of cellular shape by the extracellular matrix and its correlation with the control of cellular growth, Cancer Res., 38:4155.

Gospodarowicz, D. and Mescher, A., 1977, A comparison of the response of cultured myoblasts and chondrocytes to fibroblasts and epidermal growth factors. J. Cell Physiol., 93:117.

Gross, J.L., Krupp, M.N., Rifkin, D.B. and Lane, D., 1983, Down-regulation of epidermal growth factor receptor correlates with plasminogen activator activity in human A-431 epidermoid carcinoma cells, Proc. Natl. Acad. Sci. USA, 80:2276.

Grotendorst, G.R., 1984, Alteration of the chemotactic response of NIH/3T3 cells to PDGF by growth factor transformation and tumour promoters, Cell, 36:279

Hart, I.R. and Fidler, J.J., 1981, The implications of tumour heterogeneity for studies on the biology and therapy of cancer metastasis, Biochim. Biophys. Acta, 651:37.

Hill, R.P., Chambers, A.F., Ling, V. and Marris, J.F., 1984, Dynamic heterogeneity: rapid generation of metastatic variants in mouse B16 melanoma cells. Science, 224:998.

Hortsch, M., Schlessinger, J., Gootwine, E. and Webb, C.G., 1983, Appearance of functional EGF receptor kinase during rodent embryogenesis. EMBO Journal, 1937-1941.

Imai, Y., Leung, C.K., Friesen, H.G. and Shiu, R.P., 1982, Epidermal growth factor receptors and effect of epidermal growth factor on growth of human breast cancer cells in long term tissue culture, Cancer Res., 42:4394.

Jetten, A.M. and Goldfarb, R.H., 1983, Action of epidermal growth factor and retinoids on anchorage dependent and independent growth of non-transformed rat kidney cells, Cancer Res., 43: 3094.

Kaplan, P.L., Anderson, M. and Ozanne, B., 1982, Transforming growth factor(s) production enables cells to grow in the absence of serum: an autocrine system, Proc. Natl. Acad. Sci.USA, 79:485

Kaplan, P.L. and Ozanne, B., 1983, Cellular responsiveness to growth factors correlates with cell's ability to express the transformed phenotype. Cell, 33:931.

Kern, P., Laurent, M., Lim, A., Regnault, F. and Courtois, Y., 1983, The interaction of bovine epithelial lens cells with extracellular matrix II. Partial re-expression of the differentiated collagen distribution and phenotype, Exp. Cell Res., 149: 85.

Keski-Oja, J., De Larco, J., Rapp, U.R., Todaro, G.J., 1980, Murine sarcoma growth factors affect the growth and morphology of cultured mouse epithelial cells, J. Cell Physiol., 104:41.

Lifsmitz, A., Lazar, C.H.S., Buss, J.E. and Gill, G.N., 1983, Analysis of morphology and receptor metabolism in clonal variant A-431 cells with differing growth responses to epidermal growth factor, J. Cell Physiol. 115:235.

Lim, R.W. and Hauschka, S.D., 1984, A rapid decrease in Epidermal Growth Factor binding capacity accompanies the differentiation of mouse myoblasts in vivo, J. Cell Biol., 98:739.

Lim, R., Nagakawa, S., Arnason, B.G.W. and Turriff, D., 1981, Glia Maturation factor promotes contact inhibition in cancer cells. Proc. Natl. Acad. Sci. USA, 78:4373.

Linkhart, T.A., Clegg, C.H. and Hauschka, S.D., 1981, Myogenic differentiation in permanent clonal mouse myoblast cell lines: regulation by macromolecular growth factors in the culture medium, Develop. Biol. 86:19.

Longenecker, J.P., Kilty, L.A., Ridge, D.C., Miller, D.C. and Johnson, L.K., 1983, Proliferative variability of endothelial clones derived from adult bovine aorta: influence of fibroblast growth factor and smooth muscle cell extracellular matrix. J. Cell Physiol., 114:7

Marquardt, H., Hunkapiller, M.W., Hood, L.E., Twardzik, D.R., de Larco, J.E., Stephenson, J.R., and Todaro, G.J., 1983, Transforming growth factors produced by retrovines-transformed rodent fibroblasts and human melanoma cells: amino acid sequence homology with epidermal growth factor. Proc. Natl.Acad. Sci. USA, 88:4684.

Moczar, E., Laurent, M., Lim, A., Regnault, F. and Courtois, Y., 1983, The interaction of bovine lens epithelial cells with extracellular matrix and EDGF. III. The control of glycoproteins and proteoglycan synthesis. Exp. Cell Res., 149:95.

Moses, H.L. and Robinson, R.A., 1982, Growth factors, growth factor receptors and cell cycle control mechansims in chemically transformed cells, Fed. Proc., 41:(13) 3008.

Nicolson, G.L., 1982, Cancer metastasis organ colonization and the cell-surface properties of malignant cells, Biochim. Biophys. Acta, 695: 113.

Nicolson, G.L., 1984, Cell surface molecules and tumour metastasis, Exp. Cell Res., 150:3.

Ossowski, L. and Reich, E., 1983, Changes in malignant phenotype of a human carcinoma conditioned by growth environment, Cell, 323

Plouet, J., Barritault, D., Courtois, Y. and Lada, R., 1982, Eye-derived growth factor from retina and epidermal growth factor are immunologically distinct and bind to different receptors on human foreskin fibroblasts, FEBS Lett., 144:85

Pot-Deprun, J., Poupon, M.F., Sweeney, F.L. and Chouroulinkov, I., 1983, Growth, metastasis, immunogenicity and chromosomal content of a nickel-induced rhabdomyosarcoma and subsequent cloned cell lines in rats, J. Natl. Cancer Inst., 71:1241.

Price, J.E., Carr, D. and Tarin, D., 1984, Spontaneous and induced metastasis of naturally occurring tumors in mice: Analysis of cell shedding into the blood, J. Natl. Cancer Inst., 73:1319.

Richmond, A., Lawson, D.H., Nixon, D.W., Stevens, J.S. and Chawla, R.K., 1982, In vitro growth promotion in human malignant melanoma cells by fibroblast growth factor, Cancer Res., 42: 3175.

Robbins, K.C., Antoniades, H.N., Devare, S.G., Hunkapiller, M.W. and Aaronson, S.A., 1983, Structural and immunological similarities between simian sarcoma virus gene product(s) and human platelet-derived growth factor, Nature, 305:605.

Roberts, A.B., Frolik, C.A., Anzano, M.A., Sporn, M.B., 1983, Transforming growth factors from neoplastic and non-neoplastic tissues. Fed. Proc., 42:2621

Ross, R., Glomset, J., Kariya, B. and Karker, L., 1974, Platelet dependent serum factor that stimulates the proliferation of arterial smooth muscle cell in vitro. Proc. Natl. Acad. Sci. USA, 71:1207.

Seppa, J.T., Seppa, H.E., Liotta, L.A., Glaser, B.M., Martin, G.R. and Schiffmann, E., 1983, Cultured tumor cells produce chemotactic factors specific for endothelial cells;  a possible mechanism for tumour induced angiogenesis. Invasion Matastatis 3:139.

Sirbasku, D.A., 1978, Estrogen induction of growth factors specific for hormone responsive mammary, piuitary and kidney tumor cells, Proc. Natl. Acad. Sci. USA, 75:3786.

Shupnik, M.A. and Tasnjian, A.H., 1982, Epidermal growth factor and phorbol ester actions on human osteosarcoma cells.  Character- ization of responsive and non-responsive cell lines., J. Biol. Chem. 257:12161.

Sweeney, F.L., Pot-Deprun, J., Poupon, M.F. and Chouroulinkov, I., 1982, Heterogeneity of the growth and metastatic behaviour of cloned cell lines derived from a primary rhabdomyosarcoma, Cancer Res., 42:3772.

Tassin, J., Jacquemin, E. and Courtois, Y., 1983, The interaction of bovine lens epithelial cells with extracellular matrix and EDGF. I. Effect on short term adhesiveness and on long term organisation of the culture, Exp. Cell Res., 149:69.

Timpl, R., Rohde, H., Robey, P.G., Rennard, S.I., Foidart, J.M. and Martin, G.R., 1979, Laminin, a glycoprotein from basement membrane, J. Biol. Chem., 245:9933.

Todaro, G.J., De Larco, J. and Fryling, C.M., 1982, Sarcoma growth factor and other transforming peptides produced by human cells interaction with membrane receptors, Fed. Proc., 41:2996.

Vlodavski, I. and Gospodarowicz, D., 1981, Respective roles of laminin and fibronectin in adhesion of human carcinoma and sarcoma cells, Nature, 289:304.

Vlodavski, I., Lui, G.M. and Gospodarowicz, D., 1980, Morphological appearance, growth behaviour and migratory activity of human tumour cells maintained on extracellular matrix versus plastic, Cell, 19:607.

Westermark, B., Magnusson, A. and Heldin, C.H., 1983, Effect of epidermal growth factor on membrane mobility and cell locomotion in cultures of human clonal glioma cells, Prog.Clin. Biol. Res., 118: 491.

Zenisek, S.C. and Fernandez-Pol, J.A., 1982, Modulation of protein
    phosphorylation in human colon adenocarcinoma cell membrane
    preparations by epidermal growth factor in vitro, Int. J.Cancer,
    29:277.

# COMPARISON OF THE EFFECT OF FIBROBLAST GROWTH FACTOR

# AND EXOGENOUS EXTRACELLULAR MATRICES ON THE  PROLIFERATION

# AND PHENOTYPIC EXPRESSION OF CHONDROCYTES IN VITRO

Yukio Kato and Denis Gospodarowicz

Cancer Research Institute and the
Depts. of Medicine and Ophthalmology
Univ. of Calif., Medical Center
San Francisco, CA 94143

## INTRODUCTION

Chondrocyte cultures have been used extensively during the past 30 years to study the control of the synthesis of extracellular matrix macromolecules[1-4]. Although chondrocytes maintained on plastic tissue culture dishes initially synthesize cartilage-specific macromolecules, as they proliferate they readily lose the ability to express their phenotypic characteristics. This loss correlates with a rapid decrease in the synthesis of cartilage-characteristic proteoglycan (PG) and a switch from the synthesis of type II collagen to that of type I.[5,6] This results at confluence in a heterogeneous cell population composed of overtly differentiated chondrocytes mixed together with fibroblastic and poorly differentiated cells.[2,4] This heterogeneous cell population has impaired the analysis of the factors and mechanisms involved in the regulation of the synthesis of cartilage-matrix macromolecules.

In recent years, growth factors such as fibroblast growth factor (FGF), a mitogen for a wide variety of mesoderm-derived cells, have been shown to promote both the proliferation and phenotypic expression of target cells. This characteristic of FGF has made possible the long-term culturing of various cell types which would otherwise lose their normal phenotypes in culture when passaged repeatedly at low cell density.[7-11] It has been related to the ability of FGF to control the synthesis of various extracellular matrix components which would in turn affect cell polarity and gene expression.[7,8,11] Since FGF has been shown to be a mitogen for chondrocytes[12,13], we have in the present study analyzed its effect on the phenotypic expression of chondrocytes and have also analyzed the effect of extracellular matrices (ECMs) of defined composition produced by either cultured bovine corneal endothelial (BCE) cells or the PF-HR-9 teratocarcinoma cell line on chondrocyte proliferation and differentiation.

## EFFECT OF SUBSTRATE ON THE PROLIFERATION OF CHONDROCYTES AND PHENOTYPIC EXPRESSION

In vivo, chondrocytes are surrounded by a three-dimensional cartilage matrix which is composed of chondroitin sulfate PG and type II collagen. When cells are released from the cartilage matrix by treatment with bacterial collagenase, they their lose pericellular matrix, which may be required for the expression of their differentiated functions. If cartilage matrix is involved in supporting the phenotypic expression of chondrocytes, the ECM produced by other cell types, by promoting the production of cartilage matrix by cultured chondrocytes, may also stabilize the ability of cultured chondrocytes to express their proper phenoptype. This possibility was explored using rabbit costal chondrocytes maintained on plastic tissue culture dishes coated or not with an ECM produced by BCE cells or PF-HR-9 teratocarcinoma cells.[14,15]. Freshly isolated chondrocytes from the ribs of young rabbits seeded at low density (10 cells/mm$^2$) on plastic dishes coated or not with ECM and exposed to serum-supplemented medium started to proliferate after a 2-day lag-time. The average doubling times of cultures maintained on BCE-ECM and HR-9-ECM were shorter (14 and 17 h, respectively) than that (27 h) of cultures maintained on plastic. Cultures maintained on plastic had a fibroblastic appearance during their growing stage (Fig. 1-IA, day 6), as well as when they were in their early confluent stage (Fig. 1-IC, day 10). Over 80% of the cells failed to reexpress their spherical phenotype even after 19 days in culture (Fig. 1-IE). In contrast, when cultures were maintained on BCE-ECM, although cells adopted an epithelioid configuration during their proliferative and early confluent stages (Fig. 1-IB, day 6), after 8 days in culture cells started to round up, forming by day 10 numerous cartilage nodules (Fig. 1-ID). Similar morphological changes were observed in cultures maintained on HR-9-ECM. The number and size of cartilage nodules increased with time in culture, so that by day 14 the cells reorganized into a homogeneous cartilage-like tissue (Fig. 1-IE) which, when analyzed by transmission electron microscopy, had an ultrastructure characteristic of that seen in vivo. The chondrocytes were embedded in a three-dimensional cartilaginous matrix in which thin collagen fibrils typical of collagen type II were observed.[16] These observations suggest that, although chondrocytes maintained on ECM-coated dishes temporarily lose their phenotypic expression during their proliferative stage, they will, in contrast to cells maintained on plastic, reexpress it in the late confluent stage. The ability of chondrocytes maintained on ECM but not on plastic to reexpress their proper phenotypes once confluent was further explored by looking at the changes in the rate of $^{35}SO_4^{2-}$ incorporation into newly synthesized PGs (Fig. 1-IIA, B). During the logarithmic growth phase the rate of $^{35}SO_4^{2-}$ incorporation was extremely low, regardless of the substrate upon which cells were maintained. As soon as cells became

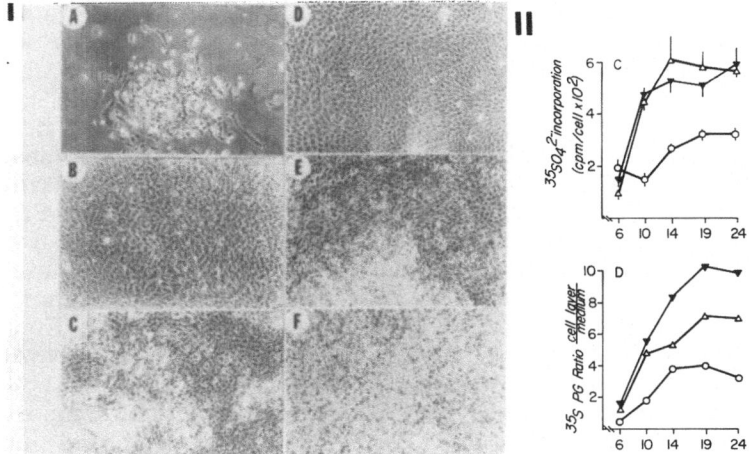

Figure 1. I. Morphological changes of chondrocytes maintained on plastic dishes coated or not with BCE-ECM. II. Changes in the rate of [35]S-sulfate incorporation into proteoglycans and distribution ratio between [35]S-labeled proteoglycans present in the cell layer versus those released into the medium in low density chondrocyte cultures maintained on plastic, BCE-ECM and HR-9-ECM and exposed to DMEM supplemented with 10% fetal calf serum.

I. Chondrocytes were seeded at $1 \times 10^4$ cells per dish and maintained on plastic dishes coated (A-C) or not (D-F) with BCE-ECM in the presence of DMEM supplemented with 10% fetal calf serum. Pictures were taken on day 6 (A, D), day 10 (B, E) and day 14 (C, F) with a Nikon phase-contrast photomicroscope (X 100).

II. Rabbit chondrocytes were seeded at $1 \times 10^4$ cells per 35 mm dish on plastic culture dishes coated or not (○) with BCE-ECM (△) or HR-9-ECM (▼) and exposed to DMEM supplemented with 10% fetal calf serum and antibiotics. After 6 to 24 days in culture, triplicate plates representing each condition were exposed to 2 µCi/ml of [35]S-sulfate in 0.8 ml of DMEM. The rate of [35]S-sulfate incorporation into total proteoglycans per cell (A) was determined as described in ref. 16. The distribution ratio between [35]S-labeled proteoglycan present in the cell layers versus those released into the medium is shown in (B).

confluent, however, the rate of $^{35}SO_4^{2-}$ incorporation in cultures maintained on ECMs increased, reaching a maximum on day 14. On the other hand, the rate of $^{35}SO_4^{2-}$ incorporation in cultures maintained on plastic, although it did increase in confluent cultures, did so to a much lower extent than with cells maintained on ECM. Fig. 1-IIB also shows the effect of BCE-ECM and HR-9-ECM on the distribution of newly synthesized PGs incorporated into the cell layers versus those released into the medium. The ratio between $^{35}$S-PGs present in the cell layers and those present in the medium increased after day 6 in all cultures, reaching a maximum on day 19. This increase was accompanied by the appearance of extensive refractile extracellular matrices, suggesting an increased deposition of PGs into a cartilaginous matrix. The proportion of $^{35}$S-labeled PGs present in the cell layers of cultures maintained on the ECMs was 3- to 5-fold higher than that of cultures maintained on plastic (Fig. 1-IIB). This observation suggests that both ECMs stimulate the incorporation of newly synthesized PGs into a cartilaginous matrix. Although BCE-ECM and HR-9-ECM had a similar effect on incorporation of $^{35}SO_4^{2-}$ into total PGs (Fig. 1-IIA), the ratio between $^{35}$S-labeled PG present in the cell layers versus those present in the medium was significantly greater during the whole length of the experiments in the case of cultures maintained on HR-9-ECM (Fig. 1-IIB), suggesting a greater efficiency in the incorporation of newly synthesized PGs into the cartilage matrix when cells were maintained on that substrate. This difference may be a result of the different chemical compositions of BCE-ECM and HR-9-ECM. The HR-9 matrix is composed mostly of collagen type IV, heparan sulfate PGs, and laminin.[17-19] It therefore has a composition very close to that seen in vivo in capillary endothelial cell basement membrane.[20, 21] In contrast, the BCE-ECM contains, in addition to the components present in the HR-9 matrix, elastin, collagen types I and III, fibronectin, as well as dermatan and chondroitin sulfate PGs[22-24].

In vivo, it has been shown that cartilage forms readily in teratocarcinoma. It is not known, however, whether cartilage formation in the tumor results from an epithelial-mesenchymal interaction mediated by ECM, as in the case of the normal chondrogenesis in vivo.[25] The results in the present study show that HR-9-ECM produced by PF-HR-9 teratocarcinoma cells markedly stimulates chondrogenesis in low density cultures of rabbit costal chondrocytes. This suggests that the HR-9-ECM could be involved in cartilage formation in teratocarcinomas.

It is unknown which components of BCE-ECM and HR-9-ECM are responsible for their stimulatory effects on chondrocyte proliferation and phenotypic expression. Preliminary studies have shown that the rate of PG synthesis by chondrocytes maintained on collagen- or fibronectin-coated dishes is higher than that of PG synthesis by chondrocytes maintained on plastic dishes. The extent of stimulation by collagen or fibronectin was, however, much lower than that observed in cultures maintained on BCE-ECM or HR-9-ECM when chondrocytes were seeded at low densities ($10^2$ to $10^3$ cells per 35 mm dish). On the other hand, the rate of PG synthesis by chondrocytes maintained on chondroitin sulfate- or hyaluronic acid-coated dishes was similar to that of cells maintained on plastic dishes. BCE-ECM which no longer contained dermatan and chondroitin sulfate PGs and whose heparan sulfate PG content was reduced by 80%[26] was also as potent as normal ECM in stimulating PG synthesis. These results suggest that, while collagen and fibronectin could be involved in supporting the phenotypic expression of chondrocytes, other components of BCE-ECM and HR-9-ECM, such as PGs, would have a lesser effect.

It has previously been shown that mesenchymal cells synthesize and accumulate fibronectin, whereas fully differentiated chondrocytes do not. West et al.[27] and Pennypacker[28] have shown that exogenously added fibronectin at relatively high concentrations (25-150 µg/ml) stimulates the attachment of chick embryo chondrocytes to the plastic substrate and suppresses their phenotypic expression in vitro. On the other hand, our results suggest that coating of dishes with fibronectin improves the ability of rabbit costal chondrocytes to reexpress cartilage phenotype in confluent cultures. The reason for this discrepancy between our results and those reported by West et al.[27] and Pennypacker[28] is unknown. Reddi has shown, however, that fibronectin plays an important role in the induction of the ectopic cartilage and bone.[29] The results of Reddi and ourselves suggest that fibronectin is somehow involved in the process of chondrogenesis. In any case, chondrocyte cultures grown on BCE-ECM or HR-9-ECM provide a model for the study of cell-substrate interactions which are responsible for the maintenance of the differentiated phenotype of chondrocytes.

## EFFECT OF FGF ON THE PROLIFERATION OF CHONDROCYTES AND THEIR PHENOTYPIC EXPRESSION

FGF purified from bovine pituitary glands and brain has been shown to be a mitogen for mesoderm-derived cells[7, 8, 11] and has been used primarily to develop new in vitro endothelial cell lines,[30] particularly of vascular and corneal origin. Previous studies have also shown that FGF markedly stimulates the proliferation of cultured rabbit ear,[12] articular,[13] and costal chondrocytes[31]. Its intraarticular administration results in a substantial stimulation of the proliferation of chondrocytes in vivo.[32] However, an effect of FGF on the phenotypic expression of chondrocytes has not been previously examined. We have therefore examined a possible effect of FGF using very low density (3 cells per mm$^2$) chondrocyte cultures maintained on plastic and exposed to DMEM supplemented with 10% fetal calf serum. Cultures exposed to FGF had an average doubling time during their logarithmic growth phase of 16 h, versus 35 h in its absence. An FGF mitogenic effect was detectable at concentrations as low as 12 pg/ml, and was maximal at 0.6 ng/ml, resulting by day 6 in a 12-fold increase in cell number over controls (Fig. 2-I). The changes in the morphology of chondrocytes maintained on plastic in the presence of FGF were similar to those observed with cells maintained in the absence of FGF on BCE-ECM or HR-9-ECM. Although both types of cultures adopted a fibroblastic or epithelioid configuration during their proliferative stages, cells did reexpress the spherical phenotype once cultures progressed into their late confluent stage (Fig. 1-IF and Fig. 2-IIB). In contrast, over 70 to 80% of chondrocytes maintained on plastic in the absence of FGF failed to reexpress the spherical phenotype once cultures had become confluent (Fig. 1-IE and Fig. 2-IIA). Transmission electron microscopy of confluent chondrocyte cultures grown in the presence of FGF showed an ultrastructure characteristic of chondrocytes in vivo, and cells were embedded in a well developed three-dimensional cartilaginous matrix in which abundant

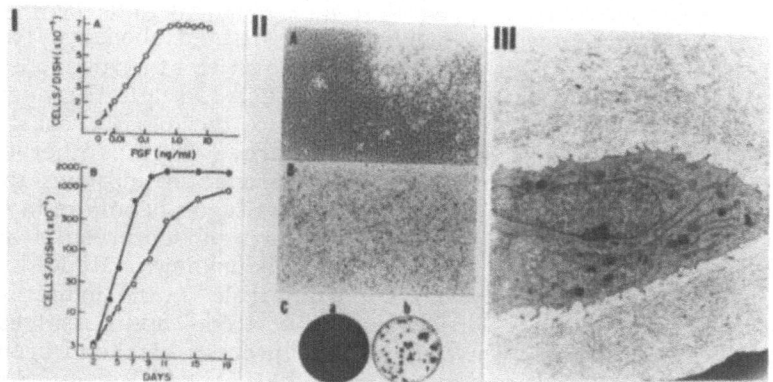

Fig. 2  I. Effect of FGF on the proliferation of low density rabbit costal chondrocytes.  II.  Morphological appearance of rabbit costal chondrocytes maintained on plastic culture dishes and exposed to DMEM supplemented with 10% fetal calf serum in the presence of FGF.  III.  Transmission electron microscopy of chondrocytes cultures maintained in the presence of FGF.

I.  (A) Rabbit costal chondrocytes were seeded at low density $(1 \times 10^4$ cells per 35 mm plastic tissue culture dish) and exposed to DMEM supplemented with 10% fetal calf serum and increasing concentrations of FGF.  After 6 days in culture, triplicate dishes were harvested and counted. (B) Rabbit costal chondrocytes were seeded at low density $(3 \times 10^3$ cells per 35 mm plastic tissue culture dish) and exposed to DMEM supplemented with 10% fetal calf serum in the presence (●) or absence (o) of FGF (0.6 ng/ml). After 2 to 19 days in culture, triplicate dishes were harvested and counted.

II.  (A-B) Rabbit costal chondrocytes were seeded at $3 \times 10^3$ cells per 35 mm plastic tissue culture dish and exposed to DMEM supplemented with 10% fetal calf serum in the presence (B) or absence (A) of FGF. FGF (0.6 ng/ml) was added every day.  Pictures were taken on day 19 (X 100). (C)  Comparison of alcian green staining of rabbit costal chondrocyte cultures grown in the presence (b) or absence (a) of FGF.  Culture conditions were as described above.  After 19 days in culture, one set of plates was fixed with 10% formalin and stained with alcian green.

III.  A cross-section of the cell layer of cultures maintained for 19 days in the presence (Bar, 2 μm X 3850) of FGF is shown.

collagen fibrils were observed (Fig.  2-III).  The ultrastructure of the cartilage-like tissue which was expressed by confluent cultures grown in the presence of FGF was strikingly similar to that seen in vivo, and was also similar to that seen with cells grown on BCE-ECM.[33] When the changes in the level of $^{35}SO_4{}^{2-}$ incorporation into PGs in cultures maintained on plastic in the presence of FGF were analyzed as a function of growth stage, they were found to be similar to those of cultures maintained on ECM-coated dishes (Fig. 3-I versus Fig. 1-II). Although by days 5-9 the level of $^{35}SO_4{}^{2-}$ incorporation into PGs per cell in cultures exposed to FGF was about 50% lower than that of cultures not exposed to it (Fig. 3-IB), the level of $^{35}SO_4{}^{2-}$ incorporation in cultures exposed to FGF markedly increased from day 11 to day 15, after which time it remained stable. In contrast, the level of $^{35}SO_4{}^{2-}$ incorporation in cultures maintained on plastic and not exposed to FGF decreased as time progressed. Rabbit costal chondrocytes maintained in vitro produce two species of PGs with high and low molecular weights. High molecular weight chondroitin sulfate PG represents a major component of cartilage matrix, while low molecular weight PGs are minor components of cartilage matrix. Recent studies have suggested that the low molecular weight PGs are involved in cell-cell and cell-substrate inter-actions and in chondrocyte differentiation.[34, 35] Addition of FGF to actively growing chondrocyte cultures resulted in a 5- to 10-fold increase in the synthesis of high molecular weight PG associated with a 2-fold increase in low molecular weight PG synthesis (Fig. 3-II), suggesting that FGF could stimulate PG synthesis directly or indirectly.

The stimulatory effect of FGF on sulfated PG synthesis was not a result of its direct action on confluent, resting cells, since it could not be observed when FGF was added to the medium only after cultures became confluent (day 12 to 18, Table I). Only when cells had been exposed to FGF during the proliferative stage of cultures (day 0 to 8) did a stimulation of PG synthesis in confluent cultures occur (Table I).

Two possibilities may account for the effect of FGF on sulfated PG synthesis in confluent chondrocyte cultures. First, FGF could have an indirect effect on chondrocyte phenotypic expression by increasing the final cell density of confluent cultures. The results from experiments with chondrocytes isolated from cartilage by prolonged collagenase treatment showed, however, that FGF could stimulate sulfated PG synthesis in confluent cultures without a concomitant increase in final cell density under certain culture conditions. It is therefore unlikely that the increase in final cell density alone accounts for the stimulation of sulfated PG synthesis in confluent cultures grown in the presence of FGF. The second possibility is that FGF, when added to actively growing chondrocytes, prevents at each cell cycle the dedifferentiation of a given percentage of the population into an irreversible fibroblastic stage. That this possiblity is the most likely is supported by the fact that cells need only to be grown in the presence of FGF in order to express their proper phenotype when confluent (Table I). A similar effect of FGF on the stabilization of phenotypic expression and prevention of dedifferentiation of vascular endothelial cells has already been reported.[7, 9] It was only when FGF was added to actively growing cells that prevention of their dedifferentiation or reversal to their proper phenotype was observed.[7, 9]

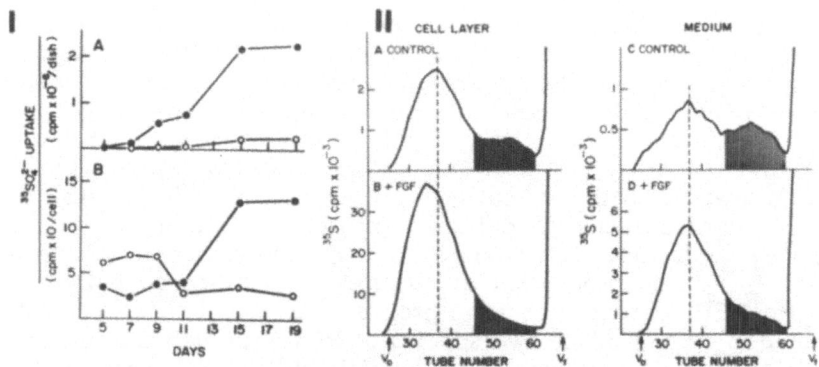

Fig. 3. I. Changes in the rate of ($^{35}$S)sulfate incorporation into proteoglycans (PGs) in low density chondrocyte cultures maintained in the
presence or absence of FGF. II. Sepharose CL-2B chromatography of PGs
present in the cell layer-matrix and in the medium from cultures grown in
the presence or absence of FGF.
    I.  Rabbit chondrocytes were seeded at 3 X 10$^3$ cells per 35 mm dish
on plastic culture dishes and exposed to DMEM supplemented with 10% fetal
calf serum alone ( o ) or DMEM supplemented with 10% fetal calf serum and
FGF (0.6 ng/ml) ( ● ). After 5 to 19 days in culture, triplicate plates representing each condition were exposed for 12 h to 10 μCi/ml of ($^{35}$S)sulfate in
1.0 ml of DMEM supplemented with 10% fetal calf serum in the presence or
absence of FGF (0.6 ng/ml), and the rate of ($^{35}$S)sulfate incorporation into
PGs present in the cell layer and in the medium per dish (A) or per cell (B)
was measured.
    II.  Cultures were seeded and maintained for 15 days as described
above. Aliquots of the 4 M guanidine HCl extract of the cell layer-matrix
(A,B) and the medium (C,D) from cultures grown in the presence (B,D) or
absence (A,C) of FGF were applied onto a Sepharose CL-2B column which
was equilibrated in 4 M guanidine HCl, 50 mM Tris HCl, pH 8.0 with
protease inhibitors. Three ml fractions were collected. Aliquots (0.3 ml) of
each fraction were mixed with 0.3 ml of ethanol and 10 ml of Aquasol.
Radioactivity was measured in a Beckmann LS-8000 scintillation counter.
Vo was determined with high molecular weight hyaluronic acid synthesized
by rabbit costal chondrocytes.

EFFECT OF FGF AND ECM ON CHONDROCYTE LIFE SPAN

    In addition to their effect on chondrocyte proliferation and phenotypic
expression, FGF or ECM markedly extended the life span of rabbit costal
chondrocytes in culture.  While cells maintained on plastic and exposed to

Table I

Effect of length of exposure on the rate of proteoglycan synthesis by 13 days cultures of chondrocytes maintained on plastic-and ECM-coated dishes

| Substrate | Addition of FGF (periods) | Cells/dish (X $10^{-5}$) | $^{35}SO_4^{2-}$ uptake | |
|---|---|---|---|---|
| | | | cpm X $10^{-3}$/dish[1] | cpm X $10^3$/cell[1] |
| Plastic | none | 10.5 ± 0.3 | 9 ± 1  (56)[2] | 9 |
| | d0 – d8 | 19.2 ± 1.2 | 111 ± 15  (90) | 58 |
| | d0 – d12 | 19.5 ± 0.3 | 133 ± 8  (92) | 68 |
| | d0 – d18 | 19.6 ± 0.7 | 150 ± 6  (88) | 77 |
| | d12 – d18 | 12.9 ± 0.2 | 8 ± 1  (63) | 6 |
| ECM | none | 17.1 ± 0.8 | 125 ± 4  (94) | 73 |
| | d0 – d18 | 21.9 ± 0.5 | 149 ± 4  (92) | 68 |

1   Incorporation of $^{35}SO_4^{2-}$ was measured on day 18.

2   Percent of the radioactivity incorporated into proteoglycans present in the cell layer versus radioactivity incorporated into proteoglycans present in the cell layer and in the culture medium.

Rabbit costal chondrocytes were seeded at 3 X $10^3$ cells per 35 mm plastic tissue culture dish and exposed to DMEM supplemented with 10% fetal calf serum. FGF (0.6 ng/ml) was added every other day during the indicated culture periods. After 18 days in culture, triplicate plates were exposed for 3 h to 2 µCi/ml of ($^{35}$S)sulfate in 0.8 ml of DMEM. Values represent averages ± standard deviation for triplicate determinations.

serum-supplemented medium undergo 10 generations, cultures maintained on plastic and exposed to FGF or maintained on ECM and not exposed to the mitogen can undergo as many as 60 generations. The mechanisms through which ECM or FGF prolong the life span of cultured cells is at present unknown. The possibility exists that specific oncogenes are activated. Three oncogenes, c ras, c myc, and c fos, have been shown to be activated by FGF.[36-38] While two of them (c ras and c myc), when inserted into normal cells, can confer immortality in vitro,[39] the activation of the third one (c fos) correlates with cell differentiation.[37,38] Interestingly enough, differentiation was defined in this study as production of ECM components (fibronectin, collagen type IV).[38] Whether or not the effects of FGF or ECM on PG production by chondrocyte cultures could be explained by activation of the c fos gene, while its effect on proliferation and cell longevity of that cell type could result from the activation of other cellular oncogenes such as c myc or c ras, remains an interesting question.

## THE DEVELOPMENT OF A SERUM-FREE CULTURE SYSTEM FOR RABBIT COSTAL CHONDROCYTES

In chondrocyte cultures, fetal calf serum is required for both cell growth and phenotypic expression. Previous studies have shown that various plasma factors affect the proliferation of cultured chondrocytes and PG synthesis. There have been no studies, however, demonstrating the hormonal requirements for cellular proliferation and PG synthesis in serum-free chondrocyte cultures. Growing cartilage cells in defined medium supplemented with hormones and growth factors would open the way for studies of factors involved not only in chondrocyte proliferation, but in differentiation as well.[40]

In an effort to maintain the differentiated state of chondrocytes grown in serum-free medium, we have taken advantage of the fact that BCE-ECM and FGF stabilize the phenotypic expression of chondrocytes grown in the presence of serum-supplemented medium. The basal medium used was a 9:1 (v/v) mixture of DMEM and F12 medium supplemented with ascorbic acid (25 µg/ml) and antibiotics (DF medium). Fig. 4-I shows the comparison of the final cell density of rabbit costal chondrocytes from primary suspension cultures when seeded at low density (30 cells/mm$^2$) on ECM-coated dishes and exposed either to DF medium supplemented with 10% FCS or to medium supplemented with high density lipoproteins (HDL), transferrin, FGF, hydrocortisone, EGF, and insulin, added either singly or in combination. In the case of chondrocytes originating from primary suspension culture, the addition of transferrin alone to the medium resulted in a 2-fold increase in cell density (Fig. 4-I). HDL, when added together with transferrin, resulted in a 20-fold increase in cell density, while the addition of FGF together with HDL and transferrin resulted in an 80-fold increase. The addition of both hydrocortisone and EGF together with HDL, transferrin, and FGF resulted in a 110-fold increase in the cell number. The final cell density of cultures exposed to a synthetic medium supplemented with all five components was much higher than that of cultures exposed to 10% fetal calf serum (Fig. 4-I). When rabbit costal chondrocytes were maintained on ECM-coated dishes in the presence of medium supplemented with transferrin, HDL, FGF, hydrocortisone, and insulin (Medium B), nearly all cells resumed a spherical configuration in confluent cultures. The spherical cells were surrounded by a refractile matrix which stained intensely with alcian green. Insulin, although it slightly decreased the final cell density (Fig. 4-I), was required for reexpression of the cartilage phenotype at confluence. On the other hand, EGF, although it was required for the optimal stimulation of chondrocyte proliferation (Fig. 4-I), had a small inhibitory effect on reexpression of cartilage phenotype at confluence. Transmission electron microscopy showed that the ultrastructure of cells maintained on ECM-coated dishes in the presence of medium supplemented with transferrin, HDL, FGF, hydrocortisone, and insulin was similar to that seen _in vivo_. The cells were embedded in a well developed three-dimensional matrix in which abundant thin collagen fibrils, characteristic of Type II collagen, were observed (Fig. 4-IIA). In contrast, the ultrastructure

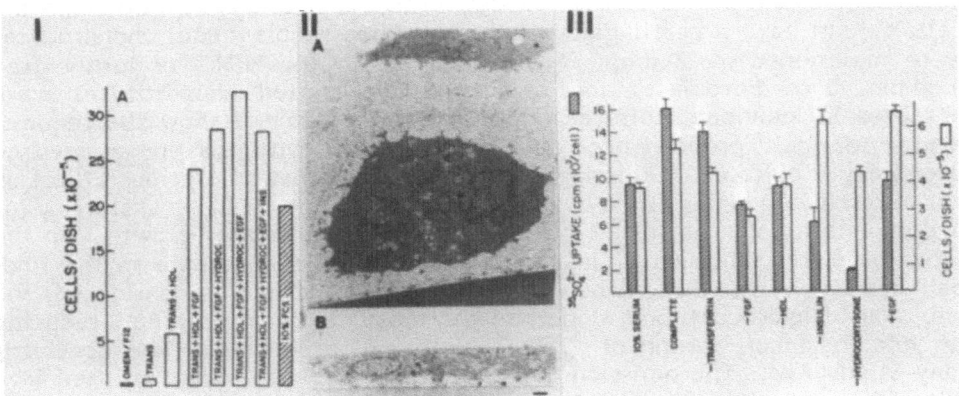

Fig. 4. I. Comparison of the final cell density of rabbit costal chondrocyte cultures originating from primary suspension cultures and exposed either to DF medium supplemented with 10% fetal calf serum or to medium supplemented with HDL, transferrin, FGF, hydrocortisone, EGF and insulin, added either singly or in combination. II. Transmission electron micrograph of chondrocyte cultures. III. Effect of the deletion of a single factor from Medium B and the effect of EGF on the final cell density (open bars) of rabbit chondrocyte cultures and their proteoglycan synthesis (cross-hatched bars).

I. Floating chondrocytes from primary suspension cultures were seeded at $3 \times 10^4$ cells per 35 mm ECM-coated dish, as described in ref. 40, and exposed to DF medium supplemented or not with 10% fetal calf serum or the following combinations of factors: transferrin 60 µg/ml), transferrin and HDL (300 µg protein/ml), transferrin-HDL and FGF (1 ng/ml), transferrin-HDL-FGF and hydrocortisone ($10^{-6}$ M), transferrin-HDL-FGF-hydrocortisone and EGF (30 ng/ml), and transferrin-HDL-FGF-hydrocortisone-FGF and insulin (1 µg/ml). After 6 days in culture, triplicate plates representing each condition were harvested and counted.

II. A cross section of the cell layer of cultures maintained for 10 days on ECM-coated dishes and exposed either to Medium B (A, Complete) or to Medium B from which FGF had been deleted is shown (Bar, 1 µm).

III. Rabbit costal chondrocytes were seeded at $1 \times 10^4$ cells per 16 mm ECM-coated dish and exposed to medium supplemented with the five components of Medium B (Complete) or Medium B from which transferrin (- Transferrin), FGF (- FGF), HDL (- HDL), insulin (- Insulin), or hydrocortisone (- Hydrocortisone) had been deleted. After 8 days in culture, cells were exposed for 3 h to 8 µCi/ml of $^{35}SO_4^{2-}$, and the final cell density (open bars) and PG synthesis (cross-hatched bars) were determined. Results were compared with those obtained with cultures exposed to Medium B supplemented with EGF (+ EGF) or cultures exposed to 10% fetal calf serum (+ Serum).

of cells maintained in the FGF-free medium containing the other components of Medium B was similar to that of fibroblasts (Fig. 4-IIB), and the cells did not have a cartilaginous matrix. When rabbit costal chondrocytes were maintained in Medium B with EGF or in the HDL- or insulin-free medium, both fibroblasts and overtly differentiated chondrocytes were observed in individual cultures. Fig. 4-III and Table II show the requirements for cell proliferation and sulfated PG synthesis in serum-free chondrocyte cultures. Omission of FGF had the most deleterious effect on cell growth, reducing it by 50%. Omission of HDL, transferrin, or hydrocortisone alone resulted in a 20% to 30% inhibition of growth. On the other hand, the omission of insulin resulted in a 20% increase in the final cell density (Fig. 4-III). When sulfated PG synthesis was considered, the omission of hydrocortisone alone had the most deleterious effect, reducing by 90% the incorporation of $^{35}SO_4^{2-}$ into PGs produced by late confluent (day 8) cultures. The omission of FGF, insulin or HDL alone resulted in a 40-60% decrease in the incorporation of $^{35}SO_4^{2-}$ into PGs in confluent cultures. On the other hand, omission of transferrin had a marginal effect on $^{35}SO_4^{2-}$ incorporation (Fig. 4-III). Although the addition of EGF to the medium resulted in a 25% increase in the final cell density of cultures, it also caused a 45% decrease in $^{35}SO_4^{2-}$ incorporation into PGs in confluent cultures. As can be seen from Fig. 5, no parallel relationship between the rate of PG synthesis and cell growth was observed. This suggests that chondrocyte proliferation and phenotypic expression are regulated by different sets of growth factors and hormones. Although transferrin, HDL, FGF, hydrocortisone, and EGF are required in order for chondrocytes to proliferate rapidly and express cartilage phenotype under serum-free culture conditions, addition of each one of these factors alone to the serum-free medium did not substantially support chondrocyte proliferation and phenotypic expression. Obviously, the interplay of these hormones and growth factors are necessary for the optimal stimulation of chondrocyte proliferation and their phenotypic expression.

Table II

The Optimal Concentrations of Growth Factors
and Hormones in Serum-Free Chondroyte Cultures

| Additions | Optimal Concentrations (per ml) | |
| --- | --- | --- |
| | Cell Proliferation | Proteoglycan Synthesis |
| Transferrin | 60 µg | (not required) |
| HDL | 300 µg protein | 300 µg protein |
| FGF | 0.25 - 1 ng | 0.25 - 1 ng |
| Hydrocortisone | $10^{-7} - 10^{-6}$ M | $10^{-7} - 10^{-6}$ M |
| Insulin | (inhibition) | 0.2 - 1.0 µg |
| EGF | 30 ng | (inhibition) |

The chondrocytes grown in serum-free medium seem to be a good experimental system for studies on the control of chondrocyte growth and their synthesis of cartilage-matrix components. In fact, using this serum-free chondrocyte system, it was demonstrated for the first time that glucocorticoids have a direct and specific stimulatory effect on cartilage-specific PG synthesis once low density chondrocyte cultures become confluent.[41] Chondrocytes grown in the presence of transferrin, HDL, FGF, insulin (medium A) and $10^{-7}$ M hydrocortisone reorganized, at confluence, into a homogeneous, cartilage-like tissue composed of round cells and surrounded by a refractile matrix in which abundant thin collagen fibrils characteristic of type II collagen were observed. The cell ultrastructure and fibrils of the pericellular matrix were similar to those seen in vivo. In contrast, cells grown in the absence of hydrocortisone, once they reached confluence, formed a fibroblastic multilayer and produced thick collagen bundles, characteristic of Type I collagen. The level of $^{35}SO_4^{2-}$ incorporated into large, cartilage-specific PGs in glucocorticoid-supplemented cultures was 33-fold higher than that of glucocorticoid-free cultures (Fig. 5-I). The level of $^{35}SO_4^{2-}$ incorporated into small, ubiquitous PGs was only 4-fold higher than that of glucocorticoid-free cultures (Fig. 5-I). A marked effect of glucocorticoids on the synthesis of extracellular-matrix macromolecules was also observed when cells were labeled with [$^3$H]glucosamine (Fig. 5-II). In the glucocorticoid-supplemented medium, confluent chondrocyte cultures produced a large amount of $^3$H-labeled chondroitin sulfate glycosaminoglycans associated with cartilage-specific PGs, which made up more than 70% of the total $^3$H-labeled glycosaminoglycans. A small population (6%) of $^3$H-labeled hyaluronic acid was present in the glucocorticoid-supplemented cultures. In contrast, confluent cultures maintained in the glucocorticoid-free medium produced a large amount of $^3$H-labeled hyaluronic acid, which made up more than 70% of the total $^3$H-labeled glycosaminoglycans synthesized in glucocorticoid-free cultures. The level of $^3$H incorporated into hyaluronic acid in glucocorticoid-free cultures was 4.5-fold higher than that of glucocorticoid-supplemented cultures, while the level of $^3$H incorporated into cartilage-specific proteoglycans in glucocorticoid-free cultures was 18-fold lower than that of glucocorticoid-supplemented cultures (Fig. 5-II). It is unclear, however, whether glucocorticoid directly stimulates PG synthesis in confluent, stationary cultures, or whether the steroid stabilizes, as does FGF, the capacity of actively growing chondrocytes to reexpress the cartilage phenotype once they reach confluence. To test for these possibilities, we have examined the effect of transient glucocorticoid exposure on PG synthesis by chondrocyte cultures grown from the sparse stage in the presence of transferrin, HDL, FGF, and insulin. When rabbit chondrocyte cultures were exposed to hydrocortisone only during their growth phase (days 0 to 4), a slight (2- to 3-fold) increase in the incorporation of $^{35}SO_4^{2-}$ into PGs was observed when measured in cultures in the late stage of confluence (day 8 or 12, Fig. 5-IIA). In contrast, when cultures were exposed to hydrocortisone during their growth phase as well as during the confluent stage (day 0 to day 5 and beyond), a marked (10- to 16-fold) increase in the incorporation of $^{35}SO_4^{2-}$ into PGs in confluent cultures was observed. The rate of $^{35}SO_4^{2-}$ incorporation into PGs,

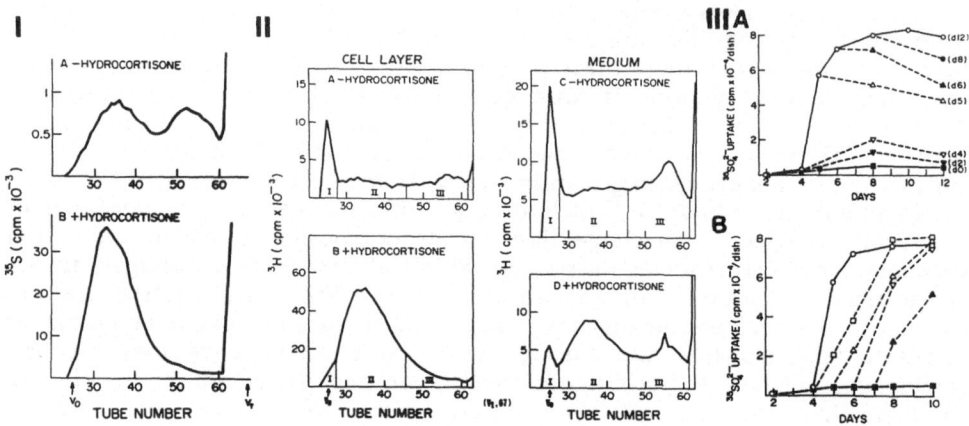

Fig. 5.   I.   Sepharose CL-2B chromatography under dissociative solvent conditions of proteoglycans from cultures grown in the presence or absence of hydrocortisone.  Rabbit costal chondrocytes were seeded at $3 \times 10^4$ cells per 35 mm ECM-coated dishes and exposed to Medium A in the absence (A) or presence (B) of hydrocortisone ($10^{-7}$ M).  After 10 days in culture, cells were labeled with $^{35}SO_4{}^{2-}$ and proteoglycans present in the cell layers and in the medium were extracted and processed as described in ref. 41.

II.   Sepharose CL-2B chromatography of hyaluronate and proteoglycans (PGs) located in the cell layers (A, B) and in the medium (C, D) from cultures maintained in the absence (A, C) or presence (B, D) of hydrocortisone.  Cultures were seeded and maintained for 10 days, and cells were then labeled with [$^3$H] glucosamine for 24 h  as described in ref.  41.  Aliquots of the 4 M guanidine HCl extract of the cell layer (A, B) or aliquots of the medium (C, D) from cultures maintained in the presence of medium A alone (A, C) or Medium A supplemented with hydrocortisone (B, D) were applied on a column of Sepharose CL-2B and analyzed as described in ref. 40.  Fraction I was identified as hyaluronic acid, Fraction II as chondroitin sulfate PG, and Fraction III as low molecular weight PG composed of chondroitin and dermatan sulfate PG.

III.   (A) Effect of length of exposure to hydrocortisone on the rate of PG synthesis by rabbit costal chondrocyte cultures maintained under serum-free conditions.  Rabbit chondrocytes were seeded at $1 \times 10^4$ cells per 16 mm ECM-coated dish and exposed to Medium A supplemented with hydrocortisone ($10^{-7}$ M).  After 0 (■), 2 (▼), 4 (▽), 5 (△), 6 (●), 8 (o), or 12 days (o) in culture, hydrocortisone alone was deleted from the complete medium.  Cultures were exposed for 3 h to 8 μCi/ml of $^{35}SO_4{}^{2-}$ on the indicated days.  (B) Effect of exposure to hydrocortisone after cultures became confluent on the rate of proteoglycan synthesis by rabbit costal chondrocytes maintained under serum-free conditions. Rabbit chondrocytes were seeded at $1 \times 10^4$ cells per 16 mm ECM-coated dish and maintained in the presence of Medium A. After 0 (o), 4 (□), 5 (△), 6 (▽), 7 (▲), and 10 days (■) in culture, hydrocortisone ($10^{-7}$ M) was added to the serum-free medium. Cultures were exposed for 3 h to 8 μCi/ml of $^{35}SO_4^{2-}$ in a 9:1 mixture of DMEM and Ham's F12 medium on the indicated days.

measured on day 8, in cultures exposed to hydrocortisone from day 0 to day 5 or 8 was 10- and 16-fold higher, respectively, than that of cultures never exposed to the glucocorticoid (Fig. 4). Fig. 5-IIIA also shows that the rate of $^{35}SO_4^{2-}$ incorporation into PGs, measured on day 12, in cultures exposed to hydrocortisone from day 0 to day 5 was 45% lower than that of cultures exposed to it from day 0 to day 12. Deletion of hydrocortisone from the medium on day 6 or 8 also resulted in a 16-34% decrease in the incorporation of $^{35}SO_4^{2-}$ into PGs, measured on day 12. These results therefore suggest that continuous exposure of confluent chondrocyte cultures to hydrocortisone is required for the maximal stimulation of PG synthesis. Confirming this conclusion is the fact that when hydrocortisone was added on day 4 to cultures previously maintained in its absence, a marked (8-fold) increase in the incorporation of $^{35}SO_4^{2-}$ into PGs was observed within 24 h (Fig. 5-IIIB). The rate of $^{35}SO_4^{2-}$ incorporation, measured on day 8, in cultures exposed to hydrocortisone from day 4 to day 8 was 16-fold higher than that of cultures never exposed to it. Furthermore, the increase in the incorporation of $^{35}SO_4^{2-}$ was accompanied by the appearance of an extensive refractile matrix. Similarly, addition of hydrocortisone to confluent, resting cultures on days 5, 6, or 7 resulted in marked increases in $^{35}SO_4^{2-}$ incorporation into PGs within 24 to 48 h (Fig. 5-IIIB), further demonstrating that glucocorticoids can revert the phenotype of confluent dedifferentiated fibroblastic cells to that of chondrocytes. It is therefore likely that, in order to promote the expression of the chondrocyte phenotype, glucocorticoids are not required during the phase of active cell proliferation but are required once cells become confluent.

CONCLUSION

By defining the conditions under which chondrocytes can proliferate and express their proper phenotype when exposed to defined medium, a means has been provided for the elucidation of the factors and environmental conditions which will control chondrocyte proliferation and differentiation in vitro. The mechanisms through which such factors operate can also be investigated. The principal question remaining is whether or not such factors are also relevant in vivo. An answer to that question requires a transition from the field of cell biology to the more difficult domain of in vivo physiology and endocrine regulation.

## REFERENCES

1.  R.D. Cahn, Factors affecting inheritance and expression of differentiation: Some methods of analysis, in "The Stability of the Differentiated State," H. Ursprung, ed., Springer-Verlag, New York (1968).

2.  W. Dessau, J. Sasse, R. Timpl, F. Jilek, and K. von der Mark, Synthesis and extracellular deposition of fibronectin in chondrocyte cultures, J. Cell Biol. 79:342 (1978).

3.  K.E. Kuettner, B.U. Pauli, G. Gall, V.A. Memoli, and R.K. Schenk, Synthesis of cartilage matrix by mammalian chondrocytes in vitro. I. Isolation, culture characteristics and morphology, J. Cell Biol. 93:743 (1982).

4.  S. Chacko, J. Abbot, and H. Holtzer, Loss of phenotypic traits by differentiated cells: VI. Behavior of the progeny of a single chondrocyte, J. Exp. Med. 130:417 (1969).

5.  P.D. Benya, S.R. Padilla, and M.E. Nimni, The progeny of rabbit articular chondrocytes synthesize collagen types I and III and type I trimer, but not type II. Verification by cyanogen bromide peptide analysis, Biochemistry 16:865 (1977).

6.  R. Mayne, M.S. Vail, P.M. Mayne, and E.J. Miller, Changes in type of collagen synthesized as clones of chick chondrocytes grow and eventually lose division capacity, Proc. Natl. Acad. Sci. USA 73:1674 (1976).

7.  D. Gospodarowicz, I. Vlodavsky, G. Greenburg, J. and L.K. Johnson, Cellular shape is determined by the extracellular matrix and is responsible for the control of cellular growth and function, in "Cold Spring Harbor Conferences on Cell Proliferation, v. 6: Hormones and Cell Culture," R. Ross and G. Sato, eds., Cold Spring Harbor, New York (1979).

8.  D. Gospodarowicz, D.C. Cohen, and D.K. Fujii, Regulation of cell growth by the basal lamina and plasma factors: Relevance to embryonic control of cell proliferation and differentiation, in "Cold Spring Harbor Conferences on Cell Proliferation, v. 9: Growth of Cells in Hormonally Defined Media," G. Sato, A. Pardee, and D. Sirbasku, eds., Cold Spring Harbor, New York (1982).

9.  I. Vlodavsky, L.K. Johnson, G. Greenburg, and D. Gospodarowicz, Vascular endothelial cells maintained in the absence of fibroblast growth factor undergo structural and functional alterations that are incompatible with their in vivo differentiated properties, J. Cell Biol. 83:468 (1979).

10. S. Tseng, N. Savion, R. Stern, and D. Gospodarowicz, Fibroblast growth factor modulates synthesis of collagen in cultured vascular endothelial cells, Eur. J. Biochem. 122:355 (1982).

11. D. Gospodarowicz, The control of mammalian cell proliferation by growth factors, extracellular matrices, and lipoproteins, J. Inv. Dermatology 519:41 (1983).

12. D. Gospodarowicz and A.L. Mescher, A comparison of the responses of cultured myoblasts and chondrocytes to fibroblast and epidermal growth factors, J. Cell. Physiol. 93:117 (1977).

13.  K.L. Jones and J. Addison, Pituitary fibroblast growth factor as a stimulator of growth in cultured rabbit articular chondrocytes, Endocrinology 97:359 (1975).

14.  D. Gospodarowicz, K. Hirabayashi, L. Giguere, and J.-P. Tauber, Factors controlling the proliferative rate, final cell density, and life span of bovine vascular smooth muscle cells, J. Cell Biol. 89:568 (1981).

15.  D. Gospodarowicz, D., Lepine, S. Massoglia, and I. Wood, Comparison of the ability of basement membranes produced by corneal endothelial and mouse-derived endodermal PF-HR-9 cells to support the proliferation and differentiation of normal diploid bovine kidney tubule epithelial cells in vitro, J. Cell Biol. 99:947 (1984).

16.  Y. Kato and D. Gospodarowicz, Effect of exogenous extracellular matrices on proteoglycan synthesis by cultured rabbit costal chondrocytes, J. Cell Biol.:in press (1984).

17.  I. Lewo, K. Alitalo, L. Riteli, A. Vaheri, R. Timpl, and J. Wartiovaara, Basal lamina glycoproteins and type IV collagen are assembled into a fine fibered matrix in cultures of a teratocarcinoma-derived endoderm cell line, Exp. Cell Res. 137:15 (1982).

18.  B.L.M. Hogan, A. Taylor, M. Kurkkinen, and J.R. Couchman, Synthesis and localization of two sulphated glycoproteins associated with basement membranes and the extracellular matrix, J. Cell Biol. 95:197 (1982).

19.  S. Strickland, K.S. Smith, and K.R. Marotti, Hormonal induction of differentiation in teratocarcinoma stem cells:  generation of parietal endoderm by retinoic acid and dibutyryl cAMP, Cell 21:347 (1980).

20.  J.M. Foidart and A.H. Reddi, Immunofluorescent localization of Type IV collagen and laminin during endochondral bone differentiation and regulation by pituitary growth hormone, Dev. Biol. 75:30 (1980).

21.  A. Martin-Hernandez, The basement membrane in the microvasculature, in "Microcirculation.  Current Physiologic, Medical, and Surgical Concepts," R.M.  Effros, H. Schmid-Schonbein, and J. Ditzel, eds., Academic Press, New York (1981).

22.  S. Tseng, N. Savion, D. Gospodarowicz, and R. Stern, Characterization of collagens synthesized by bovine corneal endothelial cell cultures, J. Biol. Chem. 256:3361 (1981).

23.  D. Gospodarowicz, G. Greenburg, J.M. Foidart, and N. Savion, The production and localization of laminin in cultured vascular and corneal endothelial cells, J. Cell. Physiol. 107:173 (1981).

24.  J. Robinson and D. Gospodarowicz, Characterization of glycosaminoglycans synthesized by cultured bovine corneal endothelial cell cultures, J. Cell. Physiol. 117:368 (1983).

25.  B.K. Hall, Epithelial-mesenchymal interactions in cartilage and bone development, in "Epithelial-mesenchymal interactions in development," R.H. Sawyer and J.F. Fallon, eds., Praeger Publishers, New York (1983).

26.   J. Robinson and D. Gospodarowicz, Effect of p-Nitrophenyl -D-xyloside on proteoglycan synthesis and extracellular matrix formation by bovine corneal endothelial cell cultures, J. Biol. Chem. 259:3818 (1984).

27.   C.M. West, R. Lanza, J. Rosenbloom, M. Lowe, H. Holtzer, and N. Avdalovic, Fibronectin alters the phenotypic properties of cultured chick embryochondroblasts, Cell 17:491 (1979).

28.   J.B. Pennypacker, Modulation of chondrogenic expression in cell culture by fibronectin, Vision Res. 21:65 (1981).

29.   A.H. Reddi, Bone induction: introduction and perspectives, in "The Chemistry and Biology of Mineralized Connective Tissues," A. Veis, ed., Elsevier North Holland, New York (1981).

30.   D. Gospodarowicz, G. Greenburg, H. Bialecki, and B. Zetter, Factors involved in the modulation of cell proliferation in vivo and in vitro: the role of fibroblast and epidermal growth factors in the proliferative response of mammalian cells, In Vitro 14:85 (1978).

31.   Y. Kato, Y. Hiraki, H. Inoue, M. Kinoshita, Y. Yutani, and F. Suzuki, Differential and synergistic actions of somatomedin-like growth factors, fibroblast growth factor and epidermal growth factor in rabbit costal chondrocytes, Eur. J. Biochem. 129:685 (1983).

32.   K.D. Jentzsch, G. Wellmitz, G. Heder, E. Petzold, P. Buntrock, and P. Oehme, A bovine brain fraction with fibroblast growth factor activity inducing articular cartilage regeneration in vivo. Acta Biol. Med.Germ. 39:967 (1980).

33.   Y. Kato and D. Gospodarowicz, Sulfated proteoglycan synthesis by confluent cultures of rabbit costal chondrocytes grown in the presence of fibroblast growth factor, J. Cell Biol.:in press (1985).

34.   A. Noro, K. Kimata, Y. Oike, T. Shinomura, N. Maeda, S. Yano, N. Takahashi, and S. Suzuki, Isolation and characteristic of a third proteoglycan (PG-Lt) from chick embryo cartilage which contains disulfide-bonded collagenous polypeptide, J. Biol. Chem. 258:9323 (1983).

35.   T. Shinomura, K. Kimata, Y. Oike, N. Maeda, S. Yano, and S. Suzuki, Appearance of distinct types of proteoglycan in a well-defined temporal and spatial pattern during early cartilage formation in the chick limb, Devel. Biol. 103:211 (1984).

36.   K. Kelly, B.H. Cochran, C.D. Stiles, and P. Leder, Cell specific regulation of the c myc by lymphocyte mitogens and platelet-derived growth factor, Cell 55:603 (1983).

37.   M.E. Greenberg, and E.B. Ziff, Stimulation of 3T3 cells induces transcription of the c fos protooncogene, Nature 311:433 (1984).

38.   R. Muller and E.F. Wagner, Differentiation of F9 teratocarcinoma stem cells after transfer of c fos protooncogenes, Nature 311:438 (1984).

39.   H. Land, L.F. Parada, and R.A. Weinberg, Tumorigenic conversion of primary embryo fibroblasts requires at least two cooperating oncogenes, Nature 304:596 (1983).

40.   Y. Kato and D. Gospodarowicz, Growth requirements of low density rabbit costal chondrocyte cultures maintained in serum free medium, J. Cell. Physiol. 120:354 (1984).

41.   Y. Kato and D. Gospodarowicz, Stimulation by glucocorticoids of the synthesis of cartilage matrix proteoglycans produced by rabbit costal chondrocytes in vitro, J. Biol. Chem.:in press (1985).

CELLS INTO ORGANS*

Lauri Saxén and Eero Lehtonen

Department of Pathology
University of Helsinki
Finland

INTRODUCTION

As illustrated by many presentations at this Symposium, progress has been fast in the field of cytodifferentiation, i.e., regulation of gene activity during development and differentiation at the molecular and cellular levels. Less has been learned recently in the field of "classic" embryology dealing, in the first place, with "supramolecular" problems related to multicellular assemblies and to the formation of complex tissues and organs from several cell lineages. Here progress has been slow, but with the development of new methods within molecular and cell biology the traditional problems might be successfully re-explored as already shown at this Symposium by the presentations of Raff and Weston.

In what follows, we will summarize some recent experimental results obtained in one model-system for organogenesis and its guiding principles. An effort will be made to bridge some observations at the cellular (molecular) and tissue (supramolecular) levels. Needless to stress, such an effort will consist not only of facts but of much speculation as well.

The model-organ

The vertebrate kidney, the metanephros, develops from three cell lineages: the epithelial collecting duct system derived from the

---

xTitle borrowed from the excellent monograph of our esteemed friend J. P. Trinkaus.

Wolffian duct, the excretory nephrons originating from the mesenchymal blastema, and the vascular endothelium from an outside origin.
The creation of a complex, yet harmonious and functional organ of the
three originally separate cell lineages requires a constant
"informative" interaction between the various cell types and within a
population of like cells as well.  In this respect, the kidney is not
unlike any other developing organ, but it has been rendered suitable
for an analytical approach in the study of interactive events.

The first stage of morphogenesis of the metanephros begins with
the ingrowth of the ureter bud into the loose metanephrogenic
mesenchyme.  Here it branches dichotomously several times and forms
the "ureter tree" and the renal pelvis. Mesenchymal condensates are
created around the tips of the branching ureter.  They soon become
converted into epithelial vesicles and, ultimately, into the entire
excretory nephron.  Constant ingrowth of the ureter and its branching
create an arcade organization of nephrons that gradually join the
collecting system.  The development of the two above cell lineages
is, as will be seen below, closely associated with the development
and organization of the third cell lineage, the vascular endothelium,
which completes the formation of functional glomeruli.

## The collecting system

The ingrowth and regular branching of the ureter seem to be the
decisive factor, the key event, for the entire creation of the kidney
architecture.  The molecular basis for this strictly regulated,
orderly branching is not known, but an interaction with the
mesenchymal component is a prerequisite for the growth and branching
of the epithelial component (Grobstein, 1955).  This type of
epithelial-mesenchymal interaction has been more thoroughly analyzed
in another model-system, the embryonic salivary gland (summarized by
Bernfield, 1981).  From these extensive investigations it may be
concluded that though the mesenchymal counterpart is definitely
required, the primary "branching program" is incorporated in the
epithelial component.  These studies have also laid the basis for our
understanding of the molecular mechanisms of such epithelial-
mesenchymal interactions and for the implementation of a branching
program.

## The excretory nephron

By separation and recombination experiments Grobstein (1955,
1967) has shown conclusively that an intimate interaction between the
collecting duct epithelium and the surrounding mesenchyme is also
required for the epithelial transformation of the latter and for the
organization of the epithelial cells into nephric tubules.  This
multistep event has been analyzed in some detail by using the

transfilter technique also devised by Grobstein (1956). By in vitro insertion of porous filter membranes between the target mesenchyme and its inductor (usually a heterotypic tissue like the embryonic spinal cord), the prerequisites and the kinetics of transmission of the inductive signals can be explored. While the molecular nature of these signals has remained unknown, some features of their action can be summarized:

1. Induction of kidney tubules is of a permissive type: the target cells seem to have only two developmental options - either to be converted into epithelial cells or to remain as stromal elements. Conversely, no other embryonic mesenchymes tested thus far will respond to the tubule inductors by epithelial transformation (Saxén, 1970).
2. Transmission of the inductive signals is cell-mediated: prevention of an intimate contact between the interactive cells hinders any inductive dialogues from taking place (Wartiovaara et al., 1974; Lehtonen, 1976; Saxén et al., 1976).
3. Induction is time-consuming: an intercellular contact of the order of 24 hours is required for an irreversible epithelial commitment (in our experimental conditions) (Saxén and Lehtonen, 1978). This relatively short pulse will program the cells all the way into segmented tubuli and glomerular podocytes (Lehtonen et al., 1983).

The vasculature

Contrary to some earlier views, the metanephric mesenchyme seems not to possess an option to develop into hematopoietic or vascular endothelial cells which have an outside origin, as already suggested by Potter (1965). This has been confirmed recently by Sariola and collaborators (1983, 1984b) by grafting experiments: when embryonic, undifferentiated and avascular mouse kidney rudiments were grafted on avian chorioallantoic membrane (CAM), both morphogenesis and vasculogenesis ensued. It was demonstrated by nuclear markers and immunohistology that the kidney vasculature was derived from the avian vessels which were guided to the murine glomerular anlagen. Here both murine podocytes and avian endothelial cells contributed to the formation of the glomerular basement membrane (GBM) (Sariola et al., 1984a).

At least three interactive events between the constituents of the actual parenchymal anlage and the invading vascular component should be considered: a release of an angiogenetic factor stimulating the sprouting of the avian vessels, creation of paths to be followed by the endothelial cells into their ultimate locations, and an interaction between the epithelial podocytes and the vascular endothelial cells ensuring a polarized formation of the GBM.

EARLY METABOLIC CHANGES

As long as the key molecules transmitting signals between the three interacting cell lineages are unknown, hints of their nature and mode of action might be found by examining the consequences of such interactions. As far as the epithelial transformation is concerned, some early metabolic events preceding morphogenesis have been detected.

As shown by incorporation experiments, one of the first signs of induction is a stimulated proliferation of the mesenchymal target cells, observed already early during the induction period and never detected in non-inductive situations (Saxén et al., 1983). It has been suggested that the effect might be brought about by rendering the cells sensitive to circulating growth factors, e.g. transferrin (Ekblom et al., 1983, 1985). Concomitant changes in the composition of the extracellular matrix of the mesenchyme have been visualized by immunohistology. Some interstitial-type proteins are lost from the induced, pretubular areas (fibronectin and collagen types I and III) and soon replaced by a set of epithelial-type components (laminin, collagen types IV and V, and heparan sulphate proteoglycan) (Ekblom et al., 1981; Lash et al., 1983; Bonadio et al., 1984). These "new" proteins are first expressed in a random, dotted fashion, but later become confined around the early renal vesicles and contribute to their basement membrane.

Invasion and migration of the endothelial cells is intimately associated with the above changes (Fig. 1). Using antibodies against avian endothelial cells, the vessels can be visualized along their migration to the glomeruli. They follow the stalk of the ureter bud, but never invade the early condensate or the renal vesicles. In fact, the endothelial cells closely follow the border-line between the pre-epithelial, laminin-expressing condensates and the interstitial stroma expressing fibronectin. It is tempting to speculate that fibronectin is involved in the formation of the paths guiding the migration of the endothelial cells (Sariola et al., 1984b) - not unlike the direction of the migration of neural crest cells (Thiery et al., 1982a). Components contributing to the basement membrane might not be involved until the endothelial cells have been trapped in the glomerular crevice and their basement membrane fuses with that of the podocytes.


CONSIDERATION OF MECHANISMS

Figure 2 summarizes the above observations and speculates their possible causal mechanisms and consequences. Stimulated proliferation - either through production of a mitogen or induction of receptors for growth factors - increases the cell mass locally, thus contributing to the condensation and to the centrifugal movement of

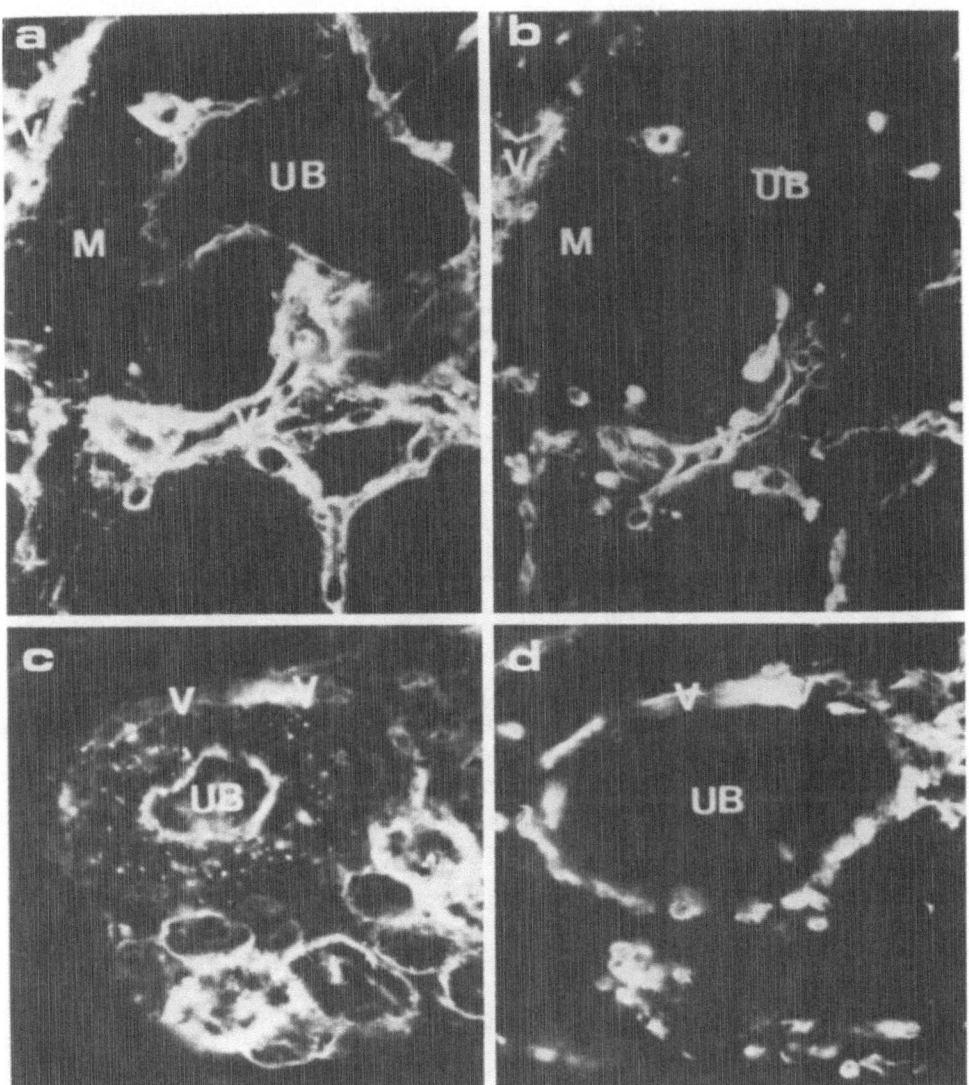

Fig. 1. Double immunofluorescence stainings of sections of murine
kidney rudiments grafted on quail chorioallantoic membrane and
invaded by blood vessels of the latter.
a and b. Section treated with antibodies against fibronectin (a)
and quail endothelial cells (b).  Codistribution is evident.
c and d. Double treatment with antibodies against laminin (c) and
quail endothelial cells (d).  Laminin is seen in the tubular basement membrane and around the ureter bud but, in a punctate fashion,
in the early condensates as well.  There is no codistribution with
the quail capillaries.  UB: ureter bud; M: mesenchyme; V: vessel.
(Sariola et al., 1984b).

INDUCTION OF THE NEPHRON

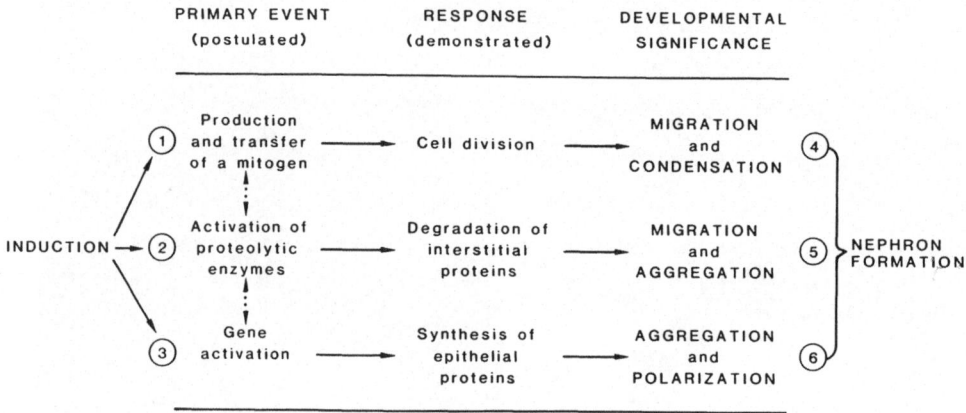

Fig. 2. Facts and speculations on the events of tubule formation after an inductive stimulus (Lehtonen and Saxén, 1985).

the induced cells as well (shown in chimaeric mouse/quail kidney recombinants by Saxén and Karkinen-Jääskeläinen, 1975). Simultaneously proteolytic enzymes are activated in the induced areas (not shown), further promoting aggregation by degrading the extracellular matrix. The actual cell-to-cell attachment could be mediated by some of the basement-membrane type proteins detected or by some other adhesive molecules, like N-CAM also shown in the condensates (Thiery et al., 1982b). Ultimately the epithelial-type proteins create the basement membrane to which the epithelialized cells adhere and become polarized.

## Cytodifferentiation versus organogenesis

In the above-described, complex development of the three cell lineages forming a kidney rudiment, cytodifferentiation and the assembly of these cells into organized tissues can be, to a certain extent, separated. This can be done by following differentiation of the mesenchymal cells in two-dimensional monolayer cultures that prevent the formation of the three-dimensional structures (Lehtonen et al., 1985).

The majority of the mesenchymal cells become irreversibly determined towards epithelial direction when induced by the transfilter technique for 24 hours (Saxén and Lehtonen, 1978). At that time, however, they are still undifferentiated according to our morphological criteria. By immunohistochemical probes, we have shown

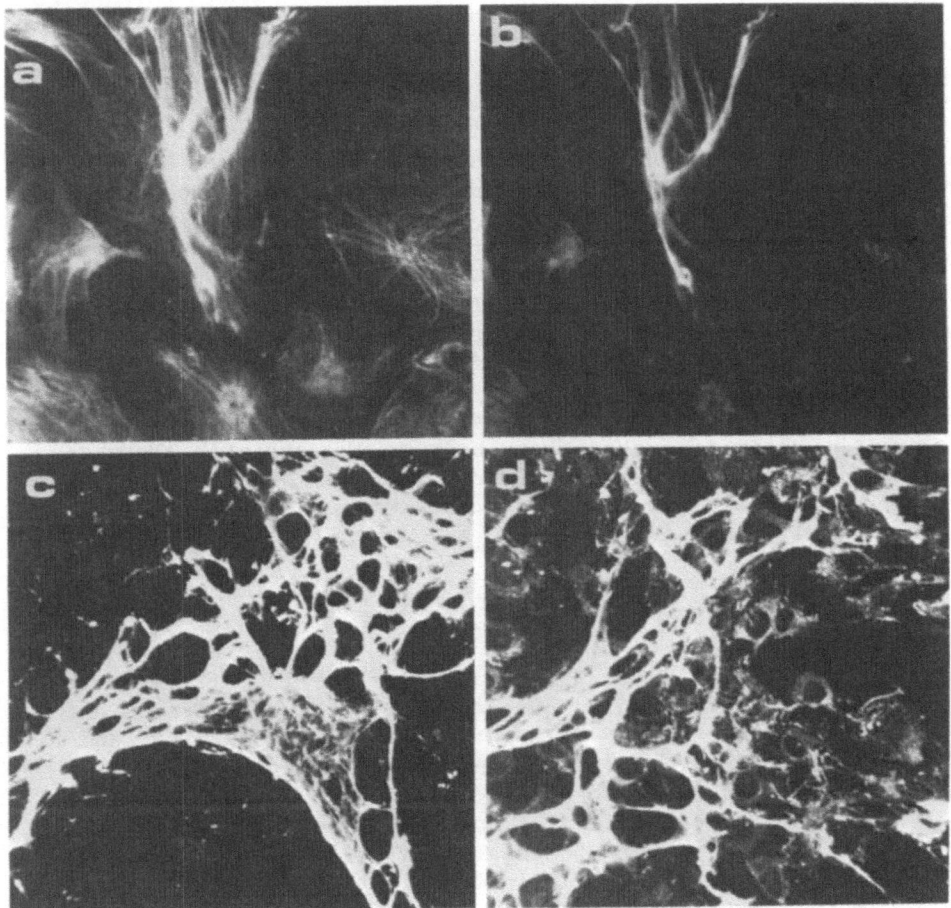

Fig. 3. Immunofluorescence localization of various components
expressed by mesenchymal cells induced for 24 h and subcultured as
monolayers.
a and b. Double staining with antibodies against vimentin (a) and
cytokeratin (b). Note partial codistribution in these cells
subcultured for 5 days.
c and d. Immunofluorescence stainings demonstrating fibronectin (c)
and laminin (d) in cells subcultured for 3 and 5 days, respectively.

that the committed cells still express mesenchymal features like
deposition of fibronectin and synthesis of vimentin-type intermediate
filaments. When the induced cells are subcultured as monolayers,
this initial phenotype is gradually converted into an epithelial type

characterized by deposition of laminin and formation of cytokeratin-type filaments (Fig. 3). While differentiation at the cellular level has been triggered and expressed in these conditions, the phenotypically altered cells show no polarization, nor do they become assembled into any recognizable histiotypic structures. Both these features are obtained, when the induced mesenchymes are allowed to develop in a three-dimensional organotypic culture where the cells adhere to the newly-formed basement membrane, become polarized and ultimately assemble into tubular structures (Saxén and Wartiovaara, 1966). Yet, the resulting "tissue" consisting of several differentiated cell types remains disorganized with abnormally shaped tubuli and with avascular glomerular bodies, even when endothelial cells are introduced in the CAM-grafts. For the spatially and temporally regulated development of the different cell lineages, the invading and orderly branching ureteric inductor is decisive. While inducing the chain of events that leads to the strictly organized nephron formation, the ureter also creates the conditions and clues for the endothelial cell migration that completes the formation of the functional glomeruli.

## References

Bernfield, M. R., 1981, Organization and remodeling of the extracellular matrix in morphogenesis, in: "Morphogenesis and Pattern Formation", T. G. Connelly, L. L. Brinkley, and B. M. Carlson, eds., p. 139, Raven Press, New York.

Bonadio, J. F., Sage, H., Cheng, F., Bernstein, J., and Striker, G. E., 1984, Localization of collagen types IV and V, laminin and heparan sulfate proteoglycan to the basal lamina of kidney epithelial cells in transfilter metanephric culture, Am. J. Pathol., 116:289.

Grobstein, C., 1955, Inductive interaction in the development of the mouse metanephros, J. Exp. Zool, 130:319.

Grobstein, C., 1956, Trans-filter induction of tubules in mouse metanephrogenic mesenchyme, Exp. Cell Res., 10:424.

Grobstein, C., 1967, Mechanisms of organogenetic tissue interactions, Nat. Cancer Inst. Monogr., 26:279.

Ekblom, P., Thesleff, I., Saxén, L., Miettinen, A., and Timpl, R., 1983, Transferrin as a growth factor for embryogenesis: acquisition of responsiveness related to embryonic induction, Proc. Natl. Acad. Sci. USA, 80:2651.

Ekblom, P., Sariola, H., and Thesleff, I., 1985, Basement membrane and organogenesis, in: Developmental Mechanisms. Normal and Abnormal, J. W. Lash, and L. Saxén, eds., Alan R. Liss, New York, in press.

Ekblom, P., Lehtonen, E., Saxén, L., and Timpl, R., 1981, Shift in collagen type as an early response to induction of the metanephric mesenchyme, J. Cell Biol., 89:276.

Lash, J., Saxén, L., and Ekblom, P., 1983, Biosynthesis of proteo-
    glycans in organ cultures of developing kidney mesenchyme,
    Exp. Cell Res., 147:85.
Lehtonen, E., 1976, Transmission of signals in embryonic induction,
    Med. Biol., 54:108.
Lehtonen, E., and Saxén, L., 1985, Control of differentiation, in:
    Human Growth: A Comprehensive Treatise, F. Falkner and J. M.
    Tanner, eds., Plenum Press, New York, in press.
Lehtonen, E., Jalanko, H., Laitinen, L., Miettinen, A., Ekblom, P.,
    and Saxén, L., 1983, Differentiation of metanephric tubules
    following a short transfilter induction pulse, Roux' Arch.
    Dev. Biol., 192:145.
Lehtonen, E., Virtanen, I., and Saxén, L., 1985, Reorganization of
    intermediate filament cytoskeleton in induced metanephric
    mesenchyme cells is independent of tubule morphogenesis, Dev.
    Biol., in press.
Potter, E. L., 1965, Development of the human glomerulus, Arch.
    Path., 80:241.
Sariola, H., Ekblom, P., Lehtonen, E., and Saxén, L., 1983,
    Differentiation and vascularization of the metanephric kidney
    grafted on the chorioallantoic membrane, Dev. Biol., 96:427.
Sariola, H., Timpl, R., von der Mark, K., Mayne, R., Fitch, J. M.,
    Linsenmayer, T. F., and Ekblom, P., 1984a, Dual origin of
    glomerular basement membrane, Dev. Biol, 101:86.
Sariola, H., Peault, B., LeDouarin, N., Buck, C., Dietèrlen, F., and
    Saxén, L., 1984b, Extracellular matrix and capillary ingrowth
    in interspecies chimaeric kidneys, Cell Differ., 15:43.
Saxén, L., 1970, Failure to demonstrate tubule induction in a
    heterologous mesenchyme, Dev. Biol., 23:511.
Saxén, L., and Karkinen-Jääskeläinen, M., 1975, Inductive inter-
    actions in morphogenesis, in: Early Development of Mammals,
    M. Balls, and A. Wild, eds., p. 319, Cambridge Univ. Press.,
    Cambridge.
Saxén, L., and Lehtonen, E., 1978, Transfilter induction of kidney
    tubules as a function of the extent and duration of inter-
    cellular contacts, J. Embryol. exp. Morphol., 47:97.
Saxén, L., and Wartiovaara, J., 1966, Cell contact and cell adhesion
    during tissue organization, Int. J. Cancer, 1:271.
Saxén, L., Lehtonen, E., Karkinen-Jääskeläinen, M., Nordling, S., and
    Wartiovaara, J., 1976, Are morphogenetic tissue interactions
    mediated by transmissible signal substances or through cell
    contacts? Nature, 259:662.
Saxén, L., Salonen, J., Ekblom, P., and Nordling, S., 1983, DNA
    synthesis and cell generation cycle during determination and
    differentiation of the metanephric mesenchyme, Dev. Biol.,
    98:130.
Thiery, J. P., Duband, J. L., and Delouvée, A., 1982a, Pathways and
    mechanisms of avian trunk neural crest cell migration and
    localization, Dev. Biol., 93:324.

Thiery, J. P., Duband, J. L., Rutishauser, U., and Edelman, G. M.,
      1982b, Cell adhesion molecules in early chicken embryogenesis,
      Proc. Natl. Acad. Sci. USA, 79:6737.
Wartiovaara, J., Nordling, S., Lehtonen, E., and Saxén, L., 1974,
      Transfilter induction of kidney tubules: correlation with
      cytoplasmic penetration into Nuclepore filters, J. Embryol.
      exp. Morphol., 31:667.

## INTRODUCTION

The increasingly complex repertoire of differentiated cell types found in higher organisms, and the capacity for flexible response to different developmental and physiological requirements, both lean upon the provision of families of molecules with similar but not identical properties. This is achieved by the evolution of gene families following a continuous process of duplication and divergence, so that a study of the evolution of proteins is essential for understanding the evolution of differentiation. We are forced to consider two different problems in thinking about this phenomenon: one is the evolutionary relationships of the structural proteins and the way in which the range of molecular properties which have become available are related to the developmental characteristics which have evolved. The second problem concerns the evolutionary changes in the regulation of these related genes since, by definition, we could not expect that they should all be transcribed simultaneously and in equal amounts. (Dayhoff, 1972; Niall, 1982; Li, 1983; Jeffreys et al., 1983).

In addition to the duplication and divergence of entire structural genes and their regulatory sequences, there are other ways of engendering diversity of proteins, such as exon shuffling (Gilbert, 1978), which must require prior duplication but which will give products with new properties overall, and methods of engendering different but related proteins from one gene, such as alternative initiation points for transcription, or alternative splicing of primary transcripts (Young et al., 1981; Rosenfeld et al., 1983): and finally the formation of alternative products by post-translational modification, such as differential scission, as in the production of ACTH and MSH, (Herbert and Uhler, 1982).

Regulation of the new products must be of several kinds to allow for the appearance of a greater diversity of differentiated cell types. These will include tissue-specific expression, expression at specific times during ontogeny and the regulation of the quantity of the product expressed. If much of cell differentiation is combinatorial and quantitative (for example Markert and Ursprung, 1962;

279

Clayton et al., 1968; Parish et al., 1981; Janeway et al., 1984;
Wilcox and Leptin, 1985; Goodman et al., 1984), then the combination
of these three variables will be sufficient to permit a range of
different cell types whose specificity does not necessarily depend on
the exclusive possession of one gene product.


REFERENCES

Clayton, R.M., Campbell, J.C. and Truman, D.E.S., 1968, A re-examina-
    tion of the organ specificity of lens antigens, Exp. Eye Res.,
    7:11.
Dayhoff, M.O., 1972, Atlas of protein sequence and structure, vol. 5,
    Natl. Biomed. Res. Found. Silver Spring, Md.
Gilbert, W., 1978, Why genes in pieces? Nature, 271:501
Goodman, C.S., Bastiani, M.J., Doe, C.G., du Lac, S., Halfand, S.L.,
    Kuwada, J.Y., and Thomas, J.B., 1984, Cell recognition during
    neuronal development, Science, 225:1271
Herbert, E. and Uhler, M., 1982, Biosynthesis of polyprotein
    precursors to regulatory peptides, Cell, 30:1
Jeffreys, A.J., Harris, S., Barrie, P.A., Wood, D., Blanchetot, A.,
    and Adams, S.M., 1983, in, Evolution From Molecules to Men,
    D.S. Bendall, ed., p.175, Cambridge University Press,
    Cambridge.
Janeway, C.A., Bottomley, K., Babich, J., Conrad, P., Lonzen, S.,
    Jones, B., Kaye, J., Katz, M., McVay, L., Murphy, D.B. and Tite,
    J., 1984, Quantitative variation in 1a antigen expression plays
    a central role in immune regulation, Immunology Today, 5:99.
Li, W-H., 1983, Evolution of duplicate genes and pseudogenes, in,
    Evolution of Genes and Proteins, M. Nei and R.K. Koehn, eds.,
    p.14, Sinamer Associates, Sunderland, Mass.
Markert, C.L. and Ursprung, H., 1962, The ontogeny of isozyme patterns
    of lactate dehydrogenase in the mouse, Dev. Biol., 5:363
Niall, H.D., 1982, The evolution of peptide hormones, Ann. Rev.
    Physiol., 44:615
Parish, C.R., Sia, D.Y. and Rylatt, D.B., 1981, Presence of receptors
    for self MHC antigens on non-T cells, Immunology Today, 2:172
Rosenfeld, M.G., Mermod, J-J, Amara, S.J., Swanson, L.W., Sawchenko,
    P.E., Rivier, J., Vale, W.W.J., and Evans, R.M., 1983, Production
    of a novel neuropeptide encoded by the calcitonin gene via tissue
    -specific RNA processing, Nature, 304:129.
Wilcox, M. and Leptin, M., 1985, Tissue-specific modulation of a
    series of related cell surface antigens in Drosophila, Nature,
    316:351
Young, R.A., Hagenbuchle, O. and Schibler, U., 1981, A single mouse α-
    amylase gene specifies two different tissue specific mRNAs, Cell,
    23:451.

# CRYSTALLINS: THE FAMILIES OF EYE LENS PROTEINS

W.W. de Jong

Department of Biochemistry
University of Nijmegen
P.O. Box 1901
6500 HB Nijmegen
The Netherlands

## GENERAL CHARACTERISTICS OF THE LENS AND ITS PROTEINS

The transparent vertebrate lens is a unique organ, compared only of elongated fibre cells and an anterior layer of epithelial cells, enclosed in a collagenous capsule. It is entirely devoid of blood vessels and innervation, and obtains all nutrients from the perifusing aqueous humor. In the process of differentiation the elongating fibre cells loose their nuclei and most organelles. The lens continues to grow throughout life, albeit at a very low rate in the adult. The fibre cells are never broken down or replaced. As a consequence the core, or nucleus, of the adult lens consists of the oldest cells, stemming from embryonic and foetal stages, while towards the periphery, or cortex, the cells become gradually younger.

The lens cells are characterised by a very high protein concentration, ranging from 20% in the relatively soft avian lenses to 50% in the very hard nuclei of fish lenses. The high protein concentration is necessary to give the required refractive power of the lens. From cortex to nucleus the protein concentration increases, which provides the proper refractive index gradient for the incident light. Changes in the aggregation state of the lens proteins and their interaction with the plasma membrane are responsible for the development of lens opacity, or cataract.

Up to 90% of the soluble protein in the lens is made up by the different types of crystallins. The crystallins can be considered as lens specific proteins, although some of them also occur in detectable amounts in other ocular tissues, and in the pineal gland and

281

adenohypophysis. The crystallins can best be described as water-soluble structural proteins, which by virtue of their dense and ordered packing in the fibre cells maintain the lens transparency. They are, as far as known, devoid of specific biological activities.

Four major types of crystallins have classically been distinguished on the basis of charge, size and immunological properties. The $\alpha$- and $\beta$-crystallins occur in all vertebrate classes, while $\delta$--crystallin is limited to reptilian and avian lenses, which in turn lack the $\gamma$-crystallins present in other vertebrates. Recent sequence studies have shown that $\beta$- and $\gamma$-crystallins are related (Diressen et al., 1981). It is becoming clear that there are additional unrelated crystallins in certain vertebrate groups. These more or less abundant crystallins are now beginning to become characterized.

Comparative studies have shown that the crystallins collectively are rather slowly evolving proteins, changing at rates between 3 and 10 amino acid replacements per 100 residues per 100 million years. At the time of evolutionary origin of the eye lens in the ancestral vertebrate lineage, more than 450 million years ago, the primordial crystallin genes must have been recruited from pre-existing suitable DNA sequences. There recently have been some surprising observations of structural similarities between crystallins and other proteins. Convincing sequence similarity exists between the C- terminal 80 to 100 residues of the $\alpha$-crystallin chains and the small heat shock proteins of Drosophila, the nematode Caenorhabditis and soy bean (Ingolia and Craig, 1982; Wistow, 1985). This clearly reflects an intriguing evolutionary relationship. The $\beta$- and $\gamma$-crystallins have considerable structural similarities with protein S. a spore surface coat-protein of the bacterium Myxococcus xanthus, (Wistow et al., 1985). Their sequences also show partial similarities with the human c-myc oncogene protein (Crabbe, 1985).

The pattern of crystallin synthesis changes considerably during development of the lens. Also between species there are enormous differences in the types and ratios of crystallin chains which are synthesized. These and other properties make the crystallins attractive objects for comparative studies of gene expression and regulation.

Several reviews dealing with the above mentioned aspects of the molecular biology of the lens and the crystallins can be found in Bloemendal (1981). Much of the following concise information about the crystallin proteins and genes can be found in more detail and will full references in the recent reviews by Harding and Crabbe (1984; lens proteins), Summers et al. (1984; tertiary structures), Piatigorsky (1984; $\delta$-crystallin), Schoenmakers et al. (1984; crystallin genes), and Piatigorsky et al. (1984a; crystallin genes).

α-CRYSTALLINS

The largest and most acidic lens protein is α-crystallin (for reviews see Bloemendal, 1981).  It occurs in almost all investigated vertebrates, at levels of up to 40% of total lens protein.  It forms aggregates of an average Mr of 800,000 in calf and 600,000 in chicken. α-crystallin is composed of two types of primary gene products, αA and αB, which are 173 and 175 residues long, respectively.  These chains have an amino acid sequence homology of 57%, reflecting their ancient origin from a common ancestral gene.  The ratio of αA and αB differs considerably from species to species, and changes also during the differentiation of lens epithelial to fibre cells.  Both αA and αB chains undergo extensive modifications during ageing, including deamidation, racemization, non-enzymatic glycation and C-terminal degradation.  Some relevant properties of α-crystallin and the other crystallins are compared in Table 1.

The structures and sequences of the genes coding for murine and hamster αA (Piatigorsky et al., 1984a; van den Heuvel et al., 1985) and αB (Quax-Jeuken et al., 1985a) are now known (Fig. 1).  They have the same pattern of introns and exons, although in the rodent αA gene a small optional exon is present in the first intron, which only is expressed in approximately 10% of the αA chains.  This is due to alternative splicing of the primary gene transcript, which leaves this exon, coding for a 23 amino acid insert peptide, in 10% of the mature mRNA (Piatigorsky et al., 1984a).  The alternative splicing may probably be attributed to the presence of the sequence AGGC at the donor splice site junction of the insert exon, instead of the consensus AGGT.  The elongated αA chain, resulting from the alternative splicing and called αA$^{Ins}$, has not been found in other animals than rat, mouse, hamster and gerbil.

The region of homology with the small heat shock proteins is confined to the last two exons of αA and αB, indicating that the ancestral α-crystallin gene has originated by exon shuffling, combining the 3' part of a heat shock gene with some unrelated 5' exon.

Both αA and αB seem to be single-copy genes in the investigated mammals (Piatigorsky et al., 1984a); Quax-Jeuken et al., 1985a). Chromosome mapping has revealed that the α-crystallin genes are not linked on the same chromosome.  The αA gene is located on human chromosome 21, and the αB gene presumably on chromosome 16 (Quax-Jeuken et al., 1985a).

In mammals the αA mRNA has a very long 3' untranslated region, of approximately 520 nucleotides, which has a high rate of evolutionary change.  There is already 20% sequence difference between the 3' untranslated regions of the mouse and hamster αA mRNA's (van den Heuvel et al., 1985), while the corresponding region of the frog αA

Table I

| | α | β | γ | δ | ε | ρ | τ |
|---|---|---|---|---|---|---|---|
| Mol. form | 30-50-mer | di-octamer | monomer | tetramer | trimer | oligomer | monomer |
| Subunit $M_r$ | 20 kDa | 23-35 kDa | 20 kDa | 48-50 kDa | 38 kDa | 35 kDa | 46-48 kDa |
| Isoelectric point | 4.8 - 5.0 | 5.7 - 7.0 | 7.1 - 8.1 | 4.9 - 5.3 | 7.5 | 8.5 | 7 - 8 |
| Sec. structure α-helix β-sheet | very low 25% | none high | none high | 30-75% 25% | 30% 23% | - - | 52% - |
| Occurrence | all vertebrates | all vertebrates | not in birds and reptiles | all birds and reptiles | some birds and reptiles | frogs | lampreys, some fishes, birds and reptiles |
| Number of gene products | 2 | ±7 | 6 | 2? | 1 | 1 | 1 |
| Synthesis during development | increase with age | increase with age | decrease after birth | mainly embryonic | late in development | - | all lens layers |

This table is composed from data in Harding and Crabbe (1984), Piatigorsky (1984; δ-crystallin), Stapel et al. (1985; ε-crystallin), Tomarev et al. (1984b; ρ-crystallin), Williams et al. (1982; τ-crystallin) and Stapel and de Jong (1983; τ-crystallin). The designations ρ- and τ-crystallin are from G.G. Gause jr and J. Piatigorsky, respectively (personal communications).

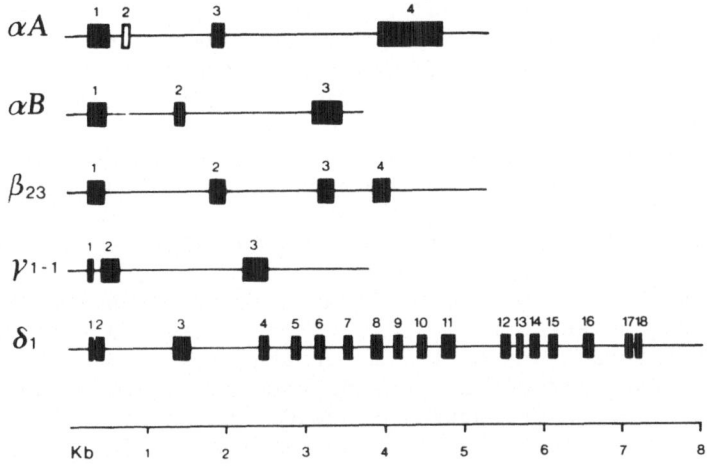

Fig. 1 Comparison of the gene structures of the crystallins. Exons are indicated by numbered boxes. The open box in the αA gene represents the exon which, by alternative splicing, codes for the insertion peptide in the rodent, αA$^{Ins}$ chain. The βB1a gene of the rat (Schoenmakers et al., 1984) differs from mouse β- 23 by the presence of a small intron in exactly the same position as the intron between exons 1 and 2 in the γ-genes (modified from Piatigorsky et al., 1984a; Y. Quax-Jeuken, 1985, Thesis, University of Nijmegen).

mRNA, which is only 130 nucleotides long, shows no detectable sequence similarity, (Tomarev et al., 1983). In remarkable contrast the 3' noncoding regions of bovine and hamster αB mRNA's are highly conserved, having less than 10% sequence difference over their length of 140 nucleotides (Quax-Jeuken et al., 1985a).

THE βγ-CRYSTALLIN SUPERFAMILY

While γ-crystallins are monomeric, basic lens proteins, the β-crystallins form dimers to octamers with somewhat lower isoelectric points (Table 1). The investigated mammalian and avian species each have at least six different β-chains, and a similar number of γ-chains. Both β- and γ-crystallins are coded by a family of duplicated genes. The γ-genes are still closely linked on a single chromosome (Schoenmakers et al., 1984), while the β-genes apparently occur dispersed in the genome (Piatigorsky et al., 1984a).

Amino acid sequence analyses revealed an unexpected homology of approximately 29% between the β- and γ-crystallins (Driessen et al., 1981). Their sequences moreover show a considerable homology between the N- and C- terminal halves, due to an ancient complete intragenic

duplication event.  This internal sequence duplication corresponds
with the two symmetrical structural domains revealed by X-ray
diffraction studies of bovine  II-crystallin (Summers et al., 1984).
Each domain again is folded into two similar "Greek key" motifs.
Model building of the other known β- and γ- crystallin sequences, by
interactive computer graphics methods, has shown that they all have
very similar tertiary structures (Summers et al., 1984).

The β-crystallins differ from the γ-crystallins by the presence
of N-terminal sequences which extend from the compact two-domain
structures (Berbers et al., 1984a; Summers et al., 1984).  These
extensions range in length from 12 to 58 residues, and are supposed to
be involved in interactions of the β- crystallins with each other and
with other cellular components.  The deduced amino acid sequence of
murine β23 has a very hydrophobic 13-residue extension, which
resembles a membrane anchor peptide (Inana et al., 1983).  The bovine
βB1a-crystallin has a very long extension of 58 residues, with a
remarkable 7-fold repeat of Pro-Ala, due to a simple C-C-C-G-C-C
repeat in the DNA (Quax-Jeuken et al., 1984).  The N-terminal
extensions of three different bovine β-crystallin subunits are, among
the soluble lens proteins, the only substrates for transglutaminase,
an endogenous lens enzyme responsible for the formation of isopeptide
linkages between polypeptides (Berbers et al., 1984b).

Whereas the domain sequences of all β-crystallins are well
conserved, the N-terminal extension sequences are extremely variable,
both within and between species (Berbers et al., 1984a; Piatigorsky et
al., 1984b).  This may be related to the fact that these extensions,
at least in rat βB1a (Schoenmakers et al., 1984), are encoded by a
separate exon.

The six γ-crystallin chains of the rat show between 80 and 98%
sequence homology (Schoenmakers et al., 1984), and similar values are
observed for four murine γ-crystallins (80-90%) (Breitman et al.,
1984).  The two completely known frog γ-sequences have 65% homology
(Tomarev et al., 1984a).  The β-crystallins show more intraspecies
sequence differences.  There is between 40 and 60% sequence similarity
between seven bovine β-crystallin subunits (Berbers et al., 1984a).
Two of the bovine β-crystallins are identical, apart from the presence
of 17 additional N-terminal residues in one of them.  It appears that
these chains are translated from the same mRNA by using two different
start codons (Gorin and Horwitz, 1984; Quax-Jeuken et al., 1984).

A rather isolated member of the βγ-superfamily is the so-called
$\beta_s$-crystallin, which has been best characterised in the bovine lens.
The sequence of this monomeric protein resembles the γ-crystallins
more than the β-crystallins (approximately 50% and 35% homology,
respectively;  Quax-Jeuken et al., 1985b).  Its very short N-
terminal extension, and its γ-like distribution of surface charges
probably explain the monomeric nature of $\beta_s$.

The structures of a number of rat and murine β- and γ-crystallin genes have been determined (Schoenmakers et al., 1984; Piatigorsky et al., 1984a).  In the γ-crystallins each structural domain is encoded by a separate exon, while a small intron places the codons for the three N-terminal residues apart in the first exon (Fig. 1).  In the β-crystallin genes there are two additional introns, corresponding in position with the boundaries between the two Greek key motifs in each domain.  This difference in exon structure may indicate that the ancestral β- and γ-genes diverged at the two-motif stage.

## δ-CRYSTALLIN

Native δ-crystallin has a molecular weight near 200,000 and is composed of four extremely similar subunits.  These δ-crystallin polypeptides range in size between 48 kDa and 50 kDa, and also display charge heterogeneity.  δ-Crystallins have a high α-helical content, even up to 80%, in contrast to α-, β- and γ-crystallins.  It has a blocked N-terminus (Yasuda et al., 1984), a low level of aromatic residues and almost no cysteines.  The leucine contents amounts to 11 -15% of the residues in the protein, which probably is related to its α-helical conformation.  δ-Crystallin is remarkably resistant to denaturation by urea and guanidine hydrochloride.

A minor part of the δ-crystallin in the chicken lens seems to be associated with the plasma membranes, as has also been observed for α-crystallin in mammalian lens cells.  Crystals of δ-crystallin have been obtained for future determination of its three-dimensional structure by X-ray analysis (Narebor et al., 1980).

The complete amino acid sequence of a chicken δ-crystallin polypeptide has been derived from the cDNA sequence (Piatigorsky, 1984; Yasuda et al., 1984).  It shows no internal duplications, nor any similarity with other crystallin sequences.

In the chicken there are at least two closely linked δ-crystallin genes.  Both genes, which are arranged head to tail, are highly interrupted with 13-15 introns.  It appears that both in vivo and in vitro one of the δ-crystallin genes is preferentially expressed (Kondoh et al., 1983).  Low levels of δ-crystallin RNA-sequences are present in other tissues than the lens (Clayton, 1982; Bower et al., 1983).

## THE NOVEL CRYSTALLINS:  EPSILON, RHO AND TAU

In the lenses of the most commonly studied species, like calf, rat, human, rabbit and chicken, the soluble proteins seem to be composed almost exclusively of the well-known α-, β-, γ- and δ-crystallins.  In other species, especially in the non-mammalian vertebrates, there are in many cases additional crystallin components present.  Some of these crystallins have recently been partially characterized.

In a number of avian and reptilian species a lens protein is present with a native molecular weight of 120,000, composed of three identical subunits of 38 kDa (Stapel et al., 1985).  This protein, designated as ε-crystallin, comprises approximately 10% of the soluble protein in duck lenses, but is absent in chicken.  Like δ-crystallin, it has a relatively high α-helical content.  No immunological cross-reactivity was found with any of the other crystallins, and partial amino acid sequence determinations likewise failed to reveal any similarities.  ε-crystallin is the latest lens protein to appear during development of the duck lens (Brahma and van der Starre, 1983).

In lamprey lens extract there is a polypeptide which, on SDS-gel electrophoresis, migrates in the position of δ-crystallin.  There has been a claim, on the basis of immunological cross- reactivity, that in the river lamprey this protein would indeed be related to chicken δ-crystallin (de Pomerai et al., 1984).  On the other hand Stapel and de Jong (1983) have characterized this 48 kDa protein from the sea lamprey, Petromyzon marinus, and showed by partial sequence analysis and immunological studies that it represents a novel and unrelated family of crystallins.  It turned out to cross-react with a previously described turtle lens protein (Williams et al., 1982), for which the name τ-crystallin (tau for turtle) has been proposed (J. Piatigorsky, personal communication).  By immunoblotting it has been demonstrated that τ-crystallin occurs also in several other reptilian, avian and fish species (Stapel and de Jong, 1983).

An oligomeric protein with a molecular weight of about 200,000 is present in lens extracts of the frog genus Rana.  It is composed of polypeptides of Mr 35 kDa, for which a partial cDNA sequence has been determined (Tomarev et al., 1984b).  About 3/4 of the amino acid sequence has been deduced, which shows no homology with other crystallins.  This protein will be designated as ρ-crystallin (rho for Rana) (G.G. Gause jr, personal communication).  According to the secondary structure prediction this protein is predominantly in the β-strand configuration, and has only few α-helical regions.

A further characterization of these newly discovered crystallins, and a continued search for additional ones, is of interest because it will extend our insight in the functional and structural requirements imposed upon the crystallins in general.

REFERENCES

Berbers, G.A.M., Hoekman, W.A., Bloemendal, H., de Jong, W.W.,
    Kleinschmidt, T., and Braunitzer, G., 1984a, Homology between the

primary structures of the major bovine β-crystallin chains,
     Eur. J. Biochem., 139:467
Berbers, G.A.M., Feenstra, R.W., van den Bos, R., Hoekman, W.A.,
     Bloemendal, H., and de Jong, W.W., 1984b, Lens transglutaminase
     selects specific β-crystallin sequences as substrate, Proc. Natl.
     Acad. Sci. USA, 81:7017
Bloemendal, H., (ed.), 1981, "Molecular and Cellular Biology of the
     Eye Lens," Wiley, New York.
Bower, D.J., Errington, L.H., Pollock, B.J., Morris, S., and Clayton,
     R.M., 1983, The pattern of expression of chick δ-crystallin genes
     in lens differentiation and transdifferentiating cultured
     tissues, EMBO J., 2:333                                    .
Brahma, S.K. and van der Starre, H., 1983, Ontogeny and localisation
     of the α-, β- and δ-crystallin antigens during lens development
     in Mallard ducks, Curr. Eye Res., 2:663
Breitman, M.L., Lok, S., Wistow, G., Piatigorsky, J., Treton, J.A.,
     Gold, R.J.M., and Tsui, L.-C., 1984, γ-crystallin family of the
     mouse lens: structural and evolutionary relationships. Proc.
     Natl. Acad. Sci. USA, 81:7762
Clayton, R.M., 1982, Cellular and molecular aspects of differentiation
     and transdifferentiation of ocular tissues in vitro, in "Differ-
     entiation in Vitro," British Society for Cell Biology Symposium
     4, Yeoman, M.M. and Truman, D.E.S., eds., p83, University
     Press, Cambridge.
Crabbe, M.J.C., 1985, Partial sequence homology of human myc oncogene
     protein to beta and gamma crystallins. FEBS Lett., 181:157
de Pomerai, D.I., Ellis, D.K. and Carr, A., 1984, A lamprey lens
     protein related to avian and reptilian crystallins, Curr.Eye
     Res., 3:729
Driessen, H.P.C., Herbrink, P., Bloemendal, H. and de Jong, W.W.,
     1981, Primary structure of the bovine β-crystallin Bp chain.
     Internal duplication and homology with γ-crystallin. Eur. J.
     Biochem., 121:83
Gorin, M.B., and Horwitz, J., 1984, Cloning and characterization of a
     cow β-crystallin cDNA, Curr. Eye Res., 3:939
Harding, J.J. and Crabbe, M.J.C., 1984, The Lens: development,
     proteins, metabolism and cataract, in "The Eye", Davson, H., ed.,
     p207, Academic Press, New York, 3rd Edition.
Inana, G., Piatigorsky, J., Norman, B., Slingsby, C. and Blundell, T.,
     1983, Gene and protein structure of a β-crystallin polypeptide in
     mutine lens: relationship of exons and structural motifs, Nature,
     302:310
Ingolia, T.D. and Craig, E.A., 1982, Four small Drosophila heat shock
     proteins are related to each other and to mammalian α-crystallin,
     Proc. Natl. Acad. Sci. USA, 79:2360
Kondoh, H., Yasuda, K. and Okada, T.S., 1983, Tissue-specific
     expression of a cloned chick δ-crystallin gene in mouse cells,
     Nature, 301:440
Narebor, E., Slingsby, C., Lindley, P.F. and Blundell, T., 1980,
     Preliminary x-ray crystallographic study of the Turkey lens

protein, δ-crystallin, J. Mol. Biol., 143:223

Piatigorsky, J., 1984, Crystallins and their nucleic acids, Molec. Cell. Biochem., 59:33

Piatigorsky, J., Chepelinsky, A.B., Hejtmancik, J.F., Borras, T., Das, G.C., Hawkins, J.W., Zelenka, P.S., King, C.R., Beebe, D.C. and Nickerson, J.M., 1984, Expression of crystallin gene families in the differentiating eye lens, in, "Molecular Biology of Development," p331, Alan R. Liss, Inc.

Piatigorsky, J., Nickerson, J.M., King, C.R., Inana, G., Hejtmancik, J.F., Hawkins, J.W., Borras, T., Shinohara, T., Wistow, G. and Norman, B., 1984, Crystallin genes: templates for lens transparency in: "Human Cataract Formation," p191, Pitman, London.

Quax-Jeuken, Y., Janssen, C., Quax, W., van den Heuvel, R. and Bloemendal, H., 1984, Bovine β-crystallin complementary DNA clones. Alternating proline/alanine sequence of B1 subunit originates from a repetitive DNA sequence, J.Mol. Biol., 180: 457

Quax-Jeuken, Y., Quax, W., van Rens, G., Meera Khan, P. and Bloemendal, H., 1985a, Complete structure of the αB-crystallin gene: conservation of the exon/intron distribution of the two non-linked α-crystallin genes, Proc. Natl. Acad. Sci. USA, 82: 5819

Quax-Jeuken, Y., Driessen, H., Leunissen, J., Quax, W., de Jong, W.W. and Bloemendal, H., 1985b, βs-crystallin: structure and evolution of a distinct member of the βγ-superfamily, EMBO Journal, 4:2597

Schoenmakers, J.G.G., den Dunnen, J.T., Moorman, R.J.M., Jongbloed, R., van Leen, R.W. and Lubsen, N.H., 1984, The crystallin gene families, in: "Human Cataract Formation", p208, Pitman, London.

Stapel, S.O. and de Jong, W.W., 1983, Lamprey 48-KDa lens protein represents a novel class of crystallins, FEBS Lett., 162:305

Stapel, S.O., Zweers, A., Dodemont, H.J., Kan, J.H. and de Jong, W.W., 1985, Epsilon crystallin. A novel avian and reptilian eye lens protein. Eur. J. Biochem., 147:129

Summers, L., Wistow, G., Narebor, M., Moss, D., Lindley, P., Slingsby, C., Blundell, T., Bartunik, H. and Bartels, K., 1984 X-ray studies of the lens specific proteins: the crystallins, in: "Peptide and Protein Reviews," vol. 3, pp147-168, Marcel Dekker, New York.

Tomarev, S.I., Zinovieva, R.D., Dolgilevich, S.M., Krayev, A.S., Skryabin, K.G. and Gause, jr, G.G., 1983, The absence of the long 3'-non-translated region in mRNA coding for eye lens αA2-crystallin of the frog (Rana temporaria), FEBS Lett., 162:47

Tomarev, S.I., Zinovieva, R.D., Chalovka, P., Krayev, A.S., Skryabin, K.G. and Gause jr., G.G., 1984a, Multiple genes coding for the frog eye lens γ-crystallin, Gene, 27:301

Tomarev, S.I., Zinovieva, R.D., Dolgilevich, S.M., Luchin, S.V., Krayev, A.S., Skryabin, K.G. and Gause jr, G.G., 1984b, A novel type of crystallin in the frog eye lens. 35-KDa polypeptide is not homologous to any of the major classes of lens crystallins, FEBS Lett., 171:297

van den Heuvel, R., Hendriks, W., Quax, W. and Bloemendal, H., 1985
     Complete sequence of the hamster αA crystallin gene; reflection
     of an evolutionary history by means of exon shuffling, J. Mol.
     Biol., (in press)
Williams, L.A., Piatigorsky, J. and Horwitz, J., 1982, Structural
     features of δ-crystallin of turtle lens, Biochim.Biophys Acta,
     708:49
Wistow, G., 1985, Domain structure and evolution in α-crystallins and
     small heat-shock proteins, FEBS Lett., 181:1
Wistow, G., Summers, L. and Blundell, T., 1985, Evidence for a
     structural relationship between protein S, a development specific
     protein of Myxococcus xanthus, and the βγ-crystallins of the
     vertebrate lens, Nature, in press.
Yasuda, K., Nakajima, N., Isobe, T., Okada, T.S. and Shimura, Y.,
     1984, The nucleotide sequence of a complete chicken δ-crystallin
     cDNA, EMBO J., 3:1397

# IMMUNOLOGICAL ANALYSIS OF δ-CRYSTALLIN EXPRESSED

# IN VARIOUS TISSUES OF THE CHICK IN VIVO AND IN VITRO

Ryuji Kodama and Goro Eguchi

Department of Developmental Biology
National Institute for Basic Biology
Okazaki, 444 Japan

## INTRODUCTION

As δ-crystallin is considered to be a major marker protein for lens cell differentiation in birds, many results have been accumulated on how the gene of δ-crystallin is transcribed and translated during normal embryonic development as well as in in vitro lens cell differentiation. Besides the enormous expression in the lens itself, δ-crystallin gene has long been claimed to be expressed in extralenticular tissues of early embryos (e.g. Clayton et al., 1968). According to recent results, retina, brain and limb bud of the chick embryo contain mRNA of δ-crystallin (Agata et al.,1983), while in adenohypophysis of the early chick embryo, accumulation of the protein is observed (Barabanov, 1977). Through in vitro culture of dissociated cells, many tissues are reported to transdifferentiate and synthesize δ-crystallin, e. g. pigmented retina (Eguchi and Okada, 1973), neural retina (Okada et al. 1975), brain (Takagi et al., 1983), pineal body (Watanabe et al., 1985), and limb bud (Kodama and Eguchi, 1982)

The relationship between the synthesis of δ-crystallin and the lens cell differentiation has become obscure because in some of the above examples (adenohypophysis in situ, cultured brain and limb bud), δ-crystallin is detected in cells without lenticular morphology. However, as minute molecular structure of δ-crystallin is still obscure, there remains a possibility that there is some subclass of δ-crystallin which is specific for normally differentiated lens fibers.

We have reported that an antiserum against feather keratin of the chick crossreacts with δ-crystallin (Kodama and Eguchi, 1983).

293

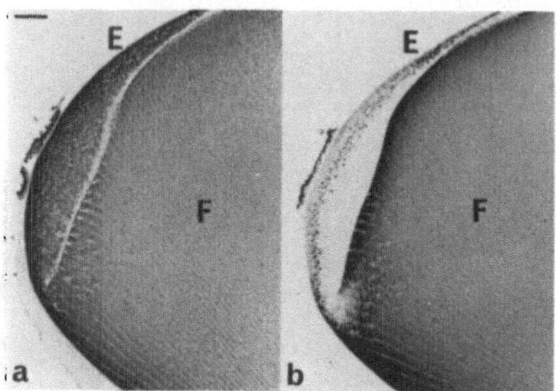

Fig. 1.  Immunohistochemical staining of day-old chick lens with
         anti-δ-crystallin antiserum (a) or anti-feather-keratin
         antiserum (b).  Specimens were fixed with Carnoy's fluid,
         paraffin-sectioned at 7 μm in thickness, and stained by
         PAP method (Kodama and Eguchi, 1983).  Dilution of anti-δ
         antiserum was 1:200, and anti-keratin antiserum 1:10.
         Lens fiber (F) shows positive dark staining in both
         specimens, while in (b) lens epithelium (E) remains
         negative.  Scale bars correspond to 100 μm in all figures.


When cells containing δ-crystallin were immunohistochemically
stained with this antiserum, the strength of staining was different
from tissue to tissue.  Here we report this result of differential
staining with anti-feather-keratin antiserum, and discuss on the
possibility that there exists a molecular subspecies of
δ-crystallin specific for lens fiber structure.


RESULTS

Differential Staining of the Lens Epithelium and the Lens Fiber

    When the paraffin section of the lens of the 4-day-old chick
embryo was immunohistochemically stained with anti-feather-keratin
antiserum, only the lens fiber was stained intensively, while the
lens epithelium was not at all stained (cf. Fig. 5a and 6a of
Kodama and Eguchi, 1983).  As we have shown that this staining is
elicited by the crossreaction of the antiserum with δ-crystallin,
this result contradicts with previous knowledge that δ-crystallin
exists both in the lens epithelium and the lens fiber.

    Lens of day-old chick also showed distinct difference in
staining between the fiber and the epithelium (Fig. 1).  In early
embryos, this staining with anti-feather-keratin antiserum becomes

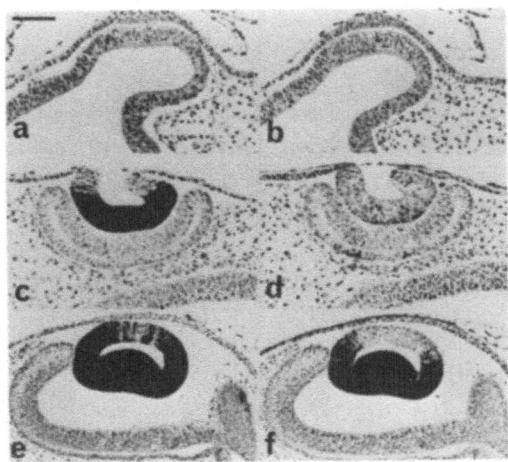

Fig. 2.   Immunohistochemical staining of eye rudiment of early
          chick embryo.  (a,b); stage 14, (c,d); stage 15, (e,f);
          stage 18, according to Hamburger and Hamilton.  (a,c,e);
          stained with anti-δ antiserum, (b,d,f); stained with
          anti-keratin antiserum.  See legend for Fig. 1 for
          details.

distinct when lens fiber formation begins at stage 18 (Fig. 2).
These results seem to show that there is a correlation between lens
fiber structure and the positive staining.

Staining of Extralenticular Cells Containing δ-Crystallin

     We further examined whether extralenticular cells reported to
contain δ-crystallin are stained with anti-feather-keratin antiserum.  Lentoid body, which has an ultrastructure characteristic to
the lens fiber, formed in the culture of neural retina cells were
stained, while the rudiment of adenohypophysis in in situ embryo
and the cultured aggregate of the limb bud cells were not (Fig. 3).

     These results, together with above observation with the lens,
seem to suggest that only those kind of δ-crystallin components
which is contained in the lens fiber or lens-fiber-like structure
(lentoid) can crossreact with anti-feather-keratin antiserum.


DISCUSSION

     By morphological criteria, the extralenticular expression of
δ-crystallin can be classified into two categories; one is accompanied with lens-like structure (lentoids) and the other is not.

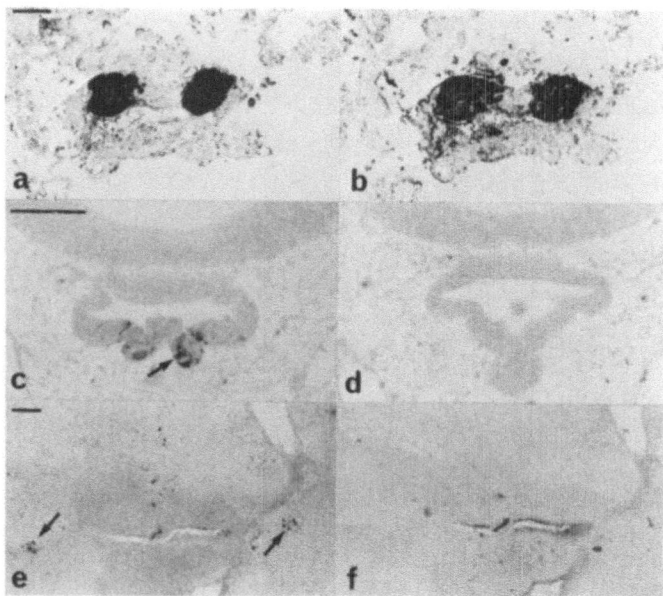

Fig. 3.   Immunohistochemical staining of tissues which show
          extralenticular accumulation of δ-crystallin.  (a,b);
          lentoids formed in the cell culture of neural retina cells
          of 8-day-old chick embryo, (c,d); rudiment of adenohypo-
          physis of 4-day-old chick embryo, (e,f); cultured
          aggregate of the limb bud cells of 4-day-old chick embryo.
          (a,c,e); stained with anti-δ antiserum, (b,d,f); stained
          with anti-keratin antiserum.  Lentoids react with both
          antiserum, while cells containing δ-crystallin without
          lens structure (arrows) react only with anti-δ antiserum.
          See legend for Fig. 1 for details.

The latter includes cultured brain cells, cultured limb bud cells
and the rudiment of adenohypophysis of <u>in situ</u> embryo.  These
examples show that the synthesis of δ-crystallin is not necessarily
accompanied with lens fiber formation and the existence of δ-crystallin alone does not mean lens differentiation.  Above results
suggest that anti-feather-keratin antiserum can be an exact probe
for lens differentiation, as it does not crossreact with δ-crystallin expressed without lens-fiber structure.

     There remains a possibility that the differential staining
shown above indicates the difference of the amount, not the quali-
ty, of δ-crystallin.  To answer this question, minute qualitative
comparison of δ-crystallin from the lens fiber and that from the
lens epithelium or other tissues without lens-fiber structure is

necessary. We have partially purified δ-crystallin from the lens fiber and the lens epithelium, and preliminarily showed that aliquots from both specimens which give the same strength of reaction with anti-δ-crystallin antiserum reacted differently with anti-feather-keratin antiserum, i. e. specimen from the fiber reacted stronger (data not shown).

Results shown above indicates a possibility that we could raise monoclonal antibodies against δ-crystallin which can distinguish the "lens-specific form" of δ-crystallin, which still is speculative.

ACKNOWLEDGEMENT

This work is supported by Grants-in-Aid for Special Project Research (Project Nos. 58119005 and 59113007) to G. E. from the Ministry of Education, Science and Culture.

REFERENCES

Agata, K., Yasuda, K., and Okada, T. S., 1983, Gene coding for a lens-specific protein, δ-crystallin, is transcribed in nonlens tissues of chicken embryos, Develop. Biol., 100:222.

Barabanov, V. M., 1977, Expression of δ-crystallin in the adenohypophysis of chick embryo, Dokl. Akad. Nauk. SSSR, 234:195.

Clayton, R. M., Campbell, J. C., and Truman, D. E. S., 1968, A re-examination of the organ specificity of lens antigens, Exptl. Eye Res., 7:11.

Eguchi, G., and Okada, T. S., 1973, Differentiation of lens tissues from the progeny of chick retinal pigment cells cultured in vitro: a demonstration of a switch of cell types in clonal cell culture, Proc. Natl. Acad. Sci. USA, 70:1495.

Kodama, R., and Eguchi, G., 1982, Dissociated limb bud cells of chick embryos can express lens specificity when reaggregated and cultured in vitro, Develop. Biol., 91:221.

Kodama, R., and Eguchi, G., 1983, Characterization of an antiserum against feather keratins of the chick: its crossreaction with a lens protein, δ-crystallin, Develop., Growth and Differ., 25:261.

Okada, T. S., Itoh, Y., Watanabe, K., and Eguchi, G., 1975, Differentiation of lens in cultures of neural retinal cells of chick embryos, Develop. Biol., 45:318.

Takagi, S., Haruguchi, M., Agata, K., Araki, M., and Okada, T. S., 1983, Expression of lens phenotype by embryonic brain cells in culture, Develop., Growth and Differ., 25:421.

Watanabe, K., Aoyama, H., Tamamaki, N., Yasujima, M., Nojyo, Y., Ueda, Y., and Okada, T. S., 1985, Oculopotency of embryonic quail pineals as revealed by cell culture studies, Cell Differ., 16:251.

# THE EVOLUTION OF CONTROL MECHANISMS IN CELLULAR DIFFERENTIATION

D.E.S. Truman

Department of Genetics
University of Edinburgh
Edinburgh EH9 3JN  U.K.

One can picture the growth of our understanding of biological phenomena as a dialogue between the theory of evolution by natural selection, on the one hand, and the ever growing range of experimental studies of living systems on the other.  Our concepts of evolution are dependent on what we know of present-day living systems, but also our appreciation of such systems can be illuminated by taking an evolutionary perspective of them.  I want to view the control of gene expression during cellular differentiation from the vantage point of biological evolution and to provide a background of geological fact and biological speculation which might help us to appreciate the control mechanisms of contemporary gene expression.

## THE GEOLOGICAL RECORD

Most of us are familiar with the scale of geological time as displayed in many text-books and on the walls of many a lecture theatre.  These tend to emphasise the more recent periods of geological history, partly because of the stress on the evidence of fossils of hard parts of large animals.  If we use a linear scale from the estimated date of the origin of the earth to the present and consider microscopic fossils and geochemical evidence we gain a different perspective (Fig. 1).  The date for the origin of the earth is about $4.65 \times 10^9$ years BP (before present).  We have the nano-fossils found in the chert of the Barberton mountains of South Africa at $3.3 \times 10^9$ years BP, and we have the oldest dated stromatolites, from Bulawayo, representing the fossilized remains of cyanobacteria and indicating flourishing populations of prokaryotes around $3.0 \times 10^9$ years BP.  The interpretation of these micro-fossils is somewhat contentious and there is no certainty about the identification of the

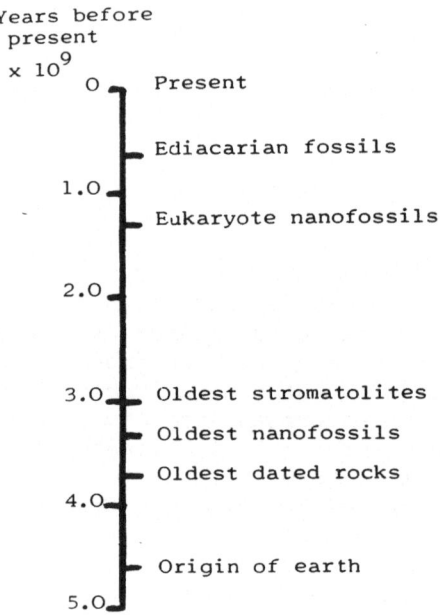

Fig. 1   The Geological Time Scale

first eukaryotes.  A critical introduction to the topic is given by
Ford (1979).  A consensus date for the earliest eukaryotes is about
1.40 x $10^9$ years BP (Schopf and Oehler, 1976).  About 0.7 x $10^9$ years
after this we find the fossils of the period now known as the
Ediacarian, towards the end of the Precambrian.  This comparatively
rich fauna was first discovered in the Ediacara Hills of South
Australia in 1946 and comparable fauna have since been discovered
around the world (Glaessner, 1984).  What we find amongst the
Ediacarian fossils are a wide variety of coelenterates, a range of
segmented organisms with strong resemblances to living annelids, and a
couple of forms that are uncertain, but which might be classified as
arthropods.  If we assume that these forms have a cellular
organisation comparable to living arthropods and annelids then we can
say that by the time of the Ediacarian cellular differentiation had
been established, that muscle cells, nerve cells and a good few more
cell types had evolved.  In a period of 0.7 x $10^9$ years (equal to the
time separating the Ediacarian from ourselves) the earliest eukaryotes
had evolved into metazoa and developed the capacity to regulate
development and to select the expression of genes.  All this occurred
in a span of time over which we have no significant fossil record.
Thus, if we are to have any idea of what happened at that time, we can
the various eukaryotic kingdoms.

obtain it only by studying contemporary organisms.

## DIFFERENTIATION IN THE LOWER INVERTEBRATES.

The phyla found in the Ediacarian fauna represent quite a range of cytological complexity. The bulk of the species are Coelenterates, which at present are moderately diverged from other metazoa in that they have musculo-epithelial cells, rather than specialized muscle cells. The annelids, however, have distinct muscle cells similar to the higher invertebrates and the chodates and represent a higher degree of cytological complexity than the coelenterates. Present day arthropods include some elaborate life forms, notably in the Insecta, but the two species found in the Ediacarian are probably primitive and may not even be true arthropods. Moreover it is not clear that the Arthropoda are monophyletic in origin (Anderson, 1973).

An understanding of the evolution of early metazoa would benefit from some clear ideas of the relationship of the various cell types concerned, and indeed from a clear definition and enumeration of the cell types (Truman, 1982). At present these numbers are very subjective, though some figures have been rather boldly stated, without specific justification, by Stebbins (1982):

| | |
|---|---|
| Coelenterates | 25 different cell types |
| Annelids | 66 |
| Insects | 100-150 |
| Mammals | 250 |

At a conservative estimate we might suppose that by the Edicarian period around 50 different types of cell had been evolved.

It is interesting to note the absence of sponges in the late Precambrian fauna. Though sponge organisation is comparatively simple the sponges do not evidently represent a primitive ancestor of other metazon forms.

## THE COMPARATIVE BIOLOGY OF GENE REGULATION

If we compare the general features of genetic orgainisation that might be associated with differential gene expression, we find much in common amongst all the major groups of living organisms. Of course the structure of DNA is the same in all organisms, and the histones are strongly conserved amongst all eukaryotes (reviewed by McGhee and Felsenfeld, 1980: Igo-Kemenes et al., 1982). Thus the organisation of eukaryotic chromatin was presumably evolved before the divergence of

It has been shown that in many cases in vertebrate species expression of a gene is correlated with modifications of chromatin structure accompanied by sensitivity to digestion by enzymes such as DNAase I (Weintraub and Groudine, 1976; Garel and Axel, 1976; Wood and Felsenfeld, 1982), and that certain specific sites within and around the structural gene may show hypersensitivity to nuclease attack (Wu et al., 1979; Elgin, 1981).  This property of active chromatin has also been found in some invertebrates, such as Drosophila  (Wu, 1980; Shermoen and Bekendorf, 1982) and echinoderms (Bryan et al., 1983), and in the protozoan Tetrahymena (Borchsenius et al., 1981).

Another feature of active chromatin that is widely distributed amongst eukaryotes is the correlation between transcriptional activity and hypomethylation of DNA (reviewed by Doerfler, 1983).  Here there are some uncertainties and anomalies, and both methylation levels and nuclease sensitivity are sparsely investigated amongst higher plants, but nevertheless the overall picture is of great similarity amongst all eukaryotes in the mechanism of control of transcription.  The conclusion we must draw is that the ability to regulate the expression of a gene by control of transcription via the modification of chromatin structure dates back to before the divergence of the great eukaryotic kingdoms of plants, animals and fungi and that the fundamentals of the mechanism have remained undiverged in all of these groups.


THE SIGNALS FOR DIFFERENTIAL GENE EXPRESSION

Whilst we are on fairly firm ground when comparing the structure of genes and chromatin and speculating on the immediate mechanism of the regulation of transcription, we move into a much more uncertain terrain when we contemplate the signals which influence gene expression - the carriers of information to the genes.  We know that in animals and plants the fate of a cell is a function both of its past history and its present position, with the relative significance of these two factors varying between species and, perhaps, between cell types. It is the cytoplasm which holds and transmits the information on past history and present position.  The evolution of the capacity to differentiate must include not only the evolution of the genes to be expressed in different cell types, and the mechanism to control their transcription, but also the evolution of the material basis for signalling to the genes.  Since this is a topic about which very little is known, our speculations must be rather general.

A basis for our understanding of tissue specificity in the control of gene expression is to be found in experiments such as those described by Walker et al., (1983).  This work indicates that sequences upstream of a gene undergo some type of tissue-specific

interaction with the environment of the gene which influences
transcription.  In this way the insulin gene is preferentially
transcribed in the endocrine cells of the pancreas, while the
chymotrypsin gene is transcribed by the exocrine cells.

Model systems have been devised which represent the upstream
regulatory systems by enhancer sequences derived from viruses (e.g.
Herz and Roizman, 1983).  One such model consists of the
chloramphenicol acetyl transferase structural gene linked to enhancer
sequences from the SV40 virus, and this construct has been used by
Scholer and Gruss (1984) to study the interaction between the
enhancers and cellular components.  The conclusion of this is that
there are a limited number of cellular components capable of binding
to the enhancers, but that the nature of the components is not clear.
The requirements for specific sequences in the enhancer DNA could,
however, be investigated.

Another study of the interactions between DNA and cellular
components has been made by Emerson and Felsenfeld (1984).  They have
characterised, to some extent, a factor binding upstream of the
chicken beta-globin gene which confers nuclease hypersensitivity on
the gene and which is found in those cells in which the gene is
transcribed, being absent when transcription does not take place.  Gel
filtration indicates that the cellular factor has a molecular weight
of about 60-kilodaltons, and it is sensitive to proteinase K.

In other systems we have better characterised proteins which
interact with specific DNA sequences to regulate transcription of
hormonally regulated genes.  The oestrogen- and progesterone-regulated
genes such as chick ovalbumin and conalbumin provide one group of
examples (Mulvihill et al., 1982; Compton et al., 1983), while the
glucocorticoid-regulated genes provide another (Payvar et al., 1981;
Pfahl, 1982; Chandler et al., 1983; Karin et al., 1984).  That similar
systems operate in invertebrates is shown by the example of the
ecdysterone receptor of Drosophila (Schaltman and Pongs, 1982).  In
these hormonally regulated systems the binding of the protein to the
upstream regulatory sequence of the gene depends on the presence of a
hormone which evidently induces some conformational change in the
hormone receptor protein, but for the moment we can regard this as an
incidental detail and take these systems as instances of cellular
factors influencing transcription.  This is indicated diagrammatically
in Fig. 2.


EVOLUTION OF A BASIC MECHANISM

The sequence of events whereby organisms can evolve a range of
proteins by gene duplication and divergence are widely known.  Ohno
(1970) has written extensively on the topic and since then many more
examples have merged (Hood et al., 1975).  The globins are a well

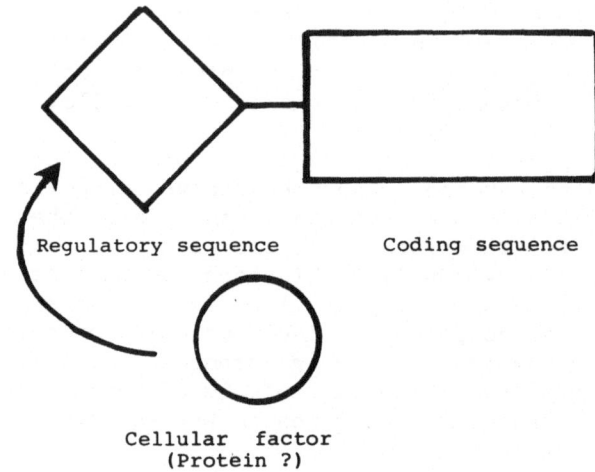

Fig. 2.    The basic mechanism of regulation

known instance (Jeffreys et al., 1983) and other examples include the
beta-crystallins (Clayton and Truman, 1974) actins and tubulins
(Cleveland et al., 1980) and keratins (Moll et al., 1982).  Sometimes
a single protein may show evidence of internal duplication, for
example ferrodoxin (Eck and Dayhoff, 1966).  The duplication of DNA
sequences can be brought about by unequal crossing-over or by gene
conversion, both giving rise on the first instance to tandem repeats.

   Whereas much has been published on the subject of gene
duplication and subsequent divergence by random mutation and natural
selection, most examples we have concern themselves with the coding
sequences of genes.  I would like to emphasise here the possible roles
of duplication of the regulatory sequences in DNA.  Fig. 3 indicates
the possible ways in which duplications and divergences might occur.
The route of duplication and divergence of structural genes while
retaining a common regulatory sequence is probably that taken to give
rise to the cluster of the genes for ovalbumin and gene X and gene Y
in the chick (Le Maur et al., 1981).  The duplication together of both
coding and regulatory sequence is presumably a common one, having taken
place many times in evolutionary history, but the pathway leading to
duplication and divergence of regulatory sequences must have been
crucial to the evolution of cellular differentiation.  Since
differentiation involves the tissue-specific regulation of the levels
of mRNA molecules common to many tissues, then we might expect to find
a variety of regulatory sequences able to respond to tissue-specific
cellular factors.

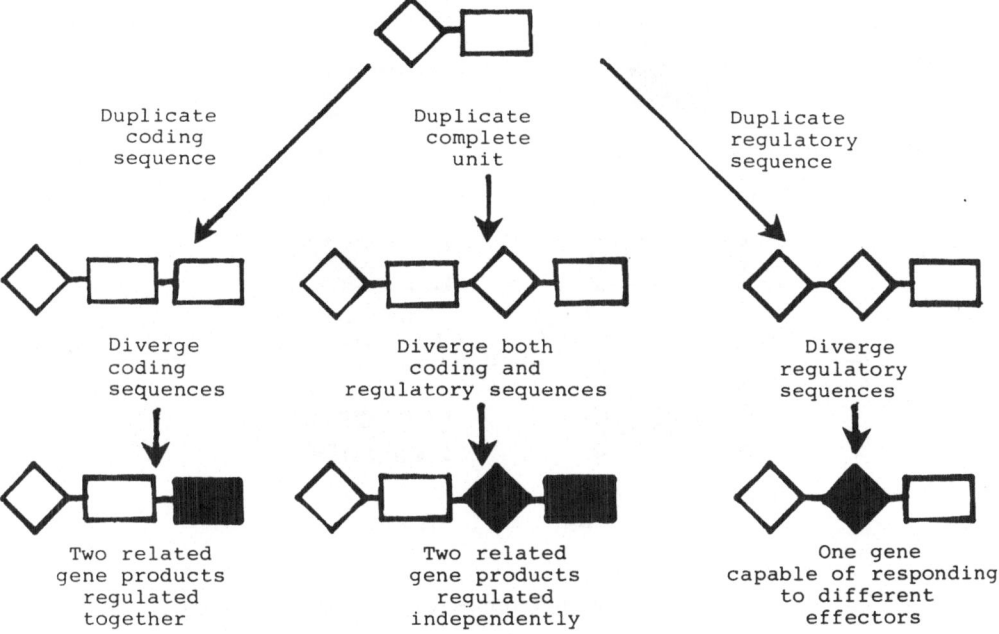

Fig. 3.   Possible duplications of the basic mechanism of duplication.


EVOLUTION OF THE SIGNALS TO THE GENES

     When we come to contemplate the events that might have occurred
to permit the evolution of cellular differentiation and consider the
signals to which the genes respond we move even further from the firm
ground of experimentation.  We can at present say so little of the
nature of these signals that it is hard to say anything of their
evolution, but at some point cells became sufficiently different to
provide a distinct environment for their genes.  It seems likely that
initially these differences may have been purely spatial, such as
those between cells on the inside or outside of a two-layered
structure, or those against a substrate and those exposed to the
medium in a bottom-dwelling form.

     In terms of gene expression we can produce some simple logical
alternatives which could be seen as differentiation.  These are set
out in Fig. 4.  The simplest situations involve on/off regulation of
gene expression, but an alternative is concerned with quantitative
regulation and this might be seen as the precursor of differentiation
as we see it today.  It is such a form of regulation which seems to
demand the presence of controlling sequences that are specific for
signals originating in a particular cell type.

     If we move forward from the most primitive form of cellular

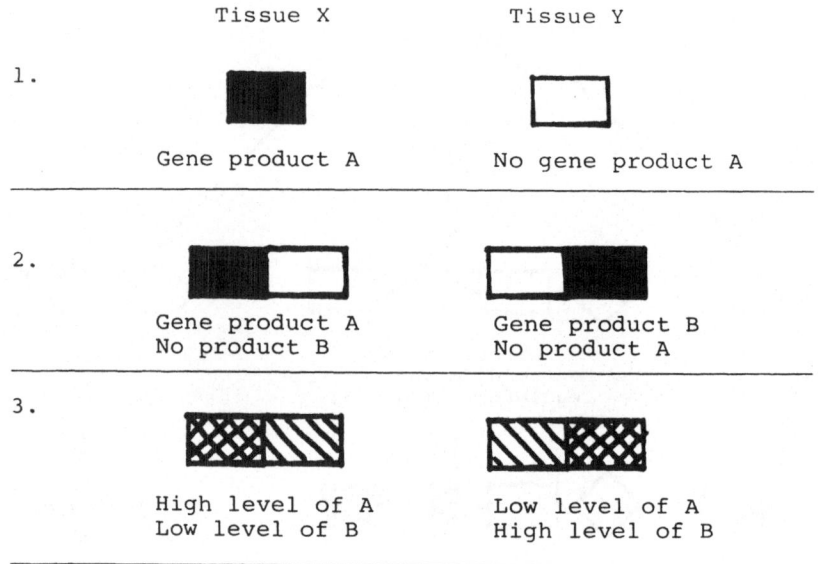

Fig. 4.    Alternative patterns of differentiation

differentiation, which might be induced by relatively simple agencies
such as mechanical factors, $CO_2$ concentration, or ionic differences, to
more sophisticated forms of differentiation regulated by specific
factors, then we have to face the difficulty of co-evolution of
signals and receptors.  In this case the signals are the postulated
cellular factors and the receptors are the regulatory DNA sequences
associated with the genes.  Now we do have a parallel to take into
consideration, namely the evolution of hormones and their receptors.

## CO-EVOLUTION OF SIGNALS AND RECEPTORS

There is a close stereochemical relationship between a hormone
and its receptor, or between a bacterial repressor and its effector.
Similarly there must be a high degree of specificity in the
interaction between the receptor or the repressor and the sequence of
DNA to which it binds.  Random changes to any of these components are
not likely to improve the fitness of the individual undergoing them.
However, as Ohno has pointed out, duplication of one of the components
in a system can break the impasse and permit changes to occur without
loss of the primary function, until such time as a new function has
fully emerged.

However there are other possibilities of evolution than the
production of new functions regulated by new effectors.  The inter-

change of regulatory sequences between genes may occur and thus old
effectors can come to influence different gene products.  Something of
this kind can be seen many times over in the world of hormonal
regulation.  As an example we can consider the hormone prolactin.  We
tend to think of this as a mammalian hormone, stimulating lactation,
but in fact it is secreted by many vertebrates, including fish,
amphibia, reptiles and birds (DeVlaming, 1979).  In all of these it
has a function related to reproduction, but its role in stimulating
transcription of the genes for casein and other milk proteins must
have arisen long after the hormone and its receptor protein had
evolved.  One of the steps involved in the evolution of the mammals
was the development of genes for casein, perhaps from keratin-like
genes (Joiles et al., 1981), and the joining of this new gene to an
existing regulatory sequence which was already responsive to the
prolactin-receptor complex.

RELATIVE RATES OF EVOLUTION OF STRUCTURAL GENES AND CONTROLLING
ELEMENTS

A number of studies in a wide range of organisms indicate that
controlling elements may evolve more rapidly than the coding sequences
that they regulate.  In bacterial systems in a chemostat exposed to a
new substrate the first response to selection pressure may be the
production of an enhanced amount of an enzyme with a marginal capacity
to metabolise the substrate, and this may be followed by selection of
the coding sequence to lead to increased ability of the enzyme to
metabolise the new substrate (Rigby et al., 1974).  At the other end
of the evolutionary scale, in the vertebrate lens there are many
instances where species divergence involves modification of the
relative proportions of different crystallin subunits without any
changes in the amino acid sequences of the subunits themselves
(Clayton, 1974).

INTEGRATION OF GENE EXPRESSION IN DIFFERENTIATION

A characteristic of cellular differentiation as seen in
contemporary animals is that large numbers of different proteins are
specifically regulated in quantitative patterns that are discrete.
This implies some mechanism which integrates the regulation of gene
expression and might involve a specific level of regulation (Truman
1982).  We can thus summarise the types of evolutionary change that
must have taken place before metazoa with cellular differentiation
could have emerged:

1.   Evolution of new proteins

2.   Evolution of control of new proteins

### 3.    Evolution of integrating systems

All this must have taken place by the late Precambrian, before that flourishing and diverse fauna could be fossilised in the seas which were to give rise to the hills of Ediacara.

REFERENCES

Anderson, D.T., 1973, "Embryology and Phylogeny in Annelids and Arthropods," Pergamon Press, Oxford.

Borschsenius, S., Bonven, B., Leer, J.C., and Westergaard, O., 1981 Nuclease-sensitive regions on the extrachromosomal r-chromatin from Tetrahymena pyriformis, Eur. J. Biochem., 117: 245.

Bryan, P.N., Olah, J., and Birnstiel, M.L., 1983, Major changes in the 5' and 3' chromatin structure of sea urchin histone genes accompany their activation and inactivation in development, Cell, 33: 843.

Chandler, V.L., Maler, B.A. and Yamamoto, K.R., 1983, DNA sequences bound specifically by glucocorticoid receptor in vitro render a heterologous promoter hormone responsive in vivo, Cell, 33:489.

Clayton, R.M., 1974, Comparative Aspects of Lens Proteins, in: "The Eye", H. Davson, ed., Academic Press, New York and London, Vol. 5, p399.

Clayton, R.M. and Truman, D.E.S., 1974, The antigenic structure of chick β-crystallin subunits, Exp. Eye Res., 18: 495.

Cleveland, D.W., Lopata, M.A., Cowan, N.J., MacDonald, R.J., Rutter, W.J. and Kirschner, M.W., 1980, A study of the number and evolutionary conservation of genes coding for α- and β-tubulin and β- and γ- cytoplasmic actin using specific cloned cDNA probes, Cell, 20: 95.

Compton, J.G., Schrader, W.T. and O'Malley, B.W., 1983, DNA sequence preference of the progesterone receptor, Proc. Natl.Acad. Sci. USA, 80: 16.

DeVlaming, V.L., 1979, Actions of prolactin among the vertebrates, in "Hormones and Evolution," E.J.W. Barrington, ed., Academic Press, New York.

Doerfler, W., 1983, DNA methylation and gene activity, Ann. Rev. Biochem., 52: 93.

Eck, R.V., and Dayhoff, M.., 1966, Evolution of the structure of ferredoxin based on living relics of primitive amino acid sequences, Science, 152: 363.

Elgin, S.C.R., 1981, DNAase 1-hypersensitive sites of chromatin, Cell, 27: 413.

Emerson, B.M. and Felsenfeld, G., 1984, Specific factor conferring nuclease hypersensitivity at the 5' end of the chicken adult β-globin gene, Proc. Natl. Acad. Sci. USA, 81: 95.

Ford, T.D., 1979, Precambrian fossils and the origin of the phanerozoic phyla, in: "The Origin of Major Invertebrate Groups," M.R. House, ed., Systematics Assoc. Special Volume 12, Academic Press, London.

Garel, A., and Axel, R., 1976, Selective digestion of transcription-
    ally active ovalbumin genes from oviduct nuclei, Proc. Natl.Acad.
    Sci. USA, 73: 3966.
Glaessner, M.F., 1984, "The Dawn of Animal Life," Cambridge University
    Press, Cambridge.
Herz, C. and Roizman, B., 1983, The $\alpha$ promoter regulator-ovalbumin
    gene resident in human cells is regulated like the authentic $\alpha 4$
    gene after infection with Herpes simplex virus 1 mutants in $\alpha 4$
    gene, Cell, 33: 145.
Hood, L., Campbell, J.H., and Elgin, S.C.R., 1975, The organisation
    and evolution of antibody genes and other multigene families,
    Ann. Rev. Genet., 9: 305.
Igo-Kemenes, T., Horz, W. and Zachau, H.G., 1982, Chromatin, Ann.Rev.
    Biochem., 51: 89.
Jeffreys, A.J., Harris, S., Barrie, P.A., Wood, D., Blanchetot, A. and
    Adams, S.M., 1983, Evolution of gene families: the globin genes,
    in: "Evolution from Molecules to Men," D.S. Bendall, ed.,
    Cambridge University Press, Cambridge.
Jolles, P., Jolles, J. and Henschen, A., 1981, Characterization of K-
    casein and keratin domains in fibrinogen, J. Mol. Evol., 17:188.
Karin, M., Haslinger, A., Holtgreve, H., Richards, R.I., Krauter, P.,
    Westphal, H.M. and Beato, M., 1984, Characterization of DNA
    sequences through which cadmium and glucocorticoid hormones
    induce human metallothionein II gene, Nature, 308:513.
LeMeur, M., Glanville, N., Mandel, J.L., Gerlinger, P., Palmiter, R.
    and Chambon, P., 1981, The ovalbumin gene family: hormonal
    control of X and Y gene transcription and mRNA accumulation,
    Cell, 23: 561.
McGhee, J.D. and Felsenfeld, G., 1982, Nucleosome structure, Ann.Rev.
    Biochem., 49: 1115.
Moll, R., Franke, W.W., Schiller, D.L., Geiger, B. and Krepler, R.
    1982, The catalog of human cytokeratins: patterns of expression
    in normal epithelia, tumours and cultured cells, Cell, 31: 11.
Mulvihill, E.R., Le Pennec, J-P., and Chambon, P., 1982, Chick oviduct
    progesterone receptor: location of specific regions of high-
    affinity binding in cloned DNA fragments of hormone-responsive
    genes, Cell, 28: 621.
Ohno, S., 1970, "Evolution by Gene Duplication," Allen and Unwin,
    London.
Payvar, F., Wrange, O., Carlstedt-Duke, J., Okret, S., Gustafsson,
    J-A., and Yamamoto, K.R., Purified glucocorticoid receptors bind
    selectively in vitro to a cloned DNA fragment whose transcription
    is regulated by glucocorticoids in vivo. Proc.Natl. Acad. Sci.
    USA, 78: 6628.
Pfahl, M., 1982, Specific binding of the glucocorticoid-receptor
    complex to the mouse mammary tumour proviral promoter region,
    Cell, 31: 475.
Rigby, P.W.J., Burleigh, B.D. and Hartley, B.S., 1974, Gene
    duplication in experimental enzyme evolution, Nature, 251: 200.

Schaltmann, K. and Pongs, O., 1982, Identification and character
    ization of the ecdysterone receptor in Drosophila melanogaster
    by photoaffinity labelling. Proc. Natl. Acad. Sci. USA, 79: 6
Scholer, H.R., and Gruss, P., 1984, Specific interaction between
    enhancer-containing molecules and cellular components, Cell,
    36: 403.
Schopf, J.W. and Oehler, D.Z., 1976, How old are the Eukaryotes?
    Science, 193: 47.
Shermoen, A.W. and Bekendorf, S.K., 1982, A complex of interacting
    DNAase I-hypersensitive sites near the Drosophila glue protein
    gene, Sgs 4, Cell, 29: 601.
Stebbins, G.L., 1982, "Darwin to DNA, Molecules to Humanity," Freeman,
    San Francisco, p210.
Truman, D.E.S., 1982, Taxonomies of differentiation, in: "Stability
    and Switching in Cellular Differentiation," R.M. Clayton and
    D.E.S. Truman, eds., Plenum Press, New York and London.
Walker, M.D., Edlund, T., Boulet, A.M. and Rutter, W.J., 1983, Cell
    -specific expression controlled by the 5'-flanking region of
    insulin and chymotrypsin genes, Nature, 306: 557.
Weintraub, H. and Groudine, M., 1976, Chromosomal subunits in active
    genes have an altered conformation, Science, 193: 848.
Wood, W.I. and Felsenfeld, G., 1982, Chromatin structure of the
    chicken β-globin gene region.  Sensitivity to DNase I, micro-
    coccal nuclease, and DNase II, J. Biol. Chem., 257: 7730.
Wu, C., 1980, The 5' ends of Drosophila heat shock genes in chromatin
    are hypersensitive to DNase I, Nature, 286: 854.
Wu, C., Bingham, P.M., Livak, K.J., Holmgren, R. and Elgin, S.C.R.
    1979, The chromatin structure of specific genes: 1. Evidence for
    higher order domains of defined DNA sequence, Cell, 16:797.

FINAL DISCUSSION


INTRODUCTION



    This final discussion is presented as a single chapter, but its
subject matter fell into two parts. The first, opened by J. Weston,
dealt with aspects of cellular decisions during differentiation,
and the difficulties of determining their nature, and when they take
place.  The second part, opened by A. Sippel, dealt with the molecular
aspects of cell differentiation, particularly the problems of gene
regulation: its complexity, and its specificity.

COORDINATED REGULATION OF GENE EXPRESSION

FINAL DISCUSSION

Weston

    In the last month, I have been to three meetings and in these
I have heard about a hundred talks. They were all good. But a few
seemed to strike a sensible note, as if two things had converged in
the same place, both the right question and the right methods. It
seems to me that the chance to turn this good conference into a
great conference, would be if we could make the right problem and
the right methodology converge in the same place. At least in the
cellular problems of development, our problem has really been to ask
the right questions. When I hear these skilful presentations of
analyses of gene regulation, I am reminded of the old story of the
drunk who lost his keys, and was looking for them under the street
light. A man came up to help, and said where did you lose them?
And he said, "Over there". "Well, why are looking over here?" And
he answered, "The light is better over here." It may be that the
light represents our intelligence, but it could be that what we are
doing is exploiting our ability to do what are routine experiments,
without trying to identify what the really crucial questions are.
The papers that we all recognise as distinguished are the ones where
the right question has been identified. For my part I would like to
try to identify what I think are the significant developmental
questions, that need to be asked at the cellular level. I hope that
people with more molecular orientations will perhaps try to think
about my problems, with their insights, and tell me how to do the
next experiment.

    To me, the most important single question that we have to deal
with is the question of lineage decisions: that is, the stable,
heritable change in developmental restrictions, or developmental
ability, in cell populations. In trying to think about lineages of
course we talk about branch points, and the question has always been
"How do you identify a branch point?" We have trouble in our lab in
thinking about what we really mean by a lineage. A whole pathway is
a lineage, but within that there are branches which you can consider
lineages, in a sense. A lot of what people work on in developmental
biology, it seems to me, are not the branches so much, as the

313

efflorescences within a branch, the individual modulations of
expression, or phenotypes that are really part of a given branch and
really don't tell us anything about the true branching decisions.
The crucial branching decisions that everyone would agree on in
vertebrate development, are the early ones; for example, between
trophectoderm and inner cell mass, between mesoderm and endoderm,
between neuroectoderm and mesoderm, or other kinds of ectoderm; where
whole areas of developmental repetoire are set out and in a sense
isolated, and are manifestly different from other areas.  The
operational problem is how to distinguish between a true branch point
in a lineage and some of these minor aspects of cellular
differentiation that occur within a branch point.  It occurred to me
that what we need to do is to identify a differentiation product that
is characteristic of one of these branch points.  Maybe the
operational way that we can use to identify the members that are
common in that branch is to do the kind of experiments that Kondoh
has done: to take the genes for a fairly common structural component
in the cells and to inject it into as many different cell types as we
can.  We might be able to operationally classify members of a lineage
by all the cell types where that particular gene can be expressed, as
you would operationally define cells of other lineages as those cells
where that gene cannot be expressed.  That of course begs the
question of what is it about that gene, or those cells, that
establishes that developmental bias, or ability.  It seems that we
have still not actually addressed the problem of how we are going to
define what are the truly important lineage decisions, where they
are, and when they occur.

If we operationally define members of the individual branches,
then we could ask what are the molecular correlates of those changes?
Are they changes in chromatin?  Or moveable genetic elements that
have somehow moved into important new places?  Once we have
identified the crucial decisions, and when they occur, we should be
able to isolate members of what I am trying to define as members of a
true lineage, so that we can identify individual sub-populations.  We
ought to be able then to characterise the responses of such lineage
populations to environmental signals.  If we can isolate such
populations, and characterise their responses to environmental cues,
we should be able to identify something about the environmental cues.
What is the identity of effective environmental signals, what are the
dose requirements, what is the mode of presentation of such a signal
to responsive cells, what is the basis of the responsiveness of the
cell or population to a given signal? In other words, what is the
nature of the receptor and how is that receptor regulated?  Finally I
think we should consider going back and considering the basis for
reversibility?  How is this reversibility maintained or prevented?
How is it elicited?  It occurs to me, on the basis of no evidence,
that oncogenes and growth factors may be concerned in the promoting
of flexibility;  whether the cell maintains a degree of stability of
the phenotypes that it expresses, or whether it may switch over to

another sub-lineage, whether the cell can respond, in other words, to
a given environmental signal and the nature of the response to the
environmental signal.  One of the most important prcblems now is to
identify what are the members of a true lineage.  How do you identify
operationally, the branch points, so that you can discover when they
occur?  Then you ought to be able to use that information to identify
and isolate members of a given lineage class.  And once you do that,
you should be able to understand how cells that are homogeneous in
the sense that they are members of a given lineage class, respond to
environmental signals.  Once you do that, in turn, you should be able
to identify the signals and understand how they are presented to the
cells and how the cells transduce those signals into regulated gene
activity.  I don't know whether I have managed to focus on questions
that are answerable or whether I have just managed to confound the
issue.  Perhaps the latter.

## Raff

I think that what you were trying to say, is that there are
major branch points that are true lineage decisions, and that then
there are minor decisions, which you might call activation.  I think
it is a dangerous distinction.  Take your own system.  If you look
at the neural crest which develops after the neuroectoderm has been
induced, some of those cells are able to form cartilage cells and
fibroblasts.  Is the decision of a neural crest cell to become a
cartilage cell a major lineage decision or a minor differentiation
event?  Are such cartilage cells different from those that arise
from mesoderm?

## Weston

In my opinion it is reasonable to believe that, (although nothing
is absolutely proved), the cells in the embryo that are involved in
producing cartilage are only operationally called neural crest cells.
These are from a population of cells that migrate just prior to the
main mass of neural crest cells.  It is conceivable that they
represent a different lineage altogether.

## Raff

Could they be mesoderm?

## Weston

You have to think where does the mesoderm come from?  It
separates out from an epithelium that exists in the embryo, the

ectoderm.  It actually drops out of this epithelial layer.  I don't want to focus too closely on a little anomaly in development but it turns out that if you look at which cells make cartilage and connective tissue cells, we thought they were neural crest, and it is true that they drop out from the junction between the medulary epithelium and the ectoderm.  But they do so in a way that is very suggestive of the way that the original mesodermal cells drop out of the ectoderm, during early gastrulation. It occurs to me that what is happening is essentially a late departure.

## Raff

So mesodermal cells are mixed in with the neuro ectodermal cells and stay as a separate population?

## Weston

I know it sounds outrageous, but you have to realise that all these years we have been identifiying the 'neural crest' essentially operationally merely as that group of cells (not necessarily a homogeneous population), that resides at the top of the neural tube. That is fairly arbitrary.  It does not really tell you anything, more than the place where the cells resided before you decided that you could identify them.

## Clayton

I think that Martin [Raff] has got a critical point though, about the possibilities of mesodermal and neural crest chondrocytes, which is that you can arrive at a characteristic differentiated cell type from different routes.  But you do have a problem about redefining the nature of the decisions.

## Weston

That is why I suggested a new operational decision.  Maybe we should take and identify the message segment of the genome and just inject it into all of these populations.  If it is expressed, then it operationally defines a member of that lineage class.

## Yaffe

But that is an oversimplification.  Why should you expect a gene that is expressed in terminal differentiation will recognise the progenitor cells, if you see for example, that an actin gene is not expressed?

Weston

    You have to choose your genes right.

Clayton

    We have a whole lot of operational problems here.  Our under-
standing of what a decision is, is actually based on the experiments
by which we decide that a decision  has been made.  In other words,
if you look at early embryology, everything we know is as a result of
transplantation, excision and grafting.  And therefore the sorts of
data that you got were always that with the graft you got this
response and without the graft you got that response, and so you say
that this tissue is an inductor, and you have got a branch point.
You tend to identify branch points.  When you look at such bits of
molecular information as there are, you may find that the genes by
which you thought you could distinguish the different products were
actually present before this decision-making event occurred.  The
difficulty is that our definition as to what makes the decision
point depends to some extent on what technology are we using and
what level are you aiming to investigate what is happening,and that
another possibility therefore is  that at some level,what is going
on is a sort of molecular population matter,and you get a series of
stochastic changes and you can eventually flip over,as judged by
microscopic evidence.

Weston

    We are talking about quantitative changes but also about the
change in a population of cells that says in this lineage, globin
is not going to be produced, but maybe neurofilament or neurofilament
related proteins is.  And in another lineage, perhaps there is some
other crucial lineage identifier.

Clayton

    Absolutely, I agree with this.  But it doesnt mean that there is
one crucial moment.

Sippel

    It is the way we think.  We always think in terms of branch
points.

Weston

Grafting experiments we now know involve mixed populations of
cells. It changes completely the way we interpret the experiments if
you are not dealing with a homogeneous population. We have to find
out how you establish a homogeneous embryonic population.

Yaffe

No doubt these are the crucial questions of developmental
biology, which you raise now. I think all the molecular biologists
will agree so. But the question is how do you go further to answer
these questions?

Weston

I am saying that operationally you need to begin with a
homogeneous population of cells. It is like when you are trying to
identify a receptor, the first thing that you need is a pure
preparation of whatever it is that the receptor binds, so that you
can measure binding constants, and things like that. In the same
way, in this case, if you want to measure developmental response,
you have got to have a pure preparation of the responding component.

Raff

You have raised the question of how one establishes lineage
relationships. Homogeneous populations is one way, but there is
another way, that is to study a single cell, and look at its progeny.
If it produces six different cell types, then you have established
at least part of its developmental potential. If you started with
two cells and end up with six, the situation is ambiguous. How can
you study the developmental potential of a single cell? One way is
cloning a single cell. Another way is marking an individual cell.
Very few experiments have been done in this way, which is why there
is so litle direct evidence about lineage relationships. It's not
good enough to mark a population of cells - as has been the main
approach in the neural crest.

Weston

I hate to say it, but they were Weston experiments. Since they
were wrong, I feel that it is right to say so. One knows that
working with a single cell is extremely difficult. So I am asking
for the next best thing. I am asking to identify members of a
population that behave as if they were all the same.

Raff

    OK. There are two other ways of doing it. You don't always
have to study single cells. Another way is to observe continuously
a population of cells, as has been done in Coenorhabditis Elegans.
There are very few examples where one can do that, but it is a direct
way of establishing lineage. Another way is to try and induce an
entire population that is dividing very little, to differentiate one
way or another, by altering the environment.


Weston

    What I was trying to assert is that I would say that the cells
you work on are already past the crucial genetic regulatory event.


Saxen

    I still have one difficulty in distinguishing between your true
lineages and what you have just called sub-lineages, and what
relationship there is between them.


Raff

    We really need some examples. Because I don't know what you mean
by modulation - other than a glial progenitor cell becoming an
oligodendrocyte or an astrocyte. What else would you put into that
category?


Weston

    Well, it may be glia or melanin, in the cases that we have
heard. Maybe cholinergic and adrenergic neurones, maybe smooth
muscle and skeletal muscle.


Raff

    OK then, what is a real decision?


Weston

    One of the ones that I mentioned. Mesoderm versus endoderm.

Saxen

That is not a very good example. Would you include ectoderm in
that? Ectoderm can be converted into mesoderm.


Weston

Except that I did not say ectoderm and mesoderm.


Raff

Give us one that could not be shot down.


Weston

I think that once a decision has been taken to be endoderm,
with all of the known derivatives of endoderm it is unlikely that
any of the cells derived from classical endoderm would ever be made
to make let us say, red blood cells, or muscle.


Raff

OK then, what can the endoderm become that is so restricted?


Weston

As far as I know it becomes all of the parts of the gut, and
any branches of the gut:  the epithelial components of the lung,
the pancreas, the liver.


Raff

So what about the neuropeptide secreting cells in the lung and
gut that are not crest derived? What I don't understand is why you
want to hold onto these divisions, when the evidence suggests that
they are not very special.


Clayton

I must say I find myself agreeing with Martin, because we have
things like Okada and Eguchi's work. If you want to say that pigment
cells and glial are really a modulation of each other, where does
that leave the lens cells which can be derived from either, in vitro,

but are far enough away in normal development.  Modulation might be
more like chromatophore exchanges.


## Weston

What I want to do is to use Okada and Eguchi's methodology in a
new way.  To set up new operational definitions of cell populations
that are indistinguishable.


## Clayton

What about erector pili which are perfectly good muscles, but
they are derived from ectoderm if I remember rightly.  You see you
always get anomalies.  Some of the anomalies are natural ones like
the erector pili and some of the anomalies are experimentally
obtained.


## Eguchi

I think it is very hard to distinguish true branching from
modulation.  We have a very good example of modulation which Ruth
proposed.  For instance the chromatophores, as shown by Dr Ide,
Tokoku University, Sendai, Japan, the melanophore is easily turned
into a xanthophore and vice versa.  In our case, it is impossible
to say 'modulation'.  It is very important what the standard is.


## Clayton

Supposing it is something like vapour pressure?  We know that
molecules in a body of water are moving at various rates.  And at
any one moment, you could pick one particular molecule and it would
have its own rate of movement.  You put in energy and you will
eventually get the whole lot boiling.  Now in the case of cell
differentiation, I suspect it might well be that what you have got
is something of this nature.  That at the molecular level perhaps
you never get zero expression of every single gene and perhaps what
it really depends on is at what point you gradually get sufficient
so that you can say, well now, this cell is not what it was before,
it has made a decision, and this again leads me to suspect that we
have first of all, not really to dismiss reversibility, because it
is just as difficult a definition in a way as decision points.  It
is the opposite image.  And if you think about it it may be that our
definition of a decision point and our definition of reversibility
depends first of all on:  can we recognise what there is in this
cell population, and at what level are we recognising it.  And
secondly, have we yet developed a technique for forcing cells to

change their recognisable expression?  Until pigment cells were
shown to be capable of turning into lens cells, one would have said
that the decision point to give you those two cell types was several
decisions away.  Perhaps we can't talk in those terms any more,
because a technique has been evolved to modify these apparent
decisions.  We are at the mercy of our technological ability, as
well as the real situation of the cells themselves.

## Weston

I would like to say two things about that.  One possibility
that you mentioned, namely that flashing phenotypes all the time, is
a remarkably similar argument to the immune system.  It may be that
embryonic cells are always trying out new tricks with their genome,
generating little bits of expression here and there.  And what we are
talking about is the continuous interaction between newly established
environments, location of individual cells and what they happen to be
doing with their genome at any particular time which may stabilised,
or amplified.

## Southern

You made a further point in your introduction which I think is
a valuable one, which is, can the molecular techniques help us to
redefine the cell types so that you can actually ask, "Are there
such things as branch points of that kind?"  We can ask "How does
it really work in a cell?  What kind of molecular phenotype can be
put on a cell and does that help  Does molecular analysis ease the
way in which you look at a cell's phenotype?  Or does it make it more
difficult?  Have we raised the molecular techniques yet to a level
where you can take a cell and say:  This is what the cell looks like
in terms of its molecular definition?  The sort of thing that
Professor Bird was talking about.

## Maitland

You are talking about introducing cellular genes back into
cells, which is what Dr Kondoh has done.  Why not think about some
of the specific cell trophisms that viruses have; for instance
Epstein-Barr virus (which we still dont understand) seems to have a
specific target B-cells.  That is a very primitive one but there are
lots of other animal viruses, for instance, papilloma virus which
are targeted in or presumably on specific differentiated cell types.

Weston

    You are saying, use them as markers?


Maitland

    Those are your transient expression markers at an early stage.
Perhaps it has never been done.  But perhaps the expression of those
genes in the early stages might define the lineage.


Sippel

    I think these approaches are dangerous because we would not know
the level of interference between viral gene expression and the host
cell.  There could be a problem of infection or a problem of
expressing the necessary mRNAs.  Before you know all of the possible
mechanisms of interrelation between virus and host this approach may
be too misleading.  The same is true for the approach in which we
use transfected marker genes as long as we haven't established the
mechanisms which regulate genes in their entire tissue and stage
specificity.


Weston

    One of the things that people do very well now is to sequence
a structural gene and regulatory elements and know what parts of the
nucleotide sequence are involved in turning the gene up or down, what
are important, and where they are located, cis-acting or whatever.
My question is:  What is it that is involved in deciding which gene
is going to be regulated during normal development.


Southern

    I think your point is that by experimenting by introducing
those genes, you actually perturbed the system.  And so what you
need is some non-interventive way of analysing cells which doesnt
require sticking in something  which is going to muck it up.  Is
that the point that you [Sippel] are making?


Sippel

    Sort of.  The warning was about an experiment in which we take
a transfected gene as an indicator for a cell lineage.  If, in order
to be expressed in the right way, genes have to go through the
entire history of a cell type, the later introduction of genes as

naked DNA may be problematic.  I believe the chromatin structure of
a particular gene is progressively developed during cell
differentiation.  If we introduce a homologue gene later in
development, and I mean for example a few steps after early
embryonal decisions, this introduced gene DNA might not be given
the same pattern of DNAase hypersensitive sites.  That would mean
it could never be regulated in the same way as its endogenous
counterpart which has gone through the total developmental history.


## Yaffe

It all depends what question you are asking.


## Sippel

Yes, I agree.


## Weston

You have to be extremely careful about which gene you are going
to use as your diagnostic reagent.  It may be that delta crystallin
is not it; maybe it happens to be a gene that isn't absolutely
required for lens differentiation but just happens to be present
in all of the cells in a particular class of cells.


## Southern

I think that our feeling as molecular biologists would be that
to answer the question as to whether you can use the molecular
approach as a way of looking at cell lineage, you really have to
answer all the questions that you are asking in the first place.
And it is not really at a stage yet when you can confidently stick
in a construct that you have made from beautiful bits of DNA
sequence and predict what the outcome of your experiment will be,
given a particular set-up in the cell.  I think that once we are at
that point we have answered all the questions you want to answer with
your experiments, or a very high proportion of them.


## Williams

I think it may be a valid approach and it is actually being
used with the immunoglobulin enhancer by coupling it up to an
essentially neutral gene and puting it into different cells in the
B-cell lineage.  Walter Schaffner has been doing this and getting
some very interesting results about the efficiency of operation of

the enhancer, in different B-cell lineages.  There is really no
reason why you should not go back as far as it is possible for the
cell biology to take things.


## Weston

What we might discover is that the classifications that result
bear remarkable resemblance to what we already know.  It would be
reassuring at least.  On the other hand, we may get completely
different classifications.


## Raff

Cell biology still will have to provide information about cell
lineage and decision points.  Take the B-lymphocyte example.  The
reason that the molecular genetic information made so much sense so
quickly was that the cell biology had been done.  It was already
clear what the general sequence of development was - from pre B-cell
to B-cell, to antibody-secreting cell.  The challenge is to try to
define as clearly as possible the lineage relationships between
cells.

You consider cells A and B as different because you have markers
that distinguish them.  But then you want to know where did A and B
come from?  Did they come from a common cell, or from two different
cells?  Ultimately you want to trace their development back to the
fertilised egg.  Then the molecular geneticist can take the clearest
examples of decision points and try to understand what the molecular
genetic basis of the decisions are.  In vertebrates, it is clear that
many of those decisions are determined by cell-cell interactions.
The cell biologist has to define the cellular basis of those
cell-cell interactions.  The molecular geneticists won't be able to do
it, although they will play a major part in determining the nature of
the molecules that mediate the interaction.


## Weston

You say cell-cell interactions, but what you are really talking
about is the mode of presentation of an appropriate signal.  It could
be on another cell, it could be attached to an extra-cellular matrix
component, it is almost certainly true that every developmental
signal that we know is spatially buffered.  It is not diffusible.  It
is not floating around accessible to all parts of the cell.

Raff

What about thyroxin in metamorphosis?


Weston

I said virtually.  OK there are some clearly humoral things.


Sippel

What about EGF or any other peptide hormone?  Why don't we stay
with the lymphocytes?  I think this is a good system because it is
a single cell system.  Here the individual cell stages can be better
defined than in other systems.  There are a number of signal peptides
involved, all of which must have their receptors.  The signals are
diffusible factors which can be isolated and can be cloned.  Here we
can see how two cell types interact with each other.  There are
several peptide factors involved in order to regulate their
respective cellular development.


Raff

But in the lymphocyte system there is almost nothing known about
lineage decisions.  In the case of the B cell, you are talking about
a cell that is already committed to becoming  an antibody secreting
cell and discussing the various steps involved in activating the
cell.  It is a very important system to study, but quite different
from asking about the decision point when a precursor cell decides to
become a T-lymphocyte or a B-lymphocyte - if there is such a cell.


Sippel

But why should these later decisions be basically different in
their mechanism than earlier ones, which are so much harder to study?


Raff

Since you don't know the mechanisms in either case, you don't
know whether they will be the same or different, but it is important
to realise that in the lymphocyte system, none of the lineage branch
points have been defined unambigously.  None of the cell-cell
interactions that influence these decisions have been defined, let
alone any of the molecules involved.  You are talking about
interactions and molecules involved in cell activation, which may be
quite different.

Clayton

There are two sorts of population problems, the molecular and the cellular. Consider for example receptors for the various peptide hormones. Quite often you get families of the peptide hormones too. So that one imagines that even if you had one specific receptor on a cell type, members of the hormone family would have different degrees of affinity for it. And similarly if you have different families of receptors, they too might have a range of affinities. If you consider possible receptors, the odds are that none of them are utterly unique to a particular cell type. It is likely that what you have got is an overlapping representation of the possible molecular populations on a number of cell types. So that again, the likelihood of a cell receiving effective signals is going to depend on what percentage of which particular receptor has it got? It may be that a cell with more of a particular receptor has a greater likelihood of responding than say, another cell that has indeed got some of that same molecular representation, but has got less of it. Some really quite ancient embryological experiments suggest there is something like a range of likelihoods that cells will be able to develop into a particular direction. Take something like a limb field or a heart field: as the region in the centre of that field becomes more and more likely to form the appropriate organ, (shall we say a limb), on explantation, so the peripheral region, which at one time had quite a measurable likelihood of doing this, declines in its capacity, until in the end (when you have really got some way into the production of a limb), the area around has lost this capacity. Now whether this is in terms of the likelihood per cell or whether it is that the cell population itself is always heterogeneous, and non-responding cells are eliminated by cell death, or diminished because they don't divide as fast, or themselves change, we don't know. But if you look at this phenomenon from a distance, you do get an impression that you have got a heterogeneous population and that this heterogeneity, in terms of the responding cell, and the markers on these cells, and in terms of the signals available to them, has got some kind of stochastic population likelihood aspect.


Saxen

To go back to what you said about the diffusible and the non-diffusible factors, there is reason to believe that they may operate together. A good example is the mammary gland, where specific testosterone receptors are induced by specific cell-cell interactions, and then when the gland is exposed to testosterone the morphogenetic change takes place.

Weston

Yes, I acknowledge that.  It is also likely that there are small
peptides that serve as signals as well.  It could even be ions that
are somehow not uniformly distributed in the embryo, and that in a
sense the proteoglycans and the glycosoaminoglycans act like ion
exchange columns and they essentially just trap some things in a
particular location.  It may be that the reason cells respond in
regions where there are particular concentrations of extra-cellular
matrix is that happens to be the particular appropriate composition
which can concentrate, by affinity, properties of a particular growth
factor that is required by a cell.  I would like to address a
particular point that Ruth made about the notion of populations.  If
you have a mixture of cell populations in an area of the embryo and
through some agency, whatever it is, a particular part of the
population of a given developmental capability gains the accendancy,
the question arises, "what happens to the other populations?"  Do
they die or do they simply hide?  Are they residing there in very
small numbers, waiting for an appropriate, happier environment?  For
the millenium?

Once again you have to have a clear way to distinguish
operationally the two populations, which is in a sense a predictor of
developmental ability but not necessarily the consequence of a
particular ability.


Southern

In asking a molecular biologist to think about a problem like
that I think you do have to focus it down to something a bit more
specific.  It is very difficult for a molecular biologist to be
presented with a problem of how in a population of cells are you
going to find something which will label it, which tells you that
that cell is destined to die.  I think it is an extremely difficult
problem.  You are going to have to give us some kind of clues, which
are going to help us along the road of finding what we call a probe
for that particular behaviour that you are looking for.


Wyllie

It might be helpful to remember the example of polyoma DNA and
the teratocarcinoma cell.  It brings in elements of what was
suggested by Norman [Maitland] shortly ago.  And for those who aren't
familiar with the story, the embryocarcinoma can be infected or
transfected with polyoma DNA and the DNA is there but it not
expressed.  Now when you allow the cell to differentiate from the
primitive embryocarcinoma stem cell and this has to be I think one of
the very major branch points, that we are discussing, then the

polyoma DNA is expressed.  And it is expressed in almost every cell
that is differentiated.  Now when one plays around with mutants to
see what it is that stops the expression, it seems to turn out that
what stops the expression in the embryocarcinoma cell is nothing to
do with the major genes that you are looking at like the T antigen.
It is the enhancer sequence.  And it may be that when we are asking
for specific gene probes to tell us what family of differentiation a
cell is capable of developing, the probes we ought to be looking for
are not the genes we understand at the moment but the very low
abundance molecules that Dr Sippel has been talking about, which may
link with the enhancer sequences.  Which is actually a degree of
complexity rather beyond what we have been considering up to now.


## Weston

Yes, I rather like that.  In a sense it is an independent marker
It has nothing to do with anything that we would commonly recognise
as the phenotype.


## Wyllie

Save in so far as it may have been borrowed from things that we
do commonly recognise.


## Weston

But that is the point, it again has to do with being very careful
about how you select your probe and maybe the rules for selecting the
probe are what we have just been talking about.


## Southern

I think that is coming to the problem from the other end.  It is
a molecular biologist sorting out a cell biology problem.  Like the
homeobox story, is possibly going to do the same sort of thing yet
again.  But what we are trying to find at the moment is how the cell
biologist can define problems in a clear way that the molecular
biologist can tackle.  And it will come later to have the molecular
biologist sort out problems from his standpoint.  But it is looking
at things from the cell end and focussing down to the molecular end
that seems to be the difficulty.

Raff

   There is a problem that we haven't discussed at this meeting very
much which I think is a critical area of development where molecular
genetics is going to play a dominant role.  So when molecular
geneticists are thinking of developmental problems to study, this one
may be worth keeping in mind.  That is the question of morphogenesis
as opposed to the question of cell diversification which we have
concentrated on at this meeting and in this discussion.  A morphogenetic question is, how is it that while the cells in the arm and
the leg are the same, they assemble into very different patterns.
Cell biologists have largely reached an impasse and there seems no
clear molecular way forward.  If you transfer a small number of
mesenchymal cells from a wing bud of a chick to the leg region, then
develop into a wing, and vice versa.  All the information for forming
a wing as opposed to a leg can be contained in a very small number
of cells.  If one could get these cells to proliferate in culture and
retain this information so that when you transplanted them back they
formed wing; now the molecular geneticists could have a go.  But the
fact is that there are no systems like that so far, so one has to
think of other ways forward.  It is likely that the way will be
through drosophila, where the combination of classical and molecular
genetics will get there long before the cell biologists have figured
out what to do.


Clayton

   There are some sorts of events which may be the consequences of
the number of cells in a population as well as their molecular
configuration, which is what we have been talking about.  For
example Rensch showed a very long time ago that if you compared
gastrulation movements in different species - whether you got it by
delamination or by invagination, depended on the available size of
the cell population.  If you had a tiny cell population, you had a
split and if you had a larger population you could afford to have
really massive gastrulation movements.  Berrill also showed the
effect of cell members on morphogenesis in Ascidians.  And I suspect
that we might find something of this kind often occurs, if we were to
really look at cell populations with that sort of question in mind.
But the other thing is this:that whether the cells can move as a
sheet, or whether they are going to make a mass is going to depend on
the number of cell-cell recognition sites of the appropriate kind on
their surfaces.  And that is something which we do know a little
about at least, because you can see (for instance) if there is a
brush border always  a particular aspect of a cell, you can ask how
do cells adhere, what sort of connections do they make, or one could,
if one had appropriate markers, whether it is lectins or antibodies,
map out the disposition of sites and look at their number.  This has
been done for cells in the immune system.  Boyse, Old and Stockert

were probably among the first to do this, they attempted to map the
relative disposition of K-sites and D-sites and other surface
antigens.  In principle, this sort of approach can be made.  One of
the difficulties is that again, for reasons of technology,
information about enzymes just accumulated a lot faster than
information about insoluble molecules which are rather hard to get
out and extract.  A quite different technical approach was needed for
that.  Basically an immunological one, which depends on whether you
can really specifically recognise something, and obviously the advent
of monoclonals now puts a new dimension into this.  But I think in
principle it should not really be such a different problem.  It is a
question again of people deciding what it is they want to ask.  One
of the problems in the study of morphogenesis is that, in the absence
of molecular techniques, in the absence of questions which could be
approached in that way, a lot of the work has been in a sense,
descriptive.  Such as: if I put these two cell types together, what
do I then see down the microscope?


Weston

    That is the exploratory phase.


Clayton

    It is necessary but I don't think that morphogenesis is going to
be either beyond our reach nor will it necessarily be explicable
exclusively in molecular terms, but we still have to be aware that
what we are dealing with is a population of cells.  Even if we look
at these positional markers on them which may not be uniformly
distributed, on the individual cells.  And of course specific cell
adhesion molecules have actually been at least obtained in some
systems haven't they?


Saxen

    What do you mean by specific?


Clayton

    I mean things like Moscona's glycoprotein which sticks retina
cells together.  I mean you can get to the point where you have
actually got one band on a gel.

Saxen

The problem with the adhesive molecules which have been so much discussed is that they seem to be highly unspecific.


Weston

That doesn't matter because the same molecule can act on two different populations of cells, providing that there is little or no chance that those two pairs of populations will normally see each other.


Clayton

In any case it doesn't really matter if something is unspecific. Because if the way you get anywhere is having a particular balance of say n non-specific characters, and then you get something else by having another particular quantitative balance of non-specific characters, some of which are shared, and some of which are not shared by that particular cell type but are shared with another, you still in the end get what you want. In other words, if you have a series of coarse seives you still get discrimination. It's just that you can't really do it if you have only one. And most of biological specificities seems to me to be a way of combining a somewhat smaller number of components than you might suppose you need, considering the number of possible responses.


Williams

Surely it is crucial to us to actually get a stem cell to make a decision. The only one that I know of is the teratocarcinoma cell. If we can get other systems like the mesenchymal cells that can make all kinds of cells, are there ways which we can go about immortalizing the stem cells, getting them in culture, so that molecular biologists can work with them?


Saxen

One obvious conclusion of this discussion is that at the moment the developmental biologist has by and large failed to provide ideal model systems for the molecular geneticist.


Sippel

I think if you want to give the molecular biologist a model, you must find that branch point which is most crucial, which is the biggest step.

## Raff

I'm not sure that there are big steps and little steps in terms of binary decisions, in the way that Jim [Weston] has suggested.  For example, the first decision in mammalian embryos is cells chosing between trophectoderm and inner cell mass pathways.  Is there any reason to think that, in molecular terms, it is different from the decision of a leucocyte progenitor makes on chosing to become a macrophage rather than a granulocyte.  I think not.

## Weston

It is as well this is being recorded, because I think you are taking the other side of that story just a few minutes ago.

## Raff

No, I am talking now about cells deciding to become one cell type or another.  It is quite different from a nesting B cell becoming actuated to secrete antibody.

## Weston

There are some significant decisions that result not so much in defining what a cell is capable of doing, as imposing some kind of restriction on what it is capable of doing.  There are cells that, no matter how hard you try to make them, they will not make globin, and there are others that no matter how hard you try, they will not make neurofilament.  Now negative experiments are extremely dangerous.  If you can't make something do something, it may be your fault, but I think it is possible to classify cells in terms of these large scale restrictions of their developmental capabilities.  Those might be the large branch points that we were talking about.

## Sippel

There are mechanisms which don't allow steps to be reversed. Once a pre-B-cell has translocated the immunoglobulin variable region to the constant region it can no longer make products from the constant region only.  This is a example of a mechanism for a "point of no return."

Raff

Well, that may be a mechanism unique to lymphocytes. In the
lymphoid system we know a lot about the different stages of
maturation of the B-cells (in the same way that we know a lot about
erythroid cell development) but what we don't know is the nature of
the decision points when cells decide to be a T-helper cell as
opposed to a cytotoxic T-cell or a T-cell versus a B-cell. We are as
much in the dark as in any other system. So for a molecular
geneticist interested in decision points, a much better system is the
granulocyte/macrophage system, where one cell can be induced by a
pure protein to become a macrophage or a granulocyte, and there are
tumours that will do it. It is a very attractive system. But to
think of it in the same terms as myoblasts fusing to become myotubes,
seems to me to be a mistake. Until we know the mechanisms, it is
useful to keep them separate.

Weston

There is a problem here. Take a lymphocyte. That is specialised
in making a particular immunoglobulin. In principle, you could take
that nucleus and put it back into an egg and get it all derepressed
and let the nucleus support development all the way up. Presumably,
all the things that had been repressed will be re-expressed and there
won't have been any changes in that genome. You will make muscle and
you will make nerve, and things like that, but when it comes to
making lymphocytes, it is going to have some serious restrictions.
And so I guess what I want to talk about, is, what are those changes
that have protected the rest of the genome during the decisions that
lead downwards?

Southern

Protected is perhaps not the right word. Perhaps nothing does
happen to the rest of the genome. No dramatic changes, no
rearrangements such as happen in the immunoglobulin genes. Nothing
happens to protect it from changes, perhaps in the normal course of
events nothing does happen to the rest of the genome other than
expressing genes that are there all the time, or suppressing those
genes. You don't actually do anything so dramatic as you do in the
lymphocytes elsewhere.

Weston

You could turn it around and say if you are going to make a Type
1 or Type 2 astrocyte or an oligodendrocyte has to do with some
genetic rearrangement that are end game for that population of cells,

and the rest of the genome is protected.  That would affect the
reversibility.


## Sippel

I would like to say something about the problem of restricting.
I have some feelings against this expression.  We look at a cell that
has acquired certain features and when it develops it can express new
genes.  It looks to me, mechanistically, as if these cells gain
something.  Restricting sets of genes to be expressed would imply
different molecular mechanisms than when a cell gains the possibility
of expressing a new set of genes.


## Southern

I agree with that.


## Sippel

There is also the problem of cell polarity.  It has a big
influence on the way tissues develop.  We need good molecular models
of how polarized cells influence other cells to develop in order to
understand organ development.  What do you think is the best cellular
model for us molecular biologists to study cell polarity?


## Raff

The best studied systems are epithelial cells, that sit on basal
laminae.  There is evidence that it is the basal lamina that is
largely responsible for planning the cells.


## Saxen

Another polarised cell is of course a moving cell, a migratory
cell.  There are some very nice studies where viruses are used as
probes.


## Raff

When such cells are put on an extra-cellular matrix they organise
their cytoskeletons in such a way that they move in a directional
way.  But I don't think there are many clues as to how cells do it.

Weston

But it does strongly suggest that there are fairly rigid
structures in the cytoskeleton, which interact with the cellular
membrane.  How the cytoskeleton components erect themselves, and how
they interact with certain points on the membrane is the question.
That would maintain the polarity once it is established, but how does
it get established?


Saxen

There are other examples of a single cell becoming polarised
without having an attachment point, or moving.


Clayton

Wasn't there an experiment by Whittaker on _Fucus_ eggs which
showed that any external discontinuity, whether it was gravity, or
light, or pH or anything else, would produce a pH gradient within the
egg and the more acidic end always became the rhizoid?


Raff

It is thought to be a carbon dioxide gradient, that is maintained
by a non-homogeneous distribution of calcium pumps in the plasma
membrane.  But how is this inhomogeneous distribution of the calcium
pumps generated in the first place?


Truman

In most animal cells, nothing starts with an entirely homogeneous
environment.  I think we may be having to look for mechanisms which
maintain an inhomogeneity which is already there.  The epithelial cell
basement lamina is one and the protozoan cells surely are.  When they
divide they perpetuate their polarity.  And it takes you back to the
beginning of creation to decide, because once they have done it they
can keep on doing it.


Raff

Yes, I think that is very likely.  Another example is seen in
some snails where the handedness of the shell is transmitted as a
maternal cytoplasmic component in the egg.

Eguchi

I think another system is very suitable for studying polarity
problems.  This is the starfish embryo.  When the fertilization
membrane is removed after fertilization in vitro, the fertilized egg
divides through cleavage stages to form a two dimensional cell
cluster.  In between the eighth cleavage stage and the ninth cleavage
stage all of the cells exhibit polarity;  half of the cell surface is
adhesive and half of the cell surface is non-adhesive and such a
polarity is easily reversed when the glass surface coated with serum.
Therefore, the starfish blastomere polarity must be determined by
some intrinsic information which is easy to manipulate by some
external signal.  Such a sort of system is extremely useful for
study.  You can easily get large quantities of starfish blastomeres
and the cell populations are very homogeneous.


Weston

Well, Martin, would you like to summarise what you think are the
most important cellular biological problems for the molecular
geneticists to address?


Raff

No.  But I could make one more point.  In some invertebrates, at
least, most of the binary decisions that occur in development are
determined by a form of cytoplasmic inheritance.  In Coenorhabdytis
elegans, most subsequent cell divisions are also asymetrical.  For
example, when the fertilised egg divides, the two daughter cells are
not equivalent, so that the fates of cells are largely determined
autonomously by their lineage.  In vertebrates, on the other hand,
cell-cell interactions seem to determine cell fate and the position
of cells relative to each other at least early in development, plays
a critical part.


Yaffe

In plants, the relationship of the cells determines the fate of
the cells, there is not such a thing as determination.  In animals
it starts like that and then the determination builds up during the
ontogenesis.  There is another approach, which is to learn the
network of control of gene expression from the end product upwards.
By which I mean how the gene is expressed in terms of
differentiation, what is the relationship between the structure of
the gene and the environment in terms of cellular environment and
what are the factors, which genes control the factors.  The scope of
molecular biology may give us a probe to see the switching point.

But the molecular biologist can give us much more. What is the
strategy of activation of genes? How is a gene activated? What is
the network of controlling the genes in the system? And from this
build up and see where we meet.

## Raff

It is too late to start from scratch. In your study of the
muscle cell development, for example, there is already a good deal of
cell biological background.

## Yaffe

I do not say we are starting from scratch. I say we are starting
from the light side, where the light is, as in Jim's [Weston] story
about the drunk man.

## Hurst

In studying differentiation we usually work backwards from the
finished article and try to guess what happened.

## Weston

The only other thing I want to say is that I hope that the
molecular types are going to talk about the possible normal role of
oncogenes in cells. Because I have the feeling that that is the key
to a lot of our problems about the interactions of cells with growth
factors and things like that.

## Yaffe

Call them growth factor genes.

## Sippel

When I started to study molecular biology, I was faced with all
the phenotypes of living nature, and I was faced with an incredible
amount of literature, which I thought I had to read. And so I made
two simplifications. One was that I ordered the nature around me by
saying that the tremendous differences in phenotypes were the result
of differences in their organs and that the development of their
organs was just the result of different cell types, and that the
basis of cell differentiation was just differential gene expression.

So I just wanted to know how genes are regulated.  And I think we can say today that we are at a point where we are beginning to understand how eukaryotic genes are regulated, what molecular mechanisms are involved in their control.  The second simplication I made was how to order the enormous flood of literature.  I left out anything that was at a higher level than the cell and I ordered the literature just as a cell is organized.  Starting from the naked DNA, to DNA plus proteins, transcription and so on, I worked my way out finally to the cell membrane and its receptors.  These two simplifications had a strong impact on the way I think about differentiation.  I feel that the complex problems cell biologists are faced with can all be solved by looking at the way regulatory elements function within a cell.  To put it in the extreme: the crucial problem of differentiation can possibly be studied with regard to the question of how phage lambda regulates its life cycle.  Whether lambda is in the lysogenic or the lytic cycle can be studied in the function of a few protein: DNA interactions and a few protein: protein interactions between the molecular components of the switching element.  The way we molecular biologists think is as follows: once we can describe the elementary switches of gene regulation we only have to multiply these events and we will find out what cell differentiation is all about.  If we understand the stage- and cell-specific expression of a couple of model genes we understand cell development.  Inherent in these problems will be the chain of events leading from the membrane receptor stimuli down to the processes at the level of the genome and back again.  We are forced to think this way by the recent discoveries about oncogenes.  Oncogene products are grouped today along this signal regulation pathway.  Some of the oncogene products are related to peptide hormones, some to membrane receptors, some are components of the second messenger pathway and a few of them are nuclear proteins involved in the regulation of replication and possibly gene expression.  Important for all this is to find the molecules which have to make contact with each other all along this signal chain.  Molecules have to make contacts between cells, between receptors and cytplasmic components, between cytoplasmic components and nuclear factors and nuclear factors and DNA signal sequences.  Without these contacts no regulation processes can be understood.  This line of thinking also leads to another important point.  Where is the substratum for cell endogenous processes and where is the substratum for the plasticity of the chain of events during cell development?  Cascades of regulatory genes rattling down their programme is one part of the story.  But if you include in this programme the expression of hormone molecules and their membrane receptors we can imagine how the extracellular stimuli come into play.  At some steps an endogenous program can only go on after it has gotten its extracellular "OK" for the next step.  Most of our problems can be put into this framework even at a time when we don't understand the molecular details of all the regulatory elements involved.

Williams

The one question that keeps arising when molecular biologists
think about cellular differentiation, is the relationship between DNA
replication and switching events.  We are all on the lookout
constantly for relationships between replication and switching.  That
is why in the first part of this session I would like to clarify the
situation with respect to the requirement for DNA replication and
cellular committment.  Does Martin Raff regard his system, where
there is very little DNA replication but where two different cell
types arise, as disproving the idea of quantal cell divisions?  Or
does he regard it as a kind of maturation process?


Raff

You certainly can't disprove the quantal mitosis hypothesis with
one system but I think our results suggest that it is unlikely to be
a general rule.  There are other examples, where you do not need to
replicate DNA to make a binary choice, and get two different cell
types.  For example, in Dictyostelium discoideum, my understanding is
that the vegetative amoebae drop out of division, chemotax,
aggregate to form a slug and within the slug or prior to the slug
formation, these cells differentiate into two different cell types,
stalk and spore.  And that decision is made after they drop out of
division.


Williams

Can I come back on that?  There is now clear evidence for a
relationship between position in the cell cycle and cell fate in
Dictyostelium.  This comes from experiments where one takes
synchronous cells and asks which population of cells they contribute
to in the slug.  The observation is that the 20 or 30% of cells which
are in S and early G2 phase form 90% of the stalk cells (MacDonald
and Durston, 1984, J. Cell Sci., 66: 195-204).  The other observation
which I think relates to this question comes from Firtels laboratory
where he has shown that the Dictyostelium and in the slug where its
expression is confined to the pre-stalk region (Raymond et al., 1984,
Cell 39: 141-148).  If there is a relationship between the position
in the cell cycle and ras gene expression in Dictyostelium - as there
is believed to be in higher eukaryotes - this suggests that position
in the cell cycle may determine the fate of the cell.


Raff

So I guess the critical experiment has not been done.  The
critical experiment would be to synchronise the cell population and

then you would expect to only get one cell population.


## Williams

You do.  You don't get only one cell population, but if you
synchronise at one particular stage in the cell cycle, you produce
either very "stalky" or very "sporey" fruit (Weijer, C.J. and David,
C.N., 1984, JEEM, 82: 183).


## Raff

You can imagine there being other interpretations.  But OK let's
throw that example out.  The question is, in making the binary
decision between the choice of two differentiation pathways, do you
always need to replicate your DNA?  That is the critical question.
And the molecular geneticists will someday be able to tell us.  I
think the evidence is no.  That it is not always necessary.  And the
case we have is not 100% certain but I would guess it is about 95%
probable that the cell can choose one pathway or another without
going through DNA replication.


## Williams

Is that a pathway with a clear committment to differentiation
into two distinct cell-types?


## Raff

An astrocyte and oligodendrocyte are very different cell types.
They don't look anything alike and they don't do any of the same
things.  One wraps its plasma membrane around axons to make myelin;
the other puts feet on blood vessels.  They are certainly more
different from each other than are T and B lymphocytes.  So it
doesn't make sense to me to consider this choice as being different
from a binary decision at any other point of development.


## Allan

Couldn't you say that the event that caused the difference
happened at a stage before you could see anything?


## Raff

No.  The reason I think that is unlikely is that you can take the

whole population and make it develop along either pathway and, for a
day or two, you can then reverse the choice.  It couldn't have made
an irrevocable decision.  It is still plastic.


## Weston

Or it could have to do with the presence of both sets of
appropriate receptors.


## Weston

One of the interesting phenomena that we note is that if you take
a population that looks by all standard criteria as homogeneous and
you give it some developmental signal which you know is meant to
elicit differentiation, you don't get homogeneous differentiation,
but rather a fraction of the population differentiating.  It could be
cell-cycle related and it could be that the population that doesn't
differentiate really has another fate, another set of receptors, let
us say, that haven't been challenged.  The question then arises
whether in fact cells must already be different before the difference
is manifest because they respond differently to a given stimulus.


## Sippel

The way I look at it is as follows:  because you can switch only
between two particular states and not between any possible
alternatives tells me that previous decisions have been made.  Every
cell has gone through a particular history of events and possibly
this history of events is somehow reflected in the way its genome is
organized.  Each gene has gone through this history of developmental
processes and this path of events very likely is reflected in the way
the DNA is organized in chromatin.  Genes very likely have not only
one enhancer but maybe several of these elements - enhancers and
suppressors.  They may have a multitude of regulators, more than we
hitherto thought.  Each of these regulatory DNA sequences could react
with one or more protein components.  We have found indications for
this complexity in the case of our model gene - the gene for chicken
lysozyme.  It is possible that, in order to finally activate the
lysozyme gene in the right cell at the right differentiation step,
the gene has to go through a particular chain of events which ensured
the final structure of its chromatin, the final structure of all
necessary stable nonhistone-protein complexes.  Maybe it is the
combinatorial system of a limited number of DNA binding proteins
which can do the job for all the thousands of genes in the genome.

Yaffe

But there are some facts which do not agree with this.  For
example, Helen Blau took myogenic cells and fused them with newly
cultivated fibroblasts or amniocytes and the non-muscle cells which
fused with the fibrils under the influence of the fibrils cytoplasm,
began to produce muscle-specific proteins.  Without cell division,
she did it in the presence of cytosine arabinoside, so without any
division, the genes in the nuclei which are programmed to produce a
different pattern of differentiation became activated, the muscle-
specific genes became activated, and produced myosin-light chains,
creatine kinase and so on.  That is a very important experiment.  If
you give it all the regulatory elements, the gene can somehow change
its regulatory proteins and without any division, will become
activated.


A. Bird

There is another example of that, which is also quite dramatic.
It concerns oocytes.  There are some experiments by John Knowland
where he has taken the oestrogen receptor from the liver and injected
it into normal Xenopus oocytes and the oocytes are full of oestrogen
anyway, and so you have oestrogen and the oestrogen receptor and the
oocyte starts making vitellogenin in large quantities, and this is
quite dramatic evidence for the idea that you can take a gene and
provided you have all the bits there, regardless of its history, you
can switch it on.  Now you can say that oocytes are totipotent, but
regardless of that I think it is a dramatic example of cytoplasmic
factors being present, and all that is necessary to activate a highly
tissue-specific gene.  With reference to something that was said
earlier, the semantic problem about whether or not maturation is
different from differentiation.  It seems to me that the problem
arises because when you take a stem cell population like a red blood
cell and you do something to it, you are actually causing a branch,
because either it can go on being a cell which you call a stem cell
and that makes it sound like an exceptional case, but you are dealing
with a dividing cell in the culture, or you can make it go and branch
off and go through these maturation steps, so it isn't as though it
is going along a straight line and it goes through irrespectively,
there is in fact a branch there.  Now in the case of the cell you
were looking at, the the branch lead not to a dividing cell
population, on one side, and a differentiated cell on the other, both
branches lead to non-dividing cells.  Since in one case, they lead to
two non-dividing cells and in the other into a dividing cell or a
differentiated cell line, does that really mean that you are dealing
with two separate phenomena?  Or does it mean that they are two
aspects of the same phenomenon?

Raff

I take your point.  The main difference is that the cell I was
talking about is bipotential; it can become one of two different
types of post-mitotic cells.  But there is another situation which is
different - where a cell stops dividing and becomes, for example, a
B-lymphocyte.  After weeks, months, or years, the cell can be
activated to secrete antibody.


Weston

But to help analyse this kind of problem it seems to me that you
do need to try to establish at first, the order of the segregations
that can occur, that give rise to the intermediate cell populations.
It could be that you have a stem cell population that drops off its
various derivatives in any order at any time, or there could be a
historical sequence in a sense.  In development there could be the
generation of intermediate cell populations, defined still as
dividing cells, but which have, somehow or other, segregated out some
of their capabilities and retained some others.  It is important to
know what the order of segregation is in order to understand what is
going on.


Sippel

When we look at the nature of the regulatory elements in the
chromatin we might get an answer to many of these questions.  There
might be two kinds of mechanism.  The first is outlined by the way it
turns out steroid receptors work.  When the hormone is present,
nuclear receptor proteins occupy DNA-binding sites in the 5' flanking
regions of genes they regulate.  However, they only can occupy their
position if pre-formed chromatin structures allow them access to
their nuclear acceptor site.  The second, more important kind of
event must involve mechanisms which allow DNAase hypersensitive site
structures to be newly created in the chromatin.  Proteins involved
in this process possibly are strong DNA binding proteins.  It is my
working hypothesis that they are not capable of pushing aside
nucleosomes once chromatin has formed, but rather build up stable
protein:DNA complexes starting from naked DNA.  The best moment to do
this might be immediately after replication.  Here you would have two
very different ways in which newly expressed regulatory factors can
switch on genes.  I see these mechanisms possibly as the molecular
basis for differentiation on the one hand and determination on the
other.

Raff

That is a very good point.  But  how do you explain the Blau
experiment, where the fusion of a fibroblast and a muscle cell and
you turn on the fibroblast nucleus to make muscle specific proteins
without DNA synthesis?


Allan

How do you know it is without DNA synthesis?  When you fuse two
cells together it would surprise me if nothing in the population
divided.


Yaffe

Everything was done in the presence of labelled thymidine and the
nuclei were unlabelled and in addition she made some experiments in
which she gave some cytosine arabinoside before the experiment and in
spite of it she got muscle protein expression.


Allan

Did she look at all the nuclei?


Raff

Because the fibroblasts were human and the myotubes were mouse or
rat, she was able to identify the muscle-specific proteins with an
antibody that reacts only with human protein in a cell in which the
nuclei did not incorporate 3H-thymidine into DNA.


Sippel

This could mean that all that a fibroblast nucleus needs in order
to turn on its muscle genes is one additional protein factor.  This
muscle cell factor could react with an already pre-formed pattern of
chromatin sites which are ready to accept this factor.


Yaffe

But this gene can never be expressed in that cell.

Sippel

   Muscle genes cannot be turned on in fibroblasts because
fibroblasts never express that last necessary regulatory factor.
Nevertheless the acceptor sites in chromatin could exist as they do
in muscle cells.  It would be my suggestion to map the DNAase
hypersensitive site pattern of muscle genes in fibroblasts.  Maybe
they are all pre-formed as in muscle cells.


Yaffe

   Again we come to the question that we raised in your lecture.
Where does the specificity come in?


Weston

   The specificity comes in with the presence or absence of the
receptor or the factor.


Yaffe

   So is the factor new and the gene and all the complex totipotent?


Weston

   No, it just happens that in fibroblasts the genes are close.


Raff

   You think fibroblasts and muscle cells are so close in lineage
that the chromatin around the muscle-specific genes is very similar.


Sippel

   Yes, but that might only be true for the muscle cells and fibroblasts.


Raff

   So now we need to repeat the experiment with various different
cell types that are even more unrelated.  Suppose the same thing
happens, then what would you say?

Southern

   There is no point in trying to answer that question until someone
has done the experiment.


A. Bird

   The oocyte and the liver you would also have to say are very
close together.


Weston

   Or that the oocyte is so very special.


Hurst

   But you do not have to propose that.  Earlier you were suggesting
that during development cells may 'flash' different phenotypes . It
that is true, it could reflect the cellular nuclei 'flashing' their
chromatin in an open configuration.  Therefore, over the whole cell
population you may not detect specific DNAase sensitive sites, for
example, because the pattern of such potential sites is continually
changing until it becomes fixed in the committed and differentiated
cell.


Sippel

   Important is that chromatin, the normal nucleosomal array, is
stripped off.  This could either happen by DNA replication or perhaps
also during transcription.  So, it could be that, even without
replication, gene domains could be remodelled in their chromatin
structure.


Weston

   Operationally, what you are doing, is taking a nucleus that is at
least not completely closed down and exposing it inside a muscle cell
either to the appropriate factors or to the receptors of those
factors.


Raff

   But the question remains whether cells normally turn on whole
genetic programmes without DNA replication?  It may never happen like

that in normal development. It may be all of those cell culture
systems. But still, we at least know that it can happen - cells
don't have to replicate their DNA in order to differentiate.


## Sippel

Maybe by an atypical type of transcription which starts more
upstream.


## Raff

But there is an alternative, and that is that cells sometimes
do chose between developmental alternatives without DNA replication.


## Sippel

My view is shaped by recent findings by Don Brown's group on the
best known regulatory elements in eukaryotes, the TFIIIA factor
binding site in the 5S genes of Xenopus laevis. Transcriptionally
active protein: DNA complexes can only be formed if the factors are
given to naked DNA in advance of the addition of nucleosomes. For
other regulatory elements of gene activity we are not that far yet to
be able to study whether they function accordingly. I think that
there is a good chance that most of the remodelling of chromatin is
done after replication, but maybe not all.


## Allan

There is also the example of the globin genes and replication,
where the evidence is very strong that you do need a cycle of
replication. You cannot induce globin gene production without a
cycle of replication in Friend cells and that is done with TS
mutants, and it is also shown that you dont have to have cell
division. All you need is replication of the DNA. You can actually
have binucleate cells or cells which have two genomes worth within
the same nucleus. But it takes that to get the genes switched on.
What I was wondering about with this experiment with the fusion is,
was it a primary fibroblast?


## Yaffe

Primary amniocytes with fibroblastic cell lines.

Allan

The point I am making is if it was a cell line, then you already
know that the epsilon globin gene is already on, in fibroblast cell
lines.


Raff

Yes, but it was done with primary cells as well.


Allan

Supposing that there are certain genes that are already switched
on rather leakily and supposing that that is what you are picking up?
I am not sure that that experiment is 100% certain.


Yaffe

She took several cell types, on the other hand there are
experiments which support your view, that the naked gene is different
from the genes which is in the cells.  For example, in several cases
you can get induction of the expression of a gene if you introduce
the naked gene when the gene in the cell itself is not active.  For
example, if you gave a cell the gene for alpha 2 globulin.  This gene
is active in the liver and it responds to corticosteroids, and if you
put this gene into L cells, which have receptors for corticosteroid
but their gene does not respond to corticosteroid but if you put in
by transfection the cloned gene, the cloned gene responds to corticosteroid though the native gene remains inactive.  So these two genes
are under different control although the receptor is there.


Sippel

Both genes, the endogenous gene and the transfected gene, are in
the same cell, but they have gone through a completely different
history.  It is an open question whether the same chromatin structure
can be formed on naked DNA which is present on the endogenous gene
DNA.  I am sure that, when naked DNA comes into the cell, some DNA
binding proteins find their binding site before any reconstitution of
nucleosomal structures is possible.


Weston

Assuming that the proteins are there.

Sippel

Assuming that they are expressed.  But some of these regulatory
proteins are not able to introduce a non histone protein:DNA complex
de novo even in case the DNA replicates.  The protein I told you
about (the TGGCA-binding protein) is one such.  This protein is
present in liver cells, and, as we found out, but its binding site
6.1 kb 5' to the promoter of the lysozyme gene is not occupied.  So,
this DNA binding protein by itself is not able to initiate a stable
nonhistone protein: DNA complex.  It looks as if it needs the help of
other proteins not present in liver cells.

Clayton

Can I ask a very naive question?  The 5' untranslated region of a
gene may be really quite long, and there are particular sites now
which can be pinpointed in it, but what about all the spaces between
these known sites? Are they occupied by other regulatory features
which we don't yet know or is it that we need spaces in order to fit
in these proteins?  For instance, if you were to clip the five prime
region and join up all the specific sites  that we know,close
together.  Would they be unable to accept any of the regulatory
proteins, because there would be no space?

Sippel

The long DNA spacer sequences between regulatory DNA signal
sequences may contain either nonfunctional DNA sequences or so far
not identified new regulatory signals.  When we first mapped 5 DNAase
hypersensitive sites in the 5' flanking chromatin of the lysozyme
gene of the induced oviduct I thought they marked all the regulatory
sites there are.  But when we looked at the same region in
macrophages, which also express lysozyme but under a different
control than in oviduct cells, we found a different set of hypersensitive sites.  So, there were in toto more regulatory sites than
I had originally expected.  At present there are a total of 6
different sites in the first 3000 bp upstream from the promoter in
different cells, roughly another signal sequence every 500 bp.  My
feeling is that these long distance acting regulatory elements act by
making protein: protein contacts with each other.  In this case it
would be unimportant what the length of DNA is between the binding
sites of regulatory proteins, the DNA would just loop out.  Such a
model would have strong evolutionary advantages because various
regulatory signals could act independently of their exact location
with respect to each other.

Bird

    Is your feeling about the spaces between the regulatory regions
and their distances apart a feeling?  Or is it something for which
you have experimental evidence that the distances are, or are not,
important?

Sippel

    We have presently only weak evidence for this model.  In case of
the mouse mammary tumor long terminal repeat promoter we have
evidence that the TGGCA protein interacts with the TATA box binding
protein.  If this is so in the MMTV promoter, in which both DNA
binding protein sites are directly adjacent to each other, why
couldn't it be so in the case of the lysozyme gene, in which the DNA
binding sites for the same two proteins are roughly 6 kb apart?
Such a DNA loop-out model for the structure of the regulatory
elements can be studied in gene transfer experiments.  We have made a
mutation of the MMTV site for the TGGCA protein.  This mutant DNA can
no longer bind the TGGCA protein in vitro and it is a strong
"promoter-down" mutation in gene transfer experiments.

Weston

    Are the mutants deletions?

Sippel

    The mutant is a 3 bp insertion.

Weston

    It suggests that there are, in a sense, forbidden locations for
these regions: if they are close enough to one another they are all
right, if they are an intermediate distance, then you cannot get the
flexibility of the intervening DNA to get them back together again.

Sippel

    The way the DNA is wrapped around these DNA complexes determines
how far the protein binding sites can be apart from each other.
Longer and longer distances may have little effect.

Weston

But there would be a distance that is too short.


Sippel

Yes, I think so.


Allan

Are you suggesting that the proteins find each other from very long distances away by affinity or is it by a mechanism?


Sippel

Maybe by facilitated diffusion. The linear structure has to fold into a three-dimensional structure.


Raff

So protein finds protein and then DNA?


Sippel

No, that's not the way I think it happens. First, the binding proteins might find their respective individual sites and then they might find each other and fold up into a more complex structure.


Clayton

If they don't diffuse readily, then you want them made near at hand. Are these proteins small or very big?


Weston

What do you mean diffuse readily?


Clayton

Well, if they are made on polysomes in the cytoplasm, they have to get back to the nucleus. You obviously need quite a lot of these in any cell, or else they can home specifically.

Weston

   They almost always have some sort of facilitated diffusion, but
very large components move very rapidly between nucleus and
cytoplasm.  So I don't think that is a problem.

Clayton

   Perhaps they can only move in after prophase.

Sippel

   Regulatory proteins would have a hard time to find their acceptor
sites on the genome if their concentration were far below 10,000
molecules per nucleus.

Clayton

   The reason why I ask if some of them are very small is that small
peptides do not need to be synthesised on the polysomes.  Can we be
sure that small peptide assembly can't happen in the nucleus?  But if
they are big, then there is the transport problem.  Can I ask another
question, which is about the other end of the molecule?  If you
consider alpha crystallins in all vertebrates, the basic chain which
is 175 aminoacids long, is coded for by a 10S message, in, I think,
every vertebrate that has ever been looked at.  The acidic chain,
which is actually a couple of aminoacids shorter, is coded for by a
much longer message, of 14S, in most vertebrates, except for
amphibians, where for some reason, it is 10S, so you have got
amphibian species in which the two proteins and their messages are
the same order of magnitude.  Yet in other species one of them, for
some function which must be very strongly conserved, has got this
immense 3' region.  Can one use comparisons of that sort?  I mean,
you have been talking about lysozyme in different tissues: maybe one
can also look at species comparisons in order to get some idea about
some of the possible functions of non-coding regions.

Williams

   I think that while there is no strong evidence yet, it becomes
clear from the sort of evidence that David Yaffe was talking about
that comparisons of 3' prime non-coding regions they are much more
conserved than one would expect.  In fact I dont think he touched on
all the examples.  There is an example from Steve Higgins in Leeds
where they looked at two genes in the seminal vesicle in which the
protein coding regions are almost totally diverged, but the 5' prime

non-coding regions and the 3' prime non-coding regions are almost
totally conserved.  So I think that in the long term we can hope to
understand what those sequences are doing, but at the present, the
best bet is that they may be involved in messenger RNA stabilisation
or in translational efficiency.  Obviously those two things are
interrelated, in that messenger RNA stability may be affected by the
intrinsic translatability of the messenger RNA.


## Clayton

May be this isn't quite the whole story because in all lenses you
have to have very stable messenger.  It can't be that the amphibians
don't need a messenger as stable for the acidic alpha chain as other
vertebrates.  You just have to have a stable message in the lens for
all the crystallins.


## Williams

Strange things happen in evolution.  Possibly the difference is
just that the polyadenelation site has been mutated in the one
instance, and not in the other.  So that you just have a much longer
3' prime non-coding region.  Is there evidence for conservation of
sequences in these 3' non-coding regions or is it just a difference
in the messenger RNA length?


## Clayton

Wilfried, [de Jong] I don't think anyone has sequenced very many
of these, have they?


## de Jong

The 3' noncoding sequences have been published for the $\alpha$-
crystallin A messenger RNAs of rat, mouse and frog (Moorman et al.,
1981, Nucl. Acid. Res. 9: 4813-4822; King et al., 1982, Science 215,
985-987; Tomarev et al., 1983, FEBS Lett. 162: 47-51).


## Yaffe

And there is no conservation at the 3' prime?


## de Jong

Yes, between rat and mouse there is conservation of the extreme

length of about 550 nucleotides in the 3' noncoding region of the
α-crystallin A messenger RNA, and they only show 32 base changes and
24 gap events in this sequence.  But the corresponding frog messenger
RNA has a much shorter 3' noncoding sequence of only 130 nucleotides,
which shows no detectable homology anymore with that of rat and
mouse.

## Williams

There is one experiment which I briefly described in the first
session that is relevant to several issues that we have discussed.
When the immunoglobulin heavy chain enhancer was linked with an
assayable gene it was expressed in two different stages of B cell
differentiation with 100% efficiency, yet the messenger RNA was
found to be present at a 20 fold different level in the two cell
types.  This says two things.  Firstly it is evidence for RNA
stabilization in the B cell lineage and this may be a role of non-
coding regions.  It also brings us back to something that we were
discussing in the first session.  Can one take tissue specific
enhancers, as they become identified, and look for the earliest
possible cell in the lineage which recognises and activates genes
under the control of that enhancer?  Is this going to be a useful
thing to the cell biologist and can we actually identify the proteins
that interact with that enhancer?

## Anon

At a branch point, the protein might be in very few cells

## Weston

Operationally you can do the experiment by taking a given gene
with its specific promoters and enhancers and just sticking it into a
variety of different cells, and asking does it work?

## Sippel

Maybe it's better to look for the presence of specific DNA
binding factors in a particular cell rather than to ask whether a
transfected indicator gene gets turned on.  The latter might demand a
lot of different factors.  If one introduces merely a single signal
sequence and asks whether it is able to create a DNAase
hypersensitive chromatin structure when transfected into the cell
to be tested, this would be a simpler assay.

Allan

If you transfect a gene into a number of different cell types,
most genes are on in most of the cell types at a very low level, so
in a transfection experiment of this sort, if you put any old gene
into a fibroblast, you can detect transcription of that gene, so I
don't really see how that approach is going to do anything.


Hurst

Not always.  You can put some genes into a lot of different cell
types and get no detectable expression.  That is certainly true for
the amylase genes.


Raff

How many experiments like that have been done?


Allan

All the early gene transfection experiments were putting genes
into L cells and everyone got low level transcription, and if you
take out mini chromosomes from a lot of cells, they have got the
specific hypersensitive sites on them. I think you have to be a bit
more selective.


Williams

It is quite obvious from what is being done that it will be
possible to identify relatively short pieces of DNA which are only
efficiently transcribed in a particular cell type.  Although there
may be low constitutive levels of expression of some genes, the
enhancer will have the property of elevating expression from
promoters to which it is coupled when introduced into the correct
cell type.


Allan

Yes, but that is slightly different from what you were saying,
that is, looking for the proteins that bind to the sites.


Raff

Everybody has been using the word enhancer.  Does that mean that

all of the DNA sequences that act in this way to enhance the
efficiency of the promoter, actually behave as enhancers in the sense
that they can work when inverted and they can work at large
distances, or are there other types of control sequences that have
already been defined?  And if so, can you tell us what they are?


## Sippel

Work in yeast has shown that there are similar elements which
suppress gene activity.  It is possible that there are such "blocker"
sequences also in the gene regions in higher eukaryotes in order to
add another level of regulation.


## Hurst

There is also some evidence from Chambon's laboratory that a
protein that stimulates transcription can, in other circumstances,
also repress expression.  In general the E1A gene of adenovirus can
act in _trans_ to increase transcription from a co-transfected  β-
globin gene, for example (Green et al., (1983) Cell, 35: 137-148).
However E1A products can also repress the activity of promoters
linked to the SV40 or polyoma virus enhancers (Borrelli et al.,
(1984) Nature 312: 608-612).  It is perhaps not entirely clear what
these observations are telling us but it seems that modulation of
gene expression may be achieved through multifunctional proteins that
can coordinately activate some promoters while suppressing others.


## A. Bird

Our knowledge of these things is very primitive.  I don't think
one can quite list all the levels of control, stop at the DNA and
say that this is the only place where one cant be fooled.  I think
one can still be fooled at that level too, and because an enhancer
is really a rather vague operational definition, which has actually
undergone a certain amount of drift since it first appeared.  Now it
is very heavily contaminated with a model about what these things do
in terms of being tissue-specific, all-important governing sites for
binding proteins.  It is probably the same in the cell biology: one
has to constantly be aware of pitfalls because we don't actually know
very much of what enhancers do.  We have a few assays, but they are
actually unreliable.


## Sippel

There are groups working on DNA binding proteins which can bind
to enhancer elements.  It is very important to get all the components

isolated so that one can study the molecular mechanism of action in vitro.

A. Bird

That is not the origin of the problem, as you sketched it at the beginning. The important question is how the hypersensitive sites or the protein actually gets there, that is the basic problem. The fact that there is a protein at a particular site is not necessarily an unambiguous piece of evidence that the gene is committed to something. I just think that our knowledge is much less that the words which we use implies.

Raff

The words "Tissue-specific" are wrong by the way, one really means cell-type specific, no?

A. Bird

Could I ask the cell biologists about how different Drosophila and nematode development are from vertebrate development and what implications that has for people studying gene regulation? When you look at the ancient stuff about mosaic eggs and regulatory eggs, do we have a fact that you can take a nematode and do a cell lineage from the fertilized egg right to the adult and count every cell and every cell division and you alluded earlier that there was something fundamentally different about the development in the nematode, and possibly you were including Drosophila. Can one say anything about what must be different at the level at which genes are controlled? Is it that in the fertilized egg of a nematode or a Drosophila the positional information in the egg which is somehow laid down archi- tecturally in the egg is soaked up by a particular cell in a particular position once, and then all its genes have their fates mapped out in a particular inflexible sequence, and that this is totally different from what happens in vertebrates, or is it a question of degree and the positional information that is in the egg in the vertebrate doesn't only occur in the egg, but you get pulses of positional information which depend on previous ones in the vertebrate, whereas you only get one in the invertebrate? When you are studying invertebrate genes and the way they are switched on, are you looking for the same things as when you are studying vertebrate genes, and is there something which suggests that you are studying things that belong to different worlds?

Raff

It depends at what level you are asking the question.  If you are
asking the question at the level of molecular genetic control then I
think there is no answer - they could be the same.  But if you are
asking the question on the cellular level, then I think in most cases
the mechanisms are different.  In nematodes, cell fate is usually
determined only by what "cytoplasmic" components the cell inherits
from the mother cell, while in vertebrates, cell fate seems to be
largely determined by cell-cell interactions.


Truman

But it is also true that there is diversity within invertebrates.


Weston

It is largely just a question of timing of the segregation from
the nuclei of a certain cytoplasmic package during cleavage.  The
implication from what Martin [Raff] said was that there is no such
thing as inductive interactions, cell-cell interactions and messages
diffusing from one cell to another in Coenorhabdytis elegans.  That
is not so.


Raff

It is true that in some cases, cell fate in Coenorhabdytis
elegans is determined by cell-cell interactions, but it is the
exception, rather than the rule.  In most cases, if you destroy a
cell's neighbours it will develop normally.


Weston

Don't you treasure your exceptions?  To go back to the egg
business, I think it is best to look in two invertebrates.  Look at
the mollusc egg and the sea urchin egg.  The mollusc and the annelid
are said to be determinative in their development where everything is
programmed on the basis of the first cell division but in the sea
urchin it is supposed to be regulative, but what that amounts to is
asking when during the initial cleavage stages does some important
cytoplasmic component become sequestered away from other nuclei.  In
the so-called regulative system, the sea urchin, it happens later,
and in the so-called determinative system - the annelid or the
mollusc, it happens earlier.

Truman

But in the annelid there is great plasticity later on.

Weston

Exactly so.  I think it is just a spectrum of partitioning of the regulatory proteins that may or may not already exist, put in there during oogenesis, and the nuclei that are going to respond to these components.  It either happens efficiently and quickly or it happens more slowly.  That is the difference between the two types.

Sippel

The Drosophila homeotic gene products must be members of an early regulatory cascade.  In the Drosophila egg, before the first cell divisions, the membrane must have some position determining function on nuclei which come close to it.

Raff

Why do you think the information is in the membrane?  It could be in the cortex, for example.

Sippel

Yes, it's the cortex.  The early segmentation genes are activated in a patterned way.  There is the suggestion that the products of these genes are DNA-binding proteins and that homologue genes make pattern formation in vertebrates.

Clayton

You do get homeotic conversions in mammals certainly, in things like the conversion of one particular vertebra type to another vertebra.

Weston

Well there is segmentation in the embryonic axis, but that is slightly different from what you were looking for.

Yaffe

It may be laid down during oogenesis.


Weston

So then you just have to go back to the follicle cells and ask
are they differentially active?


Yaffe

I would like to discuss another problem that has not been
brought up during the meeting.  It seems that the control of gene
expression is much more diversified and maybe it is still being
developed and we are used to all kinds of tricks in biology.  We know
that some genes are regulated by methylation, other genes are not.
Many genes are regulated as we discussed today, but another class of
regulation is that the same gene produces different messengers by
differential splicing.  Again it is something that is quite new, but
very fascinating I think.  There are some proteins or isozymes which
are formed by the same gene.  It is a very strange economy.  And
another protein which is manufactured in the same cell at the same
stage is produced with classical regulation.  Myosin light chain 1
and 3 are produced by the same gene, while myosin light chain 2 has
separate genes.  Troponins are the same: there is one gene which
produces 5 or 6 different troponins by different splicing, and there
is an example of calcitonin which is produced in one cell type and
another protein of apparently completely different function which is
not known yet is produced in the nervous system, and another
neuropeptide - the whole of it is produced by the same gene, so we
have to consider that maybe the regulation is much more variable
than we anticipated before.


Raff

Why do you say that there isn't the same variability or precedent
for it in cell biology?  I think there is.  If you look at the
simplest hormonal system, like epinephrin, it turns out there are 3
or 4 or 5 different receptors, two different cells having the same
receptors respond in totally different ways.  Everything suggests
enormous diversity even in the simplest systems, so I think you
would have predicted that in gene control, that everything that
could be used will be used in one way or another.

<u>Yaffe</u>

I am not denying that there is similar complexity in other
levels of organisation, but it seems that the regulation of genes is
very complex and there are many ways.  It is not a single principle
for all genes.

# QUANTITATION AND LOCALIZATION OF CHICK δ-CRYSTALLIN GENE TRANSCRIPTION IN DEVELOPING NON-LENS TISSUE

D.J. Bower[+], J-C. Jeanny[*], L.H. Errington and R.M. Clayton

Department of Genetics
University of Edinburgh
West Mains Road, Edinburgh, EH9 3JN, U.K.

+ MRC Clinical and Population Cytogenetics Unit
Western General Hospital, Crewe Road, Edinburgh

* INSERM, Unité de Recherches Gérontologiques
U.118, 29 rue Wilhem, 75016 Paris, France

The main protein of the pre-hatching chick is -crystallin. There are two -crystallin genes, (Bhat and Piatigorsky, 1979) and their sequences are similar enough to cross-hybridise under the most stringent conditions.

While the lens is the only tissue in which -crystallin is very abundant, lower levels are detectable in regions of the embryo midbrain and in the embryo epiphysis, (future pineal), and adenohypophysis (part of the future pituitary). For further discussion, see Kondoh et. al., and Clayton,(this volume). Quite substantial amounts of -crystallin RNA are found in the embryo retina, (Agata et. al., 1983, Bower et. al.,1983a); and in the 3.5 day embryo, the -crystallin RNA is localized in cells on the inner border of the retina, in the area occupied by the putative future glial cells, and is mainly, but not entirely nuclear, (Bower et. al., 1983b).

Here we show (Figures 1 and 2) that in the 4 day and 6 day embryo, δ-crystallin transcripts are still found in a subset of cells of the NR, and predominantly in the nuclei of these cells.

Smaller amounts of δ-crystallin RNA have also been detected in some non-head tissues which are not known to transdifferentiate - heart, lung, kidney and liver (Bower et al., 1983b). In contrast to

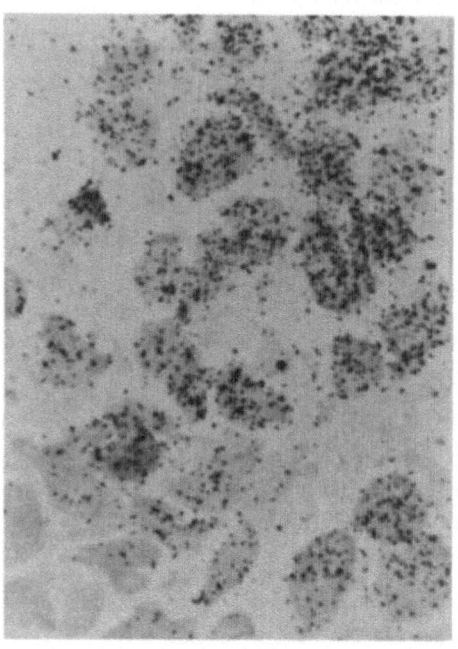

Fig. 1   Squash of 4 day chick neural retina, fixed and hybridised
         in situ to 3H pM56, a δ-crystallin cDNA clone.   Original magn.
         x 100.

the lens and other head tissues described previously, these tissues
are derived from mesoderm and endoderm.   In situ hybridisation to
squashes of embryonic heart tissue (Figures 3-5) show that δ-
crystallin transcripts are abundant in small clusters of cells,
chiefly in the nuclei, and undetectable in the surrounding cells.   The
unlabelled cells are similar in morphology and staining properties to
the labelled cells, ruling out the possibility that labelling is due
to non-specific binding of probe to cells of a particular type, as has
been reported with blood cells.   In addition, H-pBR322, the plasmid
moiety of pM56, was hybridised in parallel to squashes of heart and NF
and gave no labelling.

The relative amounts of δ-crystallin transcripts at different
points of development and their size classes were assessed from RNA
blots of embryonic chick heart, midbrain and NR, compared with day old
hatched (21 day) chick lens RNA (Figures 6 and 7).   The relative

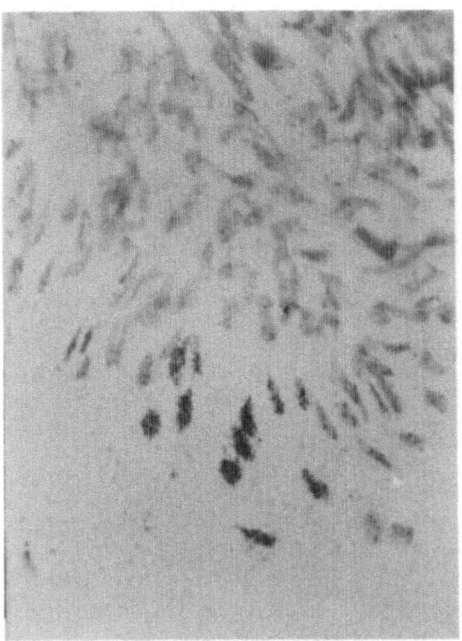

Figure 2.    Squash of 6 day chick neural retina fixed and hybridised
to 3H pM56.  Original magn. x 40.

amounts of δ-crystallin transcripts remained constant, with slight
variations between individual preparations of each age class.   In
heart and midbrain δ-crystallin transcripts were present at about 0.02
- 0.04% of the level present in 21 day lens; this allows for the
twenty-fold purification of polyA+ RNA relative to total RNA.   In NR
(Figure 7), there was about 2% of the level in 21 day lens at 17 and
23 days of development.  Preliminary results indicate that this is
very little less than in 7 day NR.  The size classes of NR δ-
crystallin transcripts at 7 days (not shown), 17 and 23 days (Figure
7) and polyA+ 7 day heart RNA were similar; the most abundant species
was 5.2kb, compared with about 1600 nucleotides for 21 day lens RNA.
In the non-lens tissues faint bands of larger material were present,
and several smaller bands including one which comigrated with the
major lens δ-crystallin mRNA (Figure 7, lane 4).

     All the RNA preparations used for data discussed thus far were
made using tissue which had been speedily extracted and immediately

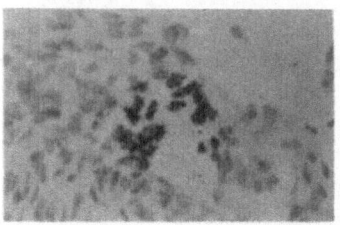

Fig. 3   Squash of 5 day chick heart fixed and hybridised to 3H pM56. x
40.

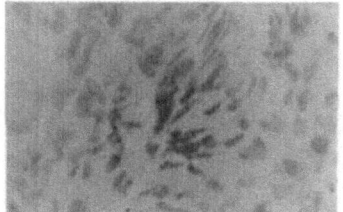

Fig. 4   As Figure 3.

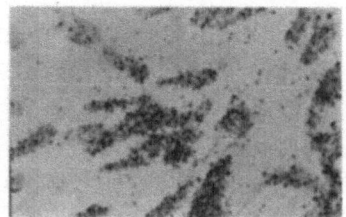

Fig. 5   Detail of Figure 4 at x 100.

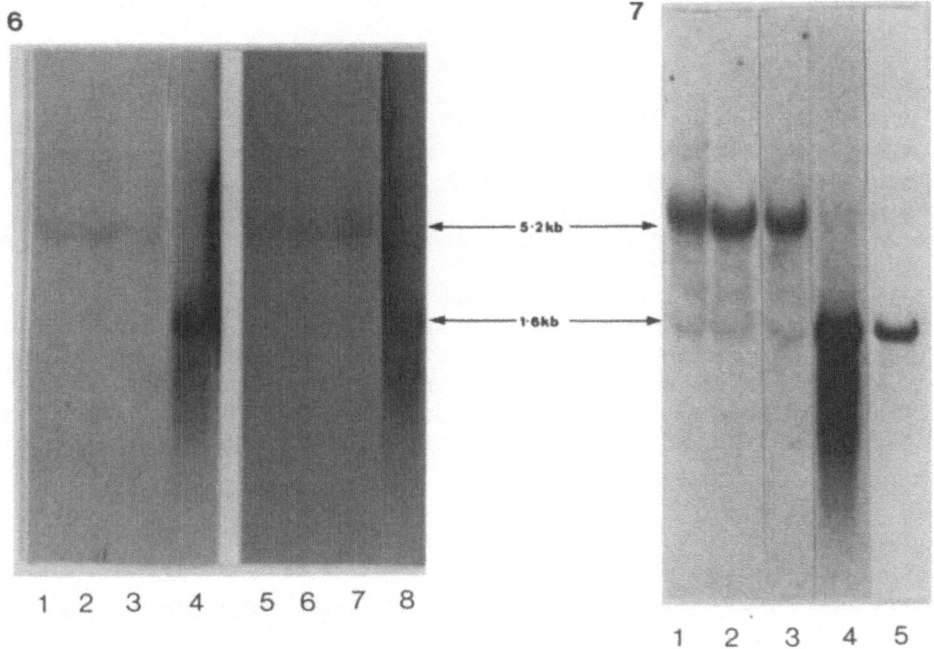

Figure 6.   RNA electrophoresed through formaldehyde-agarose gels,
blotted and hybridised to 32P-pM56.   One day exposure.
    Lane 1:   10 μg of 21 day chick heart poly A+ RNA.
    Lane 2:   10 μg of 17 day chick heart poly A+ RNA.
    Lane 3:   10 μg of 7 day chick heart poly A+ RNA.
    Lane 4:   200ng of 21 day chick lens total RNA.
    Lane 5:   10 μg of 21 day chick midbrain poly A+ RNA.
    Lane 6:   10 μg of 17 day chick midbrain poly A+ RNA.
    Lane 7:   10 μg of 7 day chick midbrain poly A+ RNA.
    Lane 8:   200ng of 21 day chick lens total RNA.

Figure 7.   RNA electrophoresed through formaldehyde-agarose gels,
blotted and hybridised to 32P-pM56.      Exposure 5 days.
    Lane 1:   10 μg of 24 day chick neural retina total RNA.
    Lane 2:   10 μg of 17 day chick neural retina total RNA.
    Lane 3:   10 μg of 7 day chick heart poly A+ RNA.
    Lane 4:   1 μg of 21 day chick lens total RNA.
    Lane 5:   10 μg of 8 day chick neural retina total RNA,
               incubated in CMF for 15 mins. before RNA extraction.

homogenised in denaturing buffer.  However, when 8 day embryo NR was
incubated in CMF medium for 15 minutes prior to RNA extraction, the
δ-crystallin RNA was processed to the size of the main δ-crystallin
mRNA of lens (Figure 7, lane 5).  This implies that NR has lens-like
δ-crystallin processing capacity, and the transcripts are processible,

but that this capacity is inhibited in vivo.

METHODS

PM56 is a chick δ-crystallin cDNA clone, containing sequence which hybridises exclusively to the two δ-crystallin genes and their transcripts (Bower et al., 1982). It contains no repetitive sequence and shows no tendency to bind weakly to ribosomal RNA or DNA (Bower et al., 1983b).

Squashes were performed according to the method of Sandritter et al., (1966). RNA extraction was by the method of Chirgwin et al., (1979). Formaldehyde-agarose gel electrophoresis, transfers and hybridisation were as described in Bower et al., (1982). In situ hybridisation and autoradiography as described in Bower et al., (1983a).

ACKNOWLEDGEMENTS

This work was supported by a programme grant from the Medical Research Council to R.M. Clayton.   J-C. Jeanny was the recipient of a Royal Society Fellowship.

REFERENCES

Agata, K., Yasuda, K. and Okada, T.S., 1983, Gene coding for a lens-specific protein, δ-crystallin is transcribed in non-lens tissues of chicken embryos. Dev. Biol., 100:222.
Bhat, S.P. and Piatigorsky, J., 1979, Molecular cloning and partial characterisation of δ-crystallin cDNA sequences in a bacterial plasmid. Proc. Natl. Acad. Sci., USA, 76: 3299-3303.
Bower, D.J., Errington, L.H., Wainwright, N.R., Sime, C., Morris, S. and Clayton, R.M. 1982, Cytoplasmic RNA sequences complementary to cloned chick δ-crystallin cDNA show size heterogeneity. Biochem. J., 204: 339-344.
Bower, D.J., Errington, L.H., Cooper, D.N., Morris, S. and Clayton, R.M., 1983a, Chicken lens δ-crystallin gene expression and methylation in several non-lens tissues. Nucleic Acids Res., 11: 2513-2527.
Bower, D.J., Errington, L.H., Pollock, B.J., Morris, S. and Clayton, R.M. 1983b, The pattern of expression of chick δ-crystallin genes in lens differentiation and transdifferentiating cultured tissues. EMBO J., 2: 333-338.
Chirgwin, J.M., Przybyla, A.E., MacDonald, R.J. and Rutter, W.J. 1979, Isolation of biologically active ribonucleic acid from sources enriched in ribonuclease. Biochemistry, 18: 5294-5299.
Clayton, R.M., Extra lenticular crystallins,(this volume.)

Kondoh, H., Hayashi, S., Okazaki, K., Yasuda, K. and Okada, T.S.,
    Tissue-specific expression of cloned chicken crystallin genes in
    mammalian cells,(this volume.)
Sandritter, W., Pilny, V., Novakova, V. and Kiefer, G., 1966, Zur
    problematic der gewebs praperation fur cytophotometrische
    messungen.  Histochemie, 7: 1-7.

# IDENTIFICATION AND CHARACTERIZATION OF A CHICK αA$_2$ CRYSTALLIN GENOMIC CLONE AND PRELIMINARY IDENTIFICATION OF A CHICK β- CRYSTALLIN cDNA CLONE

L.H. Errington, D.J. Bower,* and R.M. Clayton

Department of Genetics
University of Edinburgh
West Mains Road
Edinburgh EH9 3JN

* MRC Clinical Population and Cytogenetics Unit
Western General Hospital
Crewe Road
Edinburgh

We selected 24 clones from a λ charon 4A chicken genomic library (a gift from R.Axel) screened with cDNA made from day old chick lens total RNA. The 15 most strongly hybridizing clones carried δ-crystallin sequences overlapping each other to cover the whole 20kb region of the two tandemly arranged δ-crystallin genes.

The other nine selected clones did not hybridize to a full length cDNA δ-crystallin clone. At least one non-vector EcoR1 fragment from each of these non-δ clones cross hybridized under stringent washing conditions to one of the non-δ clones selected called L21a, showing that they all contained sequences from the same or closely related gene region.

Translations of hybrid selected RNA with two of these clones (L21a and L9a) synthesised predominantly one exogenous protein product running in the same position as the faster migrating in vitro and in vivo synthesised α-crystallin (Fig. 1). There are two α-crystallin primary gene products in vertebrates named αA$_2$ and αB$_2$ (acidic and basic referring respectively to their running positions in IEF gels). αA$_2$ migrates faster in SDS acrylamide gels in all those vertebrates characterized so far (which does not definitively include chicken). Current experiments with 2D gels (not shown here) show conclusively that the translation product from mRNA selected with these clones is αA$_2$ -crystallin.

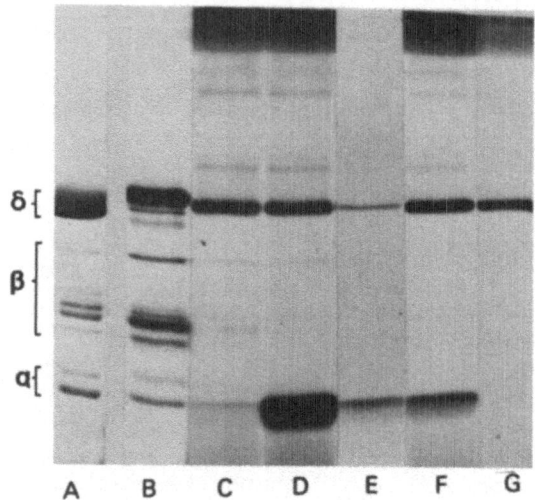

Fig. 1    Hybrid selected translation products of RNA bound and eluted
          at various temperatures from clone L21a.  Lanes A, C, D, E, F,
          G are autoradiographs of SDS acrylamide separated, $^{35}$S
          labelled translation products, (lane B is stained day old
          chick lens unlabelled accumulated protein).  Lane A, PolyA +
          day old lens RNA.  Lane C, 60$^{\circ}$C eluted RNA, lane D, 80$^{\circ}$C
          eluted RNA.  Lane E, shorter exposure of 80$^{\circ}$C eluted RNA
          autoradiograph.  Lane F, 100$^{\circ}$C elution.  Lane G, no RNA added.
          Lane E indicates the endogenous translation system product.


        Positively selected mRNA eluted at the lowest temperature (60$^{\circ}$C)
gave no $\alpha B_2$ translation products indicating relatively low cross
homology of the two $\alpha$-crystallin mRNA sequences.  This reflects the
relatively low intra species amino acid homology of the $\alpha A_2$ and $\alpha B_2$
chains (approx. 55% in chick) than interspecies homology of the $\alpha A_2$
chain (85% between calf and chick) that has resulted since $\alpha$-
crystallin gene duplication.

        Hybridisation of the non-$\delta$ clones to total lens mRNA (Fig. 2a,
lane H) always gave the same pattern, a major band of approx. 1650n.t.
and several smaller bands showing that all the nine clones are $\alpha A_2$
genomic clones (and that none of these clones detect any actively
transcribed genes other than $\alpha A_2$).  The 1650n.t. $\alpha A_2$ message compares
with the 1250/1300 $A_2/\alpha A_2^{ins}$ rat mRNA, the 1420 n.t. mouse $\alpha A$ mRNA and
the 700-800 n.t. frog $\alpha A_2$ (which lacks the long 3' non-translated
region found in the others).  Our sizing is however only approximate.
$\delta$-crystallin mRNA runs on the same gels with an apparent molecular
weight of 2000n.t. (Fig. 2b, lane H), but has since been sized at 1570
n.t. plus a short polyA tail of approx. 50-100n.t.  Since $\alpha A_2$ message
runs just below $\delta$-crystallin mRNA, its size may well be smaller than
1650n.t.

α-crystallin protein has previously been detected in freshly dissected neural retina from the same strain (Hy-1) of 8 day embryonic chicks (de Pomerai et al., 1977).  We found that hybridisation of αA2 clone L18b to neural retina RNA from 8 day chick embryos (Northern transfers, Fig. 2a, lane A) detected very small traces of the major αA2 RNA and in one single preparation, traces of an additional higher molecular weight band were just visible.  This compares to our previous finding of a relatively stronger signal with a δ-crystallin cDNA clone to the same RNA (8 day NR embryo), but this may be a result of the relatively small amount of coding sequence in the αA2 genomic clone ( 3%) separated probably by introns compared to the δ-crystallin cDNA clone pM56 coding sequence ( 12%) present in one contiguous piece.

RNA from transdifferentiating neural retina showed substantial quantities of mature αA2 crystallin mRNA at 7 days, with equal amounts of a larger probable precursor (Fig. 2a, lane B).  Later stages show no more of the precursor molecule and levels of the mature αA2 mRNA do not increase significantly even up to 42 days of culture.

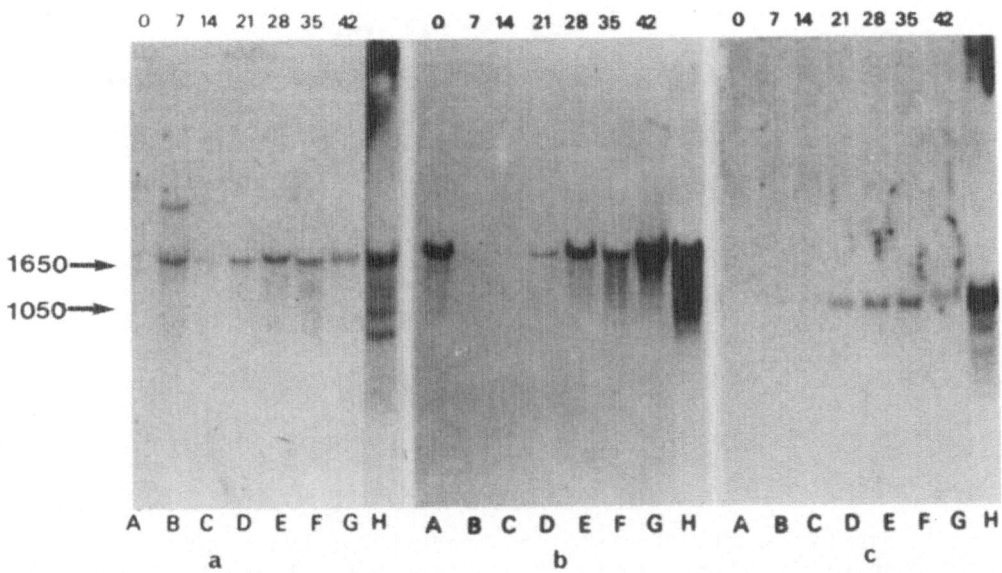

Figs. 2 a,b and c  Transdifferentiating neural retina RNA hybridised
        to αA2 - crystallin genomic clone L18b (Fig. 2a), β-crystallin
        clone pM56 (Fig. 2b) and β-crystallin cDNA clone 026 (Fig.
        2c).  In each figure lane A contains 15μg of freshly dissected
        8 day embryonic neural retina and lanes B-G contain 15μg of
        freshly dissected 8 day neural retina cultured for 7, 14, 21,
        28, 35, and 42 days.  Lane H contains day old lens RNA.

   This corresponds with the slightly later appearance ( 12 days)
and almost constant levels after 26 days of culture of α-crystallin
protein (detected by antibodies) found with cultured chick NR of the
same species and embryonic age (de Pomerai et al., 1977).  This result
compares with the relatively later appearance of δ-crystallin RNA
around 14 days (Fig. 2b, lane C) and of δ- crystallin protein around
15 days (de Pomerai et al., 1977).  Whilst in the lens itself δ-
crystallin is detectable before α- crystallin the reverse is the case
for NR derived lentoid cells.  Our results show this to be due to the
order of appearance of the RNA transcripts rather than to preferential
translation.

   A non δ-cDNA clone called 026 made from day old lens mRNA by the
method of Bower et al., (1982) has been partially characterized by
hybrid selected RNA translation (Fig. 3).  At the lowest temperature
of elution the primary translation product corresponded to the 34Kd β
(lane C) - at the highest temperature of elution the only visible
translation product corresponded to the 25Kd β (lane F).  The 80°C
eluted translated RNA (lane D, E) gave a variety of translation
products.  Short exposure of the autoradiograph (lane E) shows that

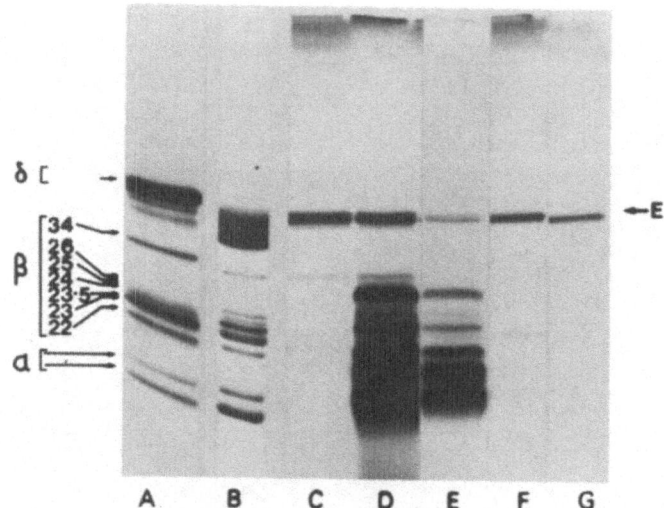

Fig. 3  Hybrid selected translation products of RNA bound and eluted
        at various temperatures from clone 026.  Lanes A, C, D, E, F,
        G are autoradiographs of SDS acrylamide separated, $^{35}$S
        labelled translation products (lane B is stained day old chick
        lens unlabelled accumulated protein).  Lane A, PolyA + day old
        lens RNA.  Lane C, 60°C eluted RNA. Lane D, 80°C eluted RNA.
        Lane E, shorter exposure of 80°C eluted RNA autoradiograph.
        Lane F, 100°C elution. Lane G, no RNA added.  E indicates the
        endogenous translation system product.

the major bands do not correspond closely to the normal in vitro products found with total polyA+ RNA. It is possible that an excessive amount of hybrid selected RNA might have resulted in incomplete translation products.

This clone probably corresponds to the 25Kd β-crystallin clone isolated by Hejtmancik and Piatigorsky (1983) which cross hybridized to other β-crystallin probes. These authors also found that a 35Kd β-crystallin clone cross-hybridised only to the 25Kd β- crystallin. Preliminary restriction analysis of this clone suggests that it is the 25Kd β-crystallin cDNA clone. Hybridisation of 026 to total lens mRNA gave a major band of approximately 1050n.t. (Fig. 2c, lane H) in accordance with the message sizes previously found for chicken β-crystallins. RNA from freshly dissected neural retina (Fig. 2c, lane A), in which low levels of β-crystallin protein have previously been detected (de Pomerai et al 1977) gave no detectable hybridisation, though this could be due to the relatively poorer hybridisation obtained with some blots. Fully processed RNA with no visible precursors appeared at 21 days of NR culture and increased gradually up to 35 days of culture (lane F) in accordance with a rise in protein levels found by de Pomerai et al. (1977). Further characterization of this clone is in progress.

REFERENCES

Bower, D.J., Errington, L.H., Wainwright, N.R., Sime, C., Morris, S. and Clayton, R.M., 1981, Cytoplasmic RNA sequences complementary to cloned chick δ-crystallin cDNA show size heterogeneity, Biochem. J., 201: 339-344.
de Pomerai, D.I., Pritchard, D.J. and Clayton, R.M., 1977, Biochemical and immunological studies of lentoid formation in cultures of embryonic chick neural retina and day-old chick lens epithelium, Dev. Biol., 60: 416-427.
Hejtmancik, J.F. and Piatigorsky, J., 1983, Diversity of β-crystallin mRNAs of the chicken lens (hybridisation, analysis, with cDNA clones). J. Biol. Chem. 258: 3382-3387.

# RETINOIC ACID IS LENTOIDIOGENIC BUT DIFFERENTIALLY AFFECTS δ-CRYSTALLIN EXPRESSION BY CHICK LENS CELLS <u>IN VITRO</u>

C.E. Patek,* and R.M. Clayton

Institute of Animal Genetics
University of Edinburgh
West Mains Road⁻
Edinburgh EH9 3JN

* Present address
Department of Pathology
University of Edinburgh Medical School
Teviot Place
Edinburgh EH8 9AG

## INTRODUCTION

Retinoids, including retinol (vitamin A) and retinoic acid, affect the early differentiation and the subsequent maintenance of a number of different types of tissue, including both mesenchymal and epithelial derivatives (reviewed Loton, 1980; Sporn and Roberts, 1983; Jetten 1984). For example both deprivation and excess of vitamin A are teratogenic, with effects on bone and cartilage differentiation, (e.g. Kocchar and Aydelotte, 1974), while vitamin A deficiency leads to a reversible keratinisation of the mammalian cornea (Hassel et al., 1980; Tseng et al., 1984), and depressed mitosis in the lens (Pirie and Overall, 1972). Retinoids also affect the differentiation <u>in vitro</u> of a number of cell types, including astrocytes, chondrocytes fibroblasts, corneal epithelium, lens epithelum and teratocarcinoma cells. Effects on the cell surface, cell contacts, the synthesis of cytoskeletal proteins, extra-cellular matrix proteins, including keratin, laminin and collagen, and several enzymes have all been reported (Shapiro and Poon, 1976; Lewis et al., 1978; Kiorpes et al., 1979; Sporn and Roberts, 1983; Wiggert et al., 1983; Tseng et al., 1984; Okarinen et al., 1985; Davies et al., 1985).

Lens epithelial cells (LEC) of the day-old chick differentiate <u>in vitro</u> to give aggregates of lens fibre cells (lentoids) and duringl

377

this process the content of the α, β, and δ crystallins change from an epithelial profile to one characteristic of fibre cells in vivo. In very long term cultures, LEC show a declining capacity for lentoid formation and a progression of changes in the crystallin profile and in the lens membrane proteins which resemble long term in vivo changes, (Patek and Clayton, 1985; and in prepn., Patek et al., accepted for publication).

Three factors led us to examine the effect of retinoic acid (RA) on lens cell differentiation in vitro: the effects on the growth of cell differentiation, outlined briefly above, an effect on mitosis of lens epithelial cells in vivo and in vitro (Pirie and Overall, 1972; Barritault et al., 1981) and the possibility that the lens may be exposed to some level of retinoids in situ, since the retina is a rich source of retinoids (Chader, 1982). We chose lens epithelia of a slow growing chick strain, NRd, because they are characterised by slow growth in vitro and a low capacity for lentoid differentiation in vitro (Patek and Clayton, 1985). It seemed likely that any effect of RA on lens cell differentiation would be most likely to be detected against this background.

MATERIALS AND METHODS

Lens epithelia from day-old post-hatch chicks of the NRd strain were cultured as described previously (Patek and Clayton, 1985). Cultures were subcultured after 28 days and seeded at the original cell density. Primary and secondary cultures were treated every 3 days with a fresh solution of β - all-trans-retinoic acid (RA; Sigma Chemical Company Ltd., Poole Dorset, England) at a concentration of $10^{-5}$ M (3.3 μg/ml) between days 3 and 27 of culture. RA was prepared in 95% Etoh and added directly to the growth medium at a final solvent concentration of o.1% v/v. Control cultures received 0.1% v/v of solvent alone. Cultures were terminated on day 28 and the cell numbers estimated using a haemocytometer. Tissues were harvested and water-soluble proteins were extracted and analysed by SDS-polyacrylamide gel electrophoresis (SDS-PAGE) as described previously (Patek and Clayton, 1985). Total cellular RNA from tissues harvested in parallel was analysed for δ-crystallin transcripts by Northern transfers using a $^{32}$P-labelled δ-crystallin cDNA clone, pM56, as described in Bower et al. (1982).

RESULTS AND DISCUSSION

Lentoids appeared several days earlier in RA treated cultures which contained about 5 times more cells and lentoids than controls (Fig. 1). RA treated cultures contained about 2.5 times more α-crystallin, 4 times more β-crystallins overall and 16.5 times more δ-crystallin than controls. Secondary cultures of the NRd strain have

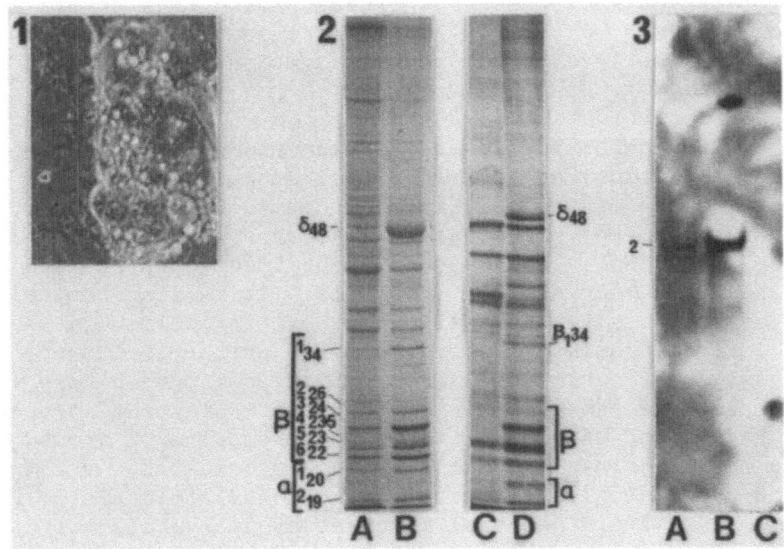

Fig. 1   Phase contrast photomicrographs, showing lentoid bodies with
         characteristic bottle cells in control and RA treated cultures
         (x 225).

Fig. 2   SDS PAGE showing water soluble proteins (60μg) present in 28
         day primary (A and B) and secondary (C and D) cultures.  A and
         C, controls, B and D, treated with RA.  Molecular sizes are
         indicated in kilodaltons.

Fig. 3   Autoradiograph of Northern transfers of a $^{32}$P labelled δ-
         crystallin cDNA probe pM56 (Bower et al., 1982) hybridised to
         total cellular RNA, 15μg , from 28 day secondary cultures:
         (A) RA treated cultures (C) control cultures,  B. polysomal
         δ-crystallin RNA, 1μg, from day old post hatch chick lens
         fibres.  Hybridisation is seen to the 2 kb (17s) species
         corresponding to fully processed δ-crystallin RNA.  No
         hybridisation was detected in duplicate filters hybridised to
         the $^{32}$p pBR322 vector.

70% fewer cells than primary cultures, less crystallin overall, and
express neither δ-crystallin protein (Fig. 2 lane C) nor δ-crystallin
mRNA (Fig 3, lane A).  Treatment of secondary cultures with RA
restores the transcription of δ-crystallin RNA and its translation
indicating that δ-crystallin expression is suppressed but not lost in
secondary culture, and that dedifferentiation appears to be reversible
at least in its initial stages.

We do not yet know whether the restoration of δ-crystallin expression in secondary LEC reflects increased transcription of genes expressed at a low level or de novo activation of completely repressed δ-crystallin DNA.

We have found that dedifferentiation and loss of δ-crystallin expression in LEC in long term or serial subculture in vitro is related to the age of the culture, and not to the lower cell density of secondary cultures, since reseeding older cultures at a high cell density or at a density equal to that obtained in RA treated cultures does not restore δ-crystallin synthesis. It is also not related to the loss of potential δ-crystallin synthesising cells, in secondary cultures derived from non lentoid cells of primary cultures, since secondary cultures established from primary cultures before lentoid formation show the same deficiency (Patek and Clayton, in prepn). A mitogenic effect of RA is implied by the promotion of growth in vitro in bovine LEC (Barritault et al., 1981) and chick LEC (this report) and by the depression of mitosis in vivo in avitaminosis A (Pirie and Overall, 1972). A differential increase of δ-crystallin synthesis also occurs in genotypes, or in growth conditions which accelerate the rate of mitosis (Clayton 1982). On the other hand, RA affects the cell membrane, the synthesis of extra cellular matrix and cytoskeletal elements (Lewis et al., 1978; Sporn and Roberts, 1983), and δ-crystallin is specifically associated with the plasma membrane (Alcalá et al. 1982; Patek et al., in press). RA has been found to affect differentially protein expression in other cell systems including effects on glycoproteins of the extra-cellular matrix, and some enzymes, (see Kiorpes et al., 1979; Davis, et al. 1985; Orkarinen, et al. 1985). These effects appear to be specific responses to retinoids rather than general responses of the cells to differentiation.

A variety of growth factors, including eye-derived growth factor (EDGF), lentropin, lenmofin and fibre differentiation factor isolated from ocular tissues, been found to affect the growth, shape and differentiation of lens cells (see Beebe, et al. 1980; Reddan, 1982;). The retina is rich in retinoids,(Chader 1982): our findings therefore raise the possibility that retinoids may also be involved in the process of lens cell development in vivo.

Our study shows that at pharmacological levels of $10^{-5}$M RA is a potent agent for lens fibre differentiation, and that it appears to have a relatively selective effect on δ-crystallin synthesis, in both primary and secondary cultures.

ACKNOWLEDGEMENTS

We thank the British Foundation for Age Research for their

financial support, Ross Poultry Products, Dumfries, Scotland for the supply of day-old chickens, Mr F. Johnston for assistance with photography, and Mrs L. Dobbie for typing the manuscript.

REFERENCES

Alcala, J., Maisel, H., Katar, M. and Ellis, M., 1982, δ-crystallin in a chick lens fiber cell membrane extrinsic protein, Exp. Eye Res., 35:379
Barritault, D., Arruti, C. and Courtois, Y., 1981, Is there a ubiquitous growth factor in the eye? Proliferation induced in different cell types by eye-derived growth factor (EDGF), Differentiation, 18:29
Beebe, D.C., Feagans, D.E. and Jebens, H.H., 1980, Lentropin: a faster in vitreous humor which promotes lens fibre cell differentiation, Proc. Natl. Acad. Sci. USA, 77:490
Beebe, D.C. and Piatigorsky, J., 1981, Translational regulation of δ-crystallin synthesis during lens development in the chicken embryo, Dev. Biol. 81:96
Bower, D.J., Errington, L.H., Wainwright, N.R., Sime, C., Morris, S. and Clayton, R.M., 1982, Cytoplasmic RNA sequences complementary to cloned chick δ-crystallin cDNA show size heterogeneity, Biochem. J., 201:339
Chader, J., 1982, Retinoids in ocular tissues: binding proteins, transport and mechanism of action. In, Cell Biology of the Eye, D.S. McDevitt, ed, p377, Academic Press, London
Clayton, R.M., 1982, Cellular and molecular aspects of differentiation and transdifferentiation of ocular tissues in vitro, In, Differentiation in Vitro, M.M. Yeoman and D.E.S. Truman, eds., p83, Cambridge University Press, Cambridge.
Davies, P.J., Murtaugh, M.P., Moore, W.T., Johnson, G.S. and Lucas, D. 1985, Retinoic-acid induced expression of tissue transglutaminase in human promyelocytic leukaemia (HL-60) cells, J. Biol. Chem., 260:5166
Hassell, J., Newsome, D. and DeLuca, L., 1980, Increased biosynthesis of specific glycoconjugates in rat corneal epithelium following treatments with vitamin A, Invest Ophthal. Vis. Sci., 19:642
Jetten, A.M., 1984, Modulations of cell growth by retinoids and their possible mechanisms of action, Febs Letts., 43:134.
Kiorpes, T., Kim, Y-C. and Watt, G., 1979, Stimulation of the synthesis of specific glycoproteins in corneal epithelium by vitamin A, Exp. Eye Res., 28:23
Kochhar, D.M. and Aydelotte, M.B., 1974, Susceptible stages and abnormal morphogenesis in the developing mouse limb analysed in organ culture after transplacental exposure to vitamin A (retinoic acid), J. Embryol. Exp. Morph., 31:721;
Lewis, C.A., Pratt, M., Pennypacker, J.P. and Hassel, J.R., 1978, Inhibition of limb chondrogenesis in vitro by vitamin A: alterations in cell surface characteristics, Dev. Biol., 64:31

Loton, R., 1980, Effects of vitamin A and its analogs (retinoids) on normal and neoplastic cells, Biochim. Biophys. Acta. 605:33

Oikarinen, H., Oikarinen, A.I., Tan, E.M., Abergel, R.P., Meeker, C.A. Chu, M-L., Prockop, D.J. and Uitto, J., 1985, Modulation of procollagen gene expression by retinoids, inhibition of collagen production by retinoic acid accompanied by reduced type 1 procollagen messenger ribonucleic acid levels in human skin fibroblasts, J. Clin. Invest., 75:1545

Patek, C.E. and Clayton, R.M., 1985, A comparison of the changing patterns of crystallin expression in vivo, in long-term primary cultures in vitro, and in response to a carcinogen, Exp. Eye Res. 40:357

Patek, C.E., Vornhagen, R., Rink, H. and Clayton, R.M., 1985, Developmental changes in membrane protein expression by chick lens cells in vivo and in vitro, and the detection of main intrinsic polypeptide (MIP), Exp. Eye Res., accepted for publication.

Pirie, A. and Overall, M., 1972, Effect of vitamin A deficiency on the lens epithelium of the rat, Exp. Eye Res., 13:105

Reddan, J.R., 1982, Control of cell division in the ocular lens retina and vitreous humor, In, Cell Biology of the Eye, D.S. McDevitt, ed., p299, Academic Press, London.

Shapiro, S.S. and Poon, J.P., 1976, Effect of retinoic acid on chondrocyte glycosaminoglycan biosynthesis, Archs. Biochem. Biophys. 174:74

Sporn, M.B. and Roberts, A.B., 1983, Role of retinoids in differentiation and carcinogenesis, Cancer Res., 43:3034

Tseng, S.C., Hatchell, D., Tierney, N., Huang, A.J.W. and Sun, T.T., 1984, Expression of specific keratin markers by rabbt corneal, conjuctival, and esophageal epithelia during vitamin A deficiency J. Cell Biol., 99:2279

Wiggert, B., Masterson, E. and Coulombre, A.J., 1983, Changes in retinoid binding levels during development of the chicken cornea, Exp. Eye Res., 37:499

# CONTRIBUTORS

M. ALLAN*        The Beatson Institute for Cancer Research,
                 Garscube Estate, Switchback Road, Glasgow G61 1BD, UK.

M.J. ARENDS      Department of Pathology, University of Edinburgh,
                 Teviot Place, Edinburgh EH8 9AG.

B. ALONI         Department of Cell Biology, The Weizmann Institute of
                 Science, Rehovot 76100, Israel.

A. BALMAIN*      The Beatson Institute for Cancer Research,
                 Garscube Estate, Switchback Road, Glasgow G61 1BD, UK.

M. BECKER        I.R.S.C. du CNRS, ER 278-94802 Villejuif Cedex,
                 France.

M.M. BENDIG      The Imperial Cancer Research Fund, Burtonhole Lane,
                 Mill Hill, London NW7, UK.

A.P. BIRD*       MRC Mammalian Genome Unit, Department of Zoology,
                 University of Edinburgh, West Mains Road, Edinburgh
                 EH9 3JT, UK.

C.C. BIRD*       Department of Pathology, University of Leeds, Leeds
                 LS2 9JT, UK.

C. BONIFER       Zentrum fur Molekulaire Biologie der Universitat
                 (ZMBH), Im Neuenheimer Feld 364, D-6900 Heidelberg,
                 West Germany.

U. BORGMEYER     Zentrum fur Molekulaire Biologie der Universitat
                 (ZMBH), Im Neuenheimer Feld 364, D-6900 Heidelberg,
                 West Germany.

D.J. BOWER*      Clinical and Population Cytogenetics Unit, Western
                 General Hospital, Crewe Road, Edinburgh, UK.

                 * Denotes those who attended the 1984 Conference.

383

P.J. BYRD*          Cancer Research Campaign Laboratories, Department of
                   Cancer Studies, University of Birmingham, Birmingham
                   B15 2TJ, UK.

R.M. CLAYTON*       Department of Genetics, University of Edinburgh,
                   West Mains Road, Edinburgh EH9 3JN, UK.

Y. COURTOIS*        INSERM, U. 118, CNRS ERA 842, Association Claude
                   Bernard, 29, rue Wilhem, 75016 Paris, France.

D.L. CRIBBS        Swiss Institute for Experimental Cancer Research,
                   Ch-1066 Epalinges, S/Lausanne, Switzerland.

G. EGUCHI*         Department of Developmental Biology, National
                   Institute for Basic Biology, Okazaki, 444 Japan

J.A. ELKINGTON     The Imperial Cancer Research Fund, Burtonhole Lane,
                   Mill Hill, London NW7, UK.

L.H. ERRINGTON*    Department of Genetics, University of Edinburgh,
                   West Mains Road, Edinburgh EH9 3JN, UK.

H.P. FRITTON       Institut fur Physiologische Chemie, Physikalische
                   Biochemie und Zellbiologie der Universitat
                   Goethestrasse 33, D-800, Munchen 2, West Germany.

P.H. GALLIMORE     Cancer Research Campaign Laboratories, Department of
                   Cancer Studies, University of Birmingham, Birmingham,
                   B15 2TJ, UK.

D. GOSPODAROWICZ   Cancer Research Institute, Departments of Medicine &
                   Ophthalmology, University of California Medical
                   Center, San Francisco, CA 94143, USA.

D. GREENBERG       Department of Cell Biology, The Weizmann Institute of
                   Science, Rehovot 76100 Israel.

G.J. GRINDLEY      The Beatson Institute for Cancer Research, Garscube
                   Estate, Switchback Road, Glasgow G61 1BD, UK.

A.R. HAAKE         Department of Biology, University of South Carolina,
                   Columbia, S. Carolina 29208, USA.

O. HAGENBUCHLE     Swiss Institute for Experimental Cancer Research,
                   1066 Epalinges, S/Lausanne, Switzerland.

S. HAYASHI         Department of Biophysics, Faculty of Science,
                   University of Kyoto, Kyoto 606, Japan.

H.C. HURST*        Swiss Institute for Experimental Cancer Research,
                   1066 Epalinges, S/Lausanne, Switzerland.

T. IGO-KEMENES      Institut fur Physiologische Chemie, Physikalische
                    Biochemie und Zellbiologie der Universitat
                    Goethestrasse 33, D-8000 Munchen 2, West Germany.

J-C. JEANNY         Institut Nationale de la Sante et de la Recherche
                    Gerontologiques, U.118, 29 Rue Wilhem, Paris 75016,
                    France.

Z. JING-DE          The Beatson Institute for Cancer Research,
                    Garscube Estate, Switchback Road, Glasgow G61 1BD, UK.

W.W. de JONG*       Laboratorium voor Biochemie, Universiteit van
                    Nijmegen,  "Heyendael" Geert Grooteplein Noord 21,
                    The Netherlands

Y. KATO             Cancer Research Institute and Departments of Medicine
                    and Ophthalmology, University of California Medical
                    Center, San Francisco, CA 94143, USA.

R. KODAMA*          Department of Developmental Biology, National
                    Institute for Basic Biology, Okazaki, 444 Japan.

H. KONDOH*          Department of Biophysics, Faculty of Science,
                    University of Kyoto, Kyoto 606, Japan.

E. LEHTONEN         Department of Pathology, University of Helsinki,
                    Finland.

N.J. MAITLAND*      Department of Pathology, University of Bristol,
                    The Medical School, University Walk, Bristol BS8 1TD.

P.J. MASON          The Imperial Cancer Research Fund, Burtonhole Lane,
                    Mill Hill, London NW7.

Y. MAYER            Department of Cell Biology, The Weizmann Institute of
                    Science, Rehovot 76100, Israel.

D. MELLOUL          Department of Cell Biology, The Weizmann Institute of
                    Science, Rehovot 76100, Israel.

P. MONTAGUE         The Beatson Institute for Cancer Research,
                    Garscube Estate, Switchback Road, Glasgow G61 1BD, UK.

R.G. MORRIS         Department of Pathology, University of Edinburgh,
                    Teviot Place, Edinburgh EH8 9AG.

J. NOWOCK           Zentrum fur Molekulaire Biologie der Universitat
                    (ZMBH), Im Neuenheimer Feld 364, D-6900 Heidelberg,
                    West Germany.

U. NUDEL            Department of Cell Biology, The Weizmann Institute of
                    Science, Rehovot, 76100, Israel.

T.S. OKADA*         Department of Biophysics, Faculty of Science,
                    University of Kyoto, Kyoto 606, Japan.

K. OKAZAKI          Department of Biophysics, Faculty of Science,
                    University of Kyoto, Kyoto 606, Japan.

C.E. PATEK*         Department of Genetics, University of Edinburgh,
                    West Mains Road, Edinburgh EH9 3JN, UK.

J. PAUL             The Beatson Institute for Cancer Research,
                    Garscube Estate, Switchback Road, Glasgow G61 1BD, UK.

M-F. POUPON         I.R.S.C. du CNRS ER 278-94802 Villejuif Cedex, France.

M. QUINTANILLA      The Beatson Institute for Cancer Research
                    Garscube Estate, Switchback Road, Glasgow G61 1BD, UK.

M.C. RAFF*          MRC Neuroimmunology Project, Zoology Department,
                    University College London, London WC1E 6BT.

M. RAMSDEN          The Beatson Institute for Cancer Research,
                    Garscube Estate, Switchback Road, Glasgow G61 1BD, UK.

R.H. SAWYER         Department of Biology, University of S. Carolina,
                    Columbia, S. Carolina 29208, USA.

L. SAXEN*           Department of Pathology, University of Helsinki,
                    Helsinki, Finland.

U. SCHIBLER         Swiss Institute for Experimental Cancer Research
                    1066 Epalinges, S/Lausanne, Switzerland.

M. SHANI            Department of Cell Biology, The Weizmann Institute
                    of Science, Rehovot 76100, Israel.

P.H. SHAW           Swiss Institute for Experimental Cancer Research,
                    1066 Epalinges, S/Lausanne, Switzerland.

A.E. SIPPEL*        Zentrum fur Molekulaire Biologie der Universitat,
                    (ZMBH), Im Neuenheimer Feld 364, D-6900 Heidelberg,
                    West Germany.

U. STRECH-JURK      Zentrum fur Molekulaire Biologie der Universitat,
                    (ZMBH), Im Neuenheimer Feld 364, D-6900 Heidelberg,
                    West Germany.

Y. TAKAHASHI        Institute for Biophysics, Faculty of Science,
                    University of Kyoto, Kyoto 606, Japan.

M. THEISEN            Zentrum fur Molekulaire Biologie der Universitat,
                     (ZMBH), Im Neuenheimer Feld 364, D-6900 Heidelberg,
                     West Germany.

D.E.S. TRUMAN*       Department of Genetics, University of Edinburgh,
                     West Mains Road, Edinburgh EH9 3JN, UK.

A.E. WATT            Department of Pathology, University of Edinburgh,
                     Teviot Place, Edinburgh EH8 9AG.

P.K. WELLAUER        Swiss Institute for Experimental Cancer Research,
                     1066 Epalinges, S/Lausanne, Switzerland.

J.G. WILLIAMS*       Imperial Cancer Research Fund, Burtonhole Lane,
                     Mill Hill, London NW7.

D. YAFFE*            Department of Cell Biology, The Weizmann Institute
                     of Science, Rehovot 76100, Israel.

K. YASUDA            Institute for Biophysics, Faculty of Science,
                     University of Kyoto, Kyoto 606, Japan.